Handbook o
Brachytheraﬁ

CW00796369

Jyoti Mayadev
Stanley H. Benedict
Mitchell Kamrava
Editors

Handbook of Image-Guided Brachytherapy

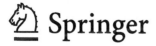 Springer

Editors
Jyoti Mayadev, MD
Associate Professor
Director of Brachytherapy
Department of Radiation
  Oncology
University of California
  Davis Medical Center
UC Davis Comprehensive
  Cancer Center
Sacramento, CA, USA

Stanley H. Benedict, PhD,
  FAAPM
Professor and Vice Chair
  of Clinical Physics
Department of Radiation
  Oncology
University of California Davis
  Medical Center
UC Davis Comprehensive
  Cancer Center
Sacramento, CA, USA

Mitchell Kamrava, MD
Assistant Clinical Professor
Chief, Division of
  Brachytherapy
Chief, Gynecologic and
  Sarcoma Services
Department of Radiation
  Oncology
University of California,
  Los Angeles
Los Angeles, CA, USA

ISBN 978-3-319-44825-1   ISBN 978-3-319-44827-5 (eBook)
DOI 10.1007/978-3-319-44827-5

Library of Congress Control Number: 2016959498

Dedicated to the mentors, practitioners, and students of brachytherapy, who continually strive for innovation, outcome improvement, and a better patient experience. I am also deeply grateful to my loving parents (Savita and Shyam), supportive sisters (Renuka and Angeli), friends, and the collective universal spirit.

Jyoti Mayadev, MD

I would like to dedicate this handbook to my clinician and scientist friends for their enlightening and enduring contributions to radiation oncology, and for their tireless efforts to advance our clinical outcomes through

clinical research and development.
I am deeply indebted to the abiding and enduring love, support, and understanding from my family (Lori, Erin, and Noelle), which strengthens me and brings me joy and purpose beyond words.

Stanley H. Benedict, PhD, FAAPM

To my greatest teachers, Sophia and Sarah.

Mitchell Kamrava, MD

Preface

It is with great enthusiasm and dedication to the art and science of brachytherapy instruction, and on behalf of our authors, that we present our image-guided brachytherapy handbook. Brachytherapy is the use of radioactive sources placed near or into a tumor to provide a high radiation dose to the area of interest and a reduced dose to surrounding normal tissues. It is this therapeutic advantage and steep dose gradient falloff that continues to make brachytherapy one of the most conformal and long-standing treatments in cancer therapeutics. Throughout the last decade, the utility of image guidance in brachytherapy has increased to enhance procedural development, treatment planning, and radiation delivery in an effort to optimize safety and clinical outcomes. Given the complexity of image guidance and required incorporation into brachytherapy skillsets, the contents of this user-friendly handbook are designed to be a practical reference for the busy and dedicated clinician. Our goal is to provide a concise compilation of brachytherapy experiences at the reader's fingertip.

After formal training in brachytherapy by pioneers in the field, continuing friendship, kinship, and association with mentors and peers of brachytherapy, my clinical practice continues to evolve. With this collaboration and direction of specific and detailed knowledge, I recognize that not all practitioners have these individual educational opportunities and that a compilation of skills and "tips" should be made available to all brachytherapists and, in turn, to their collective patients.

This image-guided brachytherapy handbook is divided into two main parts: a radiobiology and physics section led by Dr. Stanley Benedict and a clinical site-specific section directed by Dr. Mitchell Kamrava and myself. The reader will learn about the rationale and background of brachytherapy in the first section, and then review the practical application of this modality in the second section. The handbook is a combination of outline text, procedural illustrations, contour examples, treatment planning techniques, and dosimetry for the comprehensive treatment for each disease site. The handbook answers practical questions regarding the incorporation of imaging advances such as CT, MRI, and ultrasound into brachytherapy procedures. Furthermore, it presents a detailed guide on how to extrapolate these technological advances into patient contours and treatment planning. Some examples of questions we sought to answer are:

- "How shall I use MRI or CT to help in my cervical cancer brachytherapy procedures or treatment planning?"
- "How could I implant a prostate using transrectal ultrasound or MRI guidance?"
- "How do I decide which breast brachytherapy technique is better for my patient: a single multichannel catheter vs an interstitial implantation?"

I am extremely grateful to a diverse team of brachytherapy experts who tirelessly devoted their time and innovative minds to the contents of this handbook. During the handbook preparation period, I was perpetually awestruck by our authors' ability to funnel their vast and substantial practical experiences into a concise and clinically relevant brachytherapy chapter. In addition, it continues to be an honor and pleasure to work in the field of brachytherapy and have developed this handbook with my coeditors, Drs. Stanley H. Benedict and Mitchell Kamrava, whose insight, knowledge, collaboration, and expertise are invaluable to our field.

Sacramento, CA, USA   Jyoti Mayadev, MD

Contents

x   Contents

Contributors

Sushil Beriwal, MD Department of Radiation Oncology, University of Pittsburgh School of Medicine, Magee-Women's Hospital, Pittsburgh, PA, USA

Matthew Biagioli, MD, MSc Department of Radiation Oncology, University of Central Florida, Florida Hospital Cancer Institute, Orlando, FL, USA

Albert J. Chang, MD, PhD Department of Radiation Oncology, University of California, San Francisco, San Francisco, CA, USA

Jonathan Chen, MD, PhD Department of Radiation Oncology, New York Presbyterian Hospital/Weill Cornell Medicine, New York, NY, USA

J. Adam M. Cunha, PhD Department of Radiation Oncology, University of California, San Francisco, San Francisco, CA, USA

D. Jeffrey Demanes, MD, FACRO, FACR, FASTRO Division of Brachytherapy, Department of Radiation Oncology, UCLA David Geffen School of Medicine, Los Angeles, CA, USA

Brandon A. Dyer, MD Department of Radiation Oncology, Davis Comprehensive Cancer Center, University of California, Sacramento, CA, USA

Steven J. Frank, MD Department of Radiation Oncology, University of Texas MD Anderson Cancer Center, Houston, TX, USA

John Gloss, PSM Department of Radiation Oncology, Banner University Medical Center, University of Arizona, Tucson, AZ, USA

Karyn A. Goodman, MD, MS Department of Radiation Oncology, University of Colorado School of Medicine, Aurora, CO, USA

Dae Yup Han, PhD Department of Radiation Oncology, University of California, San Francisco, San Francisco, CA, USA

Alex Herskovic, MD Department of Radiation Oncology, New York Presbyterian Hospital/Weill Cornell Medicine, New York, NY, USA

I-Chow Hsu, MD, FACR, FASTRO Department of Radiation Oncology, University of California, San Francisco, San Francisco, CA, USA

Supriya K. Jain, MD, MHS Department of Radiation Oncology, University of Colorado School of Medicine, Aurora, CO, USA

Cameron Javid, MD, FACS Department of Ophthalmology, University of Arizona, Tucson, AZ, USA

Retina Associates, Tucson, AZ, USA

Mitchell Kamrava, MD Department of Radiation Oncology, University of California Los Angeles, UCLA Medical Plaza, Los Angeles, CA, USA

Taeho Kim, PhD Department of Radiation Oncology, Massey Cancer Center, Virginia Commonwealth University, Richmond, VA, USA

Rajat J. Kudchadker, PhD Department of Radiation Physics, University of Texas MD Anderson Cancer Center, Houston, TX, USA

Bruce Libby, PhD Department of Radiation Oncology, University of Virginia Health System, Charlottesville, VA, USA

Anna Likhacheva, MD, MPH Department of Radiation Oncology, Banner MD Anderson Cancer Center, Gilbert, AZ, USA

Justin Mann, MD Department of Radiation Oncology, New York Presbyterian Hospital/Weill Cornell Medicine, New York, NY, USA

Jyoti Mayadev, MD Department of Radiation Oncology, UC Davis Comprehensive Cancer Center, University of California Davis Medical Center, Sacramento, CA, USA

Amy C. Moreno, MD Department of Radiation Oncology, University of Texas MD Anderson Cancer Center, Houston, TX, USA

Alison Nielsen, MD Department of Anesthesiology and Pain Medicine, University of California, Davis Medical Center, Sacramento, CA, USA

Laura Padilla, PhD Department of Radiation Oncology, Virginia Commonwealth University Health System, Richmond, VA, USA

Bhupesh Parashar, MD Department of Radiation Oncology, New York Presbyterian Hospital/Weill Cornell Medicine, New York, NY, USA

Sang-June Park, PhD Department of Radiation Oncology, University of California, Los Angeles, Los Angeles, CA, USA

Shyamal Patel, MD Department of Radiation Oncology, University of California, Los Angeles, Lost Angeles, CA, USA

Jens Ricke, MD Department of Radiology and Nuclear Medicine, University of Magdeburg, Magdeburg, Germany

Kara D. Romano, MD Department of Radiation Oncology, University of Virginia Health System, Charlottesville, VA, USA

Kunal Saigal, MD Department of Radiation Oncology, Florida Hospital Cancer Institute, University of Central Florida College of Medicine, Orlando, FL, USA

Timothy N. Showalter, MD, MPH Department of Radiation Oncology, University of Virginia Health System, Charlottesville, VA, USA

Tijana Skrepnik, MD Department of Radiation Oncology, Banner University Medical Center, University of Arizona, Tucson, AZ, USA

Andrew W. Smith, BA University of Rochester School of Medicine and Dentistry, Rochester, NY, USA

Baldassarre Stea, MD, PhD Department of Radiation Oncology, Banner University Medical Center, University of Arizona, Tucson, AZ, USA

Shoshana Taube, BA Bar Elan Medical School, Ber Sheva, Israel

David H. Thomas, PhD Department of Radiation Oncology, University of Colorado Denver, Denver, CO, USA

Dorin A. Todor, PhD Department of Radiation Oncology, Virginia Commonwealth University Health System, Richmond, VA, USA

Daniel M. Trifiletti, MD Department of Radiation Oncology, University of Virginia Health System, Charlottesville, VA, USA

Andrew T. Vaughan, PhD Department of Radiation Oncology, Davis Medical Center, University of California, Sacramento, CA, USA

Jihong Wang, PhD Department of Radiation Physics, University of Texas MD Anderson Cancer Center, Houston, TX, USA

A. Gabriella Wernicke, MD, MS Department of Radiation Oncology, New York Presbyterian Hospital/Weill Cornell Medicine, New York, NY, USA

Yao Yu, MD Department of Radiation Oncology, University of California, San Francisco, San Francisco, CA, USA

Xiao Zhao, MD Department of Radiation Oncology, Davis Medical Center, University of California, Sacramento, CA, USA

Part I
Radiobiology and Physics
of Image-Guided Brachytherapy

Chapter 1
Radiobiology of Brachytherapy

Xiao Zhao and Andrew T. Vaughan

Basic Radiobiological Principles

DNA Damage

- Radiation therapy exerts its effects primarily through DNA damage mediated by either direct deposition of energy within DNA (~40 %) or secondarily through the generation of free radicals (~60 %)
- The free radicals may subsequently attack DNA and generate both DNA breaks and/or mutations. However, both free radical access may be restricted by the presence of chemical scavengers, such as glutathione, and chemical fixation of lesions is reduced in regions of low oxygen tension

X. Zhao, MD • A.T. Vaughan, PhD (✉)
Department of Radiation Oncology, Davis Medical Center,
University of California, 4501 X Street, Sacramento,
CA 95817, USA
e-mail: jazhao@ucdavis.edu; atvaughan@ucdavis.edu

© Springer International Publishing AG 2017   3
J. Mayadev et al. (eds.), *Handbook of Image-Guided
Brachytherapy*, DOI 10.1007/978-3-319-44827-5_1

Cell Death

- The discrete, localized, disruption of DNA generates double strand breaks that may combine with breaks on other chromosomes to produce lethal lesions that physically disrupt cell division
- Such lesions that limit cell division include chromosome rearrangements with two centromeres, a dicentric, that restricts the ability of the cell to divide. For this reason, this type of lethality is called a mitotic cell death or mitotic catastrophe and is prominent in the cells of most irradiated carcinoma
- Radiation-induced apoptosis is less common but may be observed under certain conditions, such as in endothelial cells after large single doses [1]
- Generating a lethal lesion that will lead to cell death is of key significance for both tumor control and the maintenance of normal tissues

DNA Damage Tracking

- The formation of DNA double stand breaks by irradiation may be tracked by the phosphorylation of serine 139 of multiple H2AX histones that surround the break itself
- The appearance and then removal of γH2AX phosphorylation tracks with reasonable accuracy the survival changes measured with sublethal damage repair (SLDr) consistent with their being a link between them [2]

Linear Quadratic Equation

- The required sublesions may be generated either from the same radiation event or separately. Using this understanding, the survival curves of irradiated cells have been modeled by a two component polynomial where the fraction surviving (SF) a dose (d) includes a linear component (αD) representing the simultaneous generation of DNA breaks and a quadratic component (βD^2) where the breaks are introduced as separate events

- Thus, the Linear Quadratic (LQ) equation takes the form:

$$SF = e^{-\left(\alpha d + \beta d^2\right)} \tag{1}$$

- The LQ equation therefore is more than a simple curve fitting routine in that it is based on a biological assessment of how radiation kills cells
- The relevance (or lack thereof) of the LQ relationship at large single doses (>10 Gy) is a matter of some dispute and will be discussed later
- In clinical practice, the LQ equation has often been used to estimate the effects of fraction size changes on tumor killing and tissue toxicity

Dose–Response Curves

- The shapes of acute (most tumors) and chronically (most normal tissues and some tumors such as prostate) responding tissues is quite different with the acutely responding dose response being flattened with less curvature than the chronic responders (Fig. 1.1)
- The different shapes of the dose–response curves have one immediate impact. As the dose delivered increases, the effect on late responding tissues gets progressively more significant as the dose–response curve continues to bend. Thus, large fractions delivered to critical normal tissues are to be avoided for this reason

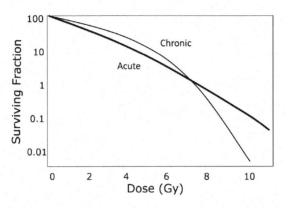

FIG. 1.1. Cell survival curves. The shapes of these two curves illustrate the predicted increased response to fraction size for chronically responding (normal tissues) targets compared to acute responders (most tumors). The difference is encapsulated in a single unit of dose, the α/β ratio derived from the linear quadratic equation where killing from the αD component equals that from the βD^2 component. Its value is high (~10 Gy) for acute responding tissues and low (~3 Gy) for most chronic reactions

Survival Curve Analysis: The α/β Ratio

- In order to provide a simple index of what constitutes an acute or chronic dose response, a unique single dose is defined where the contribution to cell killing from single event killing (αD) exactly matches that from the combination of two separate events (βD^2). This is known as the α/β ratio and is measured in dose units

- For acutely responding tissues (most tumors), the αD component predominates thus the α/β ratio equivalence point is not reached until quite high doses. Conversely, the more curved chronically responding tissues that describe most normal tissues the curved element is greater, and the equivalence point is lower

- By convention, and unless the actual numbers are determined by experiment, acute responding tissues are commonly assigned an α/β ratio of 10 Gy and chronic responders an α/β ratio of 3 Gy

The Differences Between External Beam Radiation Therapy and Brachytherapy

Brachytherapy Applications

- Brachytherapy by definition is radiation therapy in which a radioactive source is placed within or in close proximity to the area being treated.
- Traditional sites that have been treated with brachytherapy include gynecological cancers, prostate cancer, head and neck cancers, and skin cancers
- The central location of cervical tumors and their relative accessibility made brachytherapy the treatment of choice, initially using radium as the primary radiation source
- Very high, and steep dose gradients, close to the radiation source contributes to dose and dose rate heterogeneity that is not normally observed using external beams. This can be difficult to account for using traditional normal tissue tolerances
- Treatment with linear accelerators usually operates within a certain dose rate delivery range and treatment completes within minutes. However, the dose rate in brachytherapy varies from permanent implants delivering dose over months to short high dose delivery treatments in minutes. This can produce significantly different radiobiological effects

Dose Rates

- Multiple strategies have been used that are traditionally defined by the dose rate (DR) delivered. These include Very Low (VLDR <40 cGy h^{-1}), Low (LDR

<2 Gy h^{-1}), Medium (MDR 2Gy–12 Gy h^{-1}), High (HDR >12 Gy h^{-1}), and Pulsed (PDR ~ hourly)

- Modern day brachytherapy is, however, most often classified into two categories: HDR brachytherapy vs. LDR brachytherapy
- HDR is typically used to describe catheter-based procedures using non-permanent radioactive sources that complete treatment in minutes
- LDR is typically used to describe permanent implants that by definition will provide a continuous, decreasing, dose rate to the target
- Pulsed Dose Rate (PDR) Brachytherapy was designed to deliver several small HDR fractions over a shorter interval (<3–4 h) to capture more DNA lesions prior to repair, thus providing similar biologic effects to traditional LDR treatments

Radiobiological Effect of Different Dose Rates

- Alterations in the rate of dose delivery within the range likely to be encountered in the clinic have a substantial impact on cell survival
- For most tumor types irradiated in vitro, as the dose rate is decreased below ~100 cGy min^{-1} the effectiveness of the irradiation is incrementally decreased, as demonstrated by the standard clonogenic survival curve
- It is likely that all of the factors that are known to modulate the response of cells to irradiation, including the 4(5) "R's" (see below), will have some effect on both tumors and normal tissues [3] (Fig. 1.2)
- However, of these, it is the capacity to repair DNA damage and the potential for reoxygenation that are likely to show most variability during different brachytherapy protocols

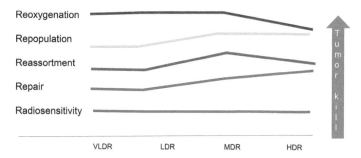

FIG. 1.2. Schematic illustrating the relative impact of brachytherapy delivery technique on biological response. Reoxygenation may be decreased if few large doses used. Repopulation of tumor will occur if small doses are delivered over a protracted period. The Reassortment of cells within the cell cycle into the more radiosensitive G_2M phase will happen at unique dose rates, but is difficult to predict clinically. Decreasing dose rates will enhance Repair and therefore survival. Decreasing dose rate will also enhance the expression of any differential Radiosensitivity, primarily through differences in DNA repair, though any specific benefit is difficult to predict

The 4(+1) "R's" of Radiobiology: Repair, Reoxygenation, Redistribution, Repopulation (and Radiosensitivity)

Repair

- The requirement for two DNA breaks, or sublesions, to generate the lethal event also provides the setting for their repair. Thus, if the individual breaks occur separated in time and/or space then one may be repaired before it has the opportunity to interact with the other
- The significance of this type of repair, called "sublethal damage repair" or SLDr, is clear in that through its activity fewer lesions will be produced if the dose is fractionated or delivered at a lower dose rate such that individual lesions are repaired and therefore cannot react with other lesions to generate a lethal event

- DNA sublethal lesions are removed by active DNA repair systems, primarily the error prone Non Homologous End Joining (NHEJ) or Homologous Recombination (HR) repair. In the latter case, increased repair fidelity is provided by using the intact homologous copy of the damaged sequence to template the repair
- The impact of the extremes of dose rate delivery is easy to describe. At very low dose rate ~0.4 cGy min^{-1} or less, such as might be observed after substantial decay of a permanent seed implant, DNA breaks have the greatest chance to be successfully repaired (few alternative breaks for interaction) and minimal toxicity will occur
- At high dose rates ~100 cGy min^{-1} and above, DNA breaks will have the greatest chance to combine with other breaks, potentially generating a lethal lesion and thus reduced survival
- Dose rates that fall between these extremes will provide an intermediate level of lethal lesion generation depending on the delivery parameters and the repair capability of the target tissue

Reoxygenation

- Multiple studies have shown that most animal and human tumors contain regions of lowered oxygen tension where the blood supply network has not kept pace with the expansion of the tumor volume
- Classical studies in radiobiology have shown that such regions of hypoxia reduce the effectiveness of irradiation by limiting the fixation of free radical damage that is best achieved in the presence of molecular oxygen
- The reduction in radiation effect is significant, approximately three fold when comparing irradiation under oxic or hypoxic conditions

- This difference is sufficiently large that it would render radiation therapy ineffective unless reoxygenation occurs during treatment
- As well-oxygenated cells die from radiation damage, hypoxic cells may have improved access to the blood supply and become more sensitive to future radiation treatments. This process can begin rapidly after treatment
- Considering the wide variation in treatment schedules that may occur within brachytherapy, it is difficult to predict the impact of hypoxia on cell kill for small variations in the rate and time of dose delivery
- However, large treatment doses that are delivered rapidly over a short time frame are least likely to ensure complete reoxygenation as the residual tumor mass may still metabolize oxygen—limiting its access to hypoxic regions

Redistribution

- Acute radiation exposures will kill the most sensitive cell populations, specifically those in $G_2M > G_1$ early $S > $ late S. The residual viable cells will then be partially synchronized
- Transition through the cell cycle is linked to checkpoints, which may be activated by genomic damage, which will provide a pause to allow DNA damage repair
- Activation of the G_2M checkpoint during a protracted exposure at a dose rate of ~0.5–1 cGy min^{-1} will stall cells at this very radiation sensitive phase of the cell cycle generating more cell kill if the dose continues
- Paradoxically, higher dose rates, ~1–2 cGy min^{-1} or greater, will freeze the progression of cells through the cell cycle such that some will remain in a relatively resistant part of the cell cycle. Here, such cells will

survive better than those irradiated at a slightly lower dose rate, ~0.5 cGy min^{-1}, that may proceed through to the radiosensitive G_2M arrest point, and continue to be irradiated. This unusual feature is called the "inverse dose rate effect."

- Interestingly, one of the original applications of brachytherapy for cervical tumors used interstitial radium implants delivering a dose rate of ~40 cGy h^{-1}. This dose rate is consistent with the inverse dose rate effect described, potentially contributing to the efficacy of this treatment method

Repopulation

- After protracted exposure to radiation, residual tumor cells may increase their rate of cell division. This is one of the principle reasons why delays in any protracted irradiation schemes are to be avoided
- This parameter was initially described by key studies of Withers et al. Here, in a head and neck cancer setting, the dose to achieve tumor control (TCD$_{50}$) increased after 30 days of treatment [4]. The explanation for this finding was the accelerated repopulation of tumor clonogens
- The effect of repopulation is related more to total treatment duration than dose rate. This effect is not seen in treatment delivery times less than 1 week. After 1 week, there can be increased repopulation of high turnover normal tissues such as the skin and mucosa. For treatment delivery times greater than 3 weeks, there could be repopulation effects of fast growing tumors
- In terms of brachytherapy, faster treatments will mitigate this effect. However, faster treatment times may limit successful reoxygenation of the tumor—how this balance impacts outcome within the same or different tumor types is not known

Radiosensitivity

- Individual tumor types vary substantially as to their response to irradiation. Thus, clonogens from a radiation unresponsive tumors are also likely to be radiation resistant; however, this is only one factor in the ability of radiation to control an individual tumor [5]
- The role of radiation sensitivity followed a number of studies that showed a correlation between the radiation response of individual tumor types and the in vitro clonogenic sensitivity of their tumor cells, particularly as measured by the fraction surviving 2 Gy (SF_2) [6]
- The relative differences in tumor cell survival after irradiation is reduced at higher doses as the slopes of the survival curves become increasingly similar
- Thus, relative differences in intrinsic radiation sensitivity, either between tumors of the same type or between tumors with different radiation response profiles, may be of lesser importance following large doses of brachytherapy than multiple smaller doses of conventional (1.8–2 Gy) fractionation

How Are 4R(5)s Affected by the Interval Between Fractions?

- Repair—Most repair happens between the first few hours after irradiation so unless a very short interval is used between fractions such as in PDR, the interval between fractions will not affect the degree of repair
- Redistribution—There is likely no measurable clinical impact of redistribution, based on the interval between fractions, due to the clonal heterogeneity of tumor composition
- Repopulation—As discussed previously, this effect typically does not occur until after 2–3 weeks and can be considered negligible for most brachytherapy fractionation schemes

- Reoxygenation—The process of reoxygenation may be rapid; however, complete reoxygenation after large single doses may not be as effective as multiple small fractions
- Radiosensitivity effects, if present, are more likely dependent on fraction number and/or dose rate than the interval between fractions

Timing with EBRT

- Given the effects of repopulation beginning after several weeks of treatment, it is important to not allow a prolonged break from treatment prior to initiation of brachytherapy
- Brachytherapy treatments can be given before the completion of external beam radiation therapy. In these cases, it is important to consider the cumulative dose of radiation on a daily and weekly basis to the tumor and normal tissues. This can be calculated using BED and EQD_2 equations
- It is not recommended to give both EBRT and brachytherapy treatments on the same day to ensure enough time is allowed for repair of sublethal damage in normal tissue

Modeling the Dose Response

Effect of Varying the Dose Size

BED Equations

- Using the linear quadratic equation, it is possible to estimate the biological effect of changing the fraction size of the delivered radiation using a concept first proposed by Dr. Jack Fowler [7]. This is the Biologically Effective Dose (BED)

- Its goal was to illustrate the effect of changing fraction size on the likely effectiveness of the new fractionation scheme
- It was derived only as tool to estimate such effects and was never intended to be used to prescribe actual clinical doses

$$\text{BED} = n \times d \times \left(1 + \frac{d}{\alpha / \beta}\right) \qquad (2)$$

- Here, using the defined α/β ratio for the tissue and n fractions of d Gy are given. This equation, however, does not account for the effect of repopulation. While this effect may be negligible for treatments less than 3 weeks in duration, it can be significant for longer treatments especially permanent LDR implants
- To account for the effect of repopulation, the equation can be expanded to:

$$\text{BED} = n \times d \times \left(1 + \frac{d}{\alpha / \beta}\right) - \frac{0.693 \times (T - T_\text{k})}{\alpha \times T_\text{p}} \qquad (3)$$

- Here, an overall time of T days and repopulation (with a cell doubling time T_p) is delayed until day T_k of treatment

EQD2 Equations

- In order to provide a more direct basis for comparison, the BEDs calculated above may be readily converted into doses that are equivalent to a conventional fraction scheme using 2 Gy fractions. This is the equivalent dose in 2 Gy fractions (EQD_2) equation
- This conversion generates doses that are comparable to those seen using conventional 2 Gy per day fractions

$$\text{EQD}_2 = n \times d \times \left(\frac{d + (\alpha / \beta)}{2 + (\alpha / \beta)}\right) \qquad (4)$$

- This equation can be used when both external beam and IGBT are being employed in order to generate a composite dose for comparison

Radiobiological Effects of Large Single Doses

- In the context of IGBT, the use of refined imaging techniques to locate both the tumor and organs at risk has enabled the delivery of larger fraction sizes to better defined target areas
- This development, matching changes in the delivery of external beam radiation, has raised questions over the utility of the LQ formula as being the most appropriate tool as it predicts a continuously bending cell survival curve at elevated doses rather than a simple exponential that is normally observed
- This will have the effect of overestimating the potency of LQ-based calculations of BED or EQD_2
- To address this discrepancy, two groups of thought have emerged. One group proposes the continued use of the LQ formulae, citing its long and successful use in the clinic [8]. Others have advised caution, suggesting that the LQ formula does not adequately model biological effects at high doses, such as the introduction of damage to the vascular system [9]
- For this reason, models such as the Universal Cell Survival Curve (USC) have been described that address the practical reality by adding an exponential dose–response element to the LQ model [10]
- Such models, however, negate the biological rationale of using the LQ formulae and its BED and EQD_2 derivatives though not necessarily its practical utility

References

1. Garcia-Barros M, Paris F, Cordon-Cardo C, Lyden D, Rafii S, Haimovitz-Friedman A, et al. Tumor response to radiotherapy regulated by endothelial cell apoptosis. Science (New York, NY). 2003;300(5622):1155–9.
2. Mariotti LG, Pirovano G, Savage KI, Ghita M, Ottolenghi A, Prise KM, et al. Use of the gamma-H2AX assay to investigate DNA repair dynamics following multiple radiation exposures. PLoS One. 2013;8(11):e79541.
3. Hall EJ, Giaccia AJ. Radiobiology for the radiologist. Philadelphia: Wolters Kluwer Health; 2012.
4. Withers HR, Taylor JM, Maciejewski B. The hazard of accelerated tumor clonogen repopulation during radiotherapy. Acta Oncol (Stockholm, Sweden). 1988;27(2):131–46.
5. Steel GG, McMillan TJ, Peacock JH. The 5Rs of radiobiology. Int J Radiat Biol. 1989;56(6):1045–8.
6. Deacon J, Peckham MJ, Steel GG. The radio responsiveness of human tumours and the initial slope of the cell survival curve. Radiother Oncol. 1984;2(4):317–23.
7. Fowler JF. 21 years of biologically effective dose. Br J Radiol. 2010;83(991):554–68.
8. Brown JM, Carlson DJ, Brenner DJ. The tumor radiobiology of SRS and SBRT: are more than the 5 Rs involved? Int J Radiat Oncol Biol Phys. 2014;88(2):254–62.
9. Park HJ, Griffin RJ, Hui S, Levitt SH, Song CW. Radiation-induced vascular damage in tumors: implications of vascular damage in ablative hypofractionated radiotherapy (SBRT and SRS). Radiat Res. 2012;177(3):311–27.
10. Park C, Papiez L, Zhang S, Story M, Timmerman RD. Universal survival curve and single fraction equivalent dose: useful tools in understanding potency of ablative radiotherapy. Int J Radiat Oncol Biol Phys. 2008;70(3):847–52.

Chapter 2
General Physics Principles in Brachytherapy

Sang-June Park and David H. Thomas

Classifications of Brachytherapy

Types of Brachytherapy Implants

- Interstitial: Radiation sources or catheters are surgically inserted into or near the targets (e.g., prostate, gynecological, breast, rectum, and head and neck cancer)
- Intracavitary: Radiation sources are placed into the body cavity in close proximity to the target tissue using applicators (e.g., breast balloon applicators, gynecological vaginal cylinders, multichannel vaginal balloon applicators, tandem and ovoids, tandem and ring, endometrial Y applicator, and rectum mold applicator, etc.)
- Intracavitary + Interstitial hybrid, GYN: Intracavitary hybrid applicators (e.g., tandem and ovoids with

S.-J. Park, PhD (✉)
Department of Radiation Oncology, University of California, Los Angeles, 200 UCLA Medical Plaza, Suite B265, Lost Angeles, CA 90095, USA
e-mail: spark@mednet.ucla.edu

D.H. Thomas, PhD
Department of Radiation Oncology, University of Colorado Denver, 1665 Aurora Ct, Campus Mail Stop F706, Aurora, CO, USA
e-mail: david.h.thomas@ucdenver.edu

© Springer International Publishing AG 2017
J. Mayadev et al. (eds.), *Handbook of Image-Guided Brachytherapy*, DOI 10.1007/978-3-319-44827-5_2

interstitial needles through the ovoids (Utrecht applicator, Elekta, Veenendaal, The Netherlands) and tandem and ring with interstitial needles through the ring (Vienna applicator, Elekta), tandem and ovoids/ring with interstitial needles through the ring combined with interstitial template (Venezia applicator, Elekta)), or a freehand hybrid placement of supplemental needles with a standard intracavitary applicator

- Interstitial + Intracavitary, Breast: Single-entry hybrid applicators placed in the lumpectomy cavity for accelerated partial breast irradiation (e.g., Strut Adjusted Volume Implant (SAVI, Cianna Medical, Aliso Viejo, CA, USA), ClearPath (North American Scientific, Chatsworth, CA, USA), Contura, and MammoSite (Hologic, Bedford, MA, USA) applicators)
- Surface/contact: Radiation sources are inserted into applicators positioned on a skin surface lesion (e.g., tungsten shielded skin applicators with and without flattening filter, the Freiburg flap (Elekta), end Catheter Flap set (Varian, Palo Alto, CA, USA), custom-mold applicators, plaque applicators, surface electronic brachytherapy applicators (Elekta Esteya® system; and iCAD Xoft® system, Nashua, NH, USA))
- Intraluminal: Sources are loaded into a lumen to treat its surface and adjacent tissue (e.g., esophageal, tracheal, bronchial tubes, bile duct applicator)
- Intravascular: Sources are brought intravascularly into or near a lesion
- Intraoperative: Sources are brought surgically into the tumor bed or near the tumor volume (e.g., Harrison-Anderson-Mick (HAM) applicator (Mick Radio-Nuclear Instruments, NY), Freiburg flap applicator (Elekta), the intrabeam system (Carl Zeiss, Oberkochen, Germany), the Axxent® electronic brachytherapy system (Xoft®, iCAD, Nashua, NH, USA))
- Figure 2.1 summarizes the main types of brachytherapy implants

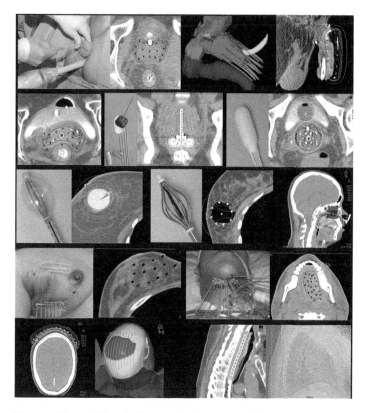

FIG. 2.1. Types of brachytherapy implant. From *left* to *right*, prostate interstitial brachytherapy CT image, implant photo, prostate 3D image, and penile interstitial in the *first row*; gynecological interstitial, tandem and ovoid applicator and CT image, Capri™ vaginal balloon applicator (Varian Medical Systems, Palo Alto, CA, USA), and CT in the *second row*; Contura® breast balloon applicator (Hologic, Bedford, MA, USA) and CT, SAVI applicator (Cianna Medical Group, Aliso Viego, CA, USA) and CT, and nasopharynx intracavitary CT image in the *third row*; breast interstitial (breast tube and button) CT image and photo, head and neck interstitial for base of tongue and implant photo in the *fourth row*; surface/contact brachytherapy for skin (scalp) and 3D image, and esophagus intracavitary CT and scout images in the *fifth row*

Types of Implant Duration

- Temporary implant: Dose is delivered over a period of time that is short in comparison with the half-life of the radiation sources. Sources are removed when the prescribed dose has been reached
- Permanent implant: Dose is delivered over the lifetime of the sources. The sources undergo complete radioactive decay

Types of Source Loading

- Preloading or hot loading: The applicator is preloaded and contains radioactive sources at time of placement into the patient
- Afterloading: The applicator is placed first into the patient, and the radioactive sources are loaded later either by hand (manual afterloading) or by computer controlled machine (automatic remote afterloading) to minimize radiation exposure to hospital personnel

Types of Dose Rate

- Very low dose rate (VLDR): <0.4 Gy/h
- Low dose rate (LDR): 0.4–2 Gy/h
- Medium dose rate (MDR): 2–12 Gy/h
- High-dose rate (HDR): >12 Gy/h [1]
- Pulsed dose rate (PDR) delivers the dose in a large number of small fractions with short intervals in order to achieve a radiobiological effect similar to low dose rate over the same treatment time. PDR treatments are delivered on the same hardware and applicators as the HDR modality [2–4]

Radioactive Sources

Characteristics of Radioactive Source

- Half-life: The time required for the source strength to decay to half of its initial value
- Specific activity: The amount of radioactivity for a given mass of the radioactive source
- Energy spectrum: The energies and types of the radiation particles that are emitted from the source
- Half value layer: Thickness of the material required to decrease the intensity of the incident beam to half of its original value
- Exposure rate constant (Gamma ray constant): The exposure in R/h at a point 1 cm from a 1 mCi point source

Ideal Radioisotopes for Brachytherapy

- Easily available inexpensive materials
- Easily filter emitted charged particles or the absence of charged particle emission
- No gaseous decay product to avoid source contamination by leaking
- Moderate half-life for minimal decay correction during treatment
- Moderate gamma ray constant which determines activity, output, and shielding requirements
- High specific activity to produce smaller size sources with higher output
- Nontoxic and insoluble materials

Source Forms

- Needles, tubes, wires, seeds, cylinder, spherical, beads, pellets, and micro pellets

Brachytherapy Radioisotopes

- Photon sources emit gamma rays through gamma decay and possibly characteristic x-rays through electron capture and internal conversion
- Beta sources emit electrons following beta decay
- Neutron sources emit neutrons following spontaneous nuclear fission reaction
- Historical sources: ^{222}Rn and ^{226}Ra
- Currently used sources: ^{32}P, ^{60}Co, ^{90}Sr/^{90}Y, ^{103}Pd, ^{125}I, ^{137}Cs, ^{192}Ir, and ^{198}Au, and electronic brachytherapy sources [5]
- Developmental sealed sources: ^{131}Cs, ^{145}Sm, ^{169}Yb, ^{241}Am, and ^{252}Cf
- Table 2.1 summarizes physical characteristics of brachytherapy radioisotopes

Treatment Planning

Historically, dosimetry systems such as the Manchester, Paris, Quimby, and Stockholm systems were derived from rich clinical experience used to deliver a specified dose to the tumor accurately in the absence of computerized treatment planning systems.

Dosimetric Systems

- Dosimetric systems are a set of rules to deliver a defined dose to a designated region
- Prior to the development of computerized treatment planning techniques, several classical implant systems were developed to calculate, for a given target volume
  - The total activity of the sources
  - Number of sources
  - The source distribution within the target volume
- Each system is specific to a radioisotope and its spatial distribution within the applicator

TABLE 2.1 Brachytherapy radioisotopes and characteristics

Radionuclide	Half-life	Average energy (MeV)	HVL (mm-lead)	Exposure rate constant (R cm^2 mCi^{-1} h^{-1})
High energy photon sources				
^{60}Co	5.25 years	1.25	11.0	13.07
^{137}Cs	30.0 years	0.662	6.2	3.26
^{192}Ir	73.8 days	0.38	2.5	4.69
^{198}Au	2.7 days	0.412	3.3	2.35
^{222}Rn	3.83 years	0.83	12	8.25
^{226}Ra	1600 years	0.83	14	8.25
Low energy photon sources				
^{103}Pd	17.0 days	0.021	0.0085	1.48
^{125}I	59.4 days	0.028	0.025	1.46
^{131}Cs	9.96 days	0.030	0.022	0.64
Beta sources				
^{32}P	14.3 days	0.695	–	–
^{90}Sr/^{90}Y	28.9 years	0.564	–	–
Developmental sources				
^{145}Sm	340 days	0.043	0.060	0.885
^{169}Yb	32 days	0.093	0.48	1.80
^{241}Am	432 years	0.060	0.12	0.12
^{252}Cf	2.65 years	2.1 neutron	–	–

- Each system therefore specifies the following:
  - Type of radioisotope to be used
  - The geometrical arrangement of radioisotope
  - Explicit details of the treatment including dose, time, and administration

- Usually, a system provides a set of tables to allow simple and reproducible calculation in most of the encountered clinical scenarios
- These classical systems have, for the most part, been replaced by computerized treatment planning systems, but remain useful as tools of independent quality assurance (QA) of the computer treatment plans

Manchester System or Paterson–Parker System for Interstitial Implants

- Paterson and Parker developed the Manchester system in 1934 [6, 7]
- The aim of this system is to deliver a uniform dose (within ±10 % from the prescribed dose) within a volume or planar implant
- In order to deliver homogeneous dose distribution, sources are distributed nonuniformly with more source strength concentrated in the periphery of the target volume in comparison to the center
- Different linear activities, 0.33, 0.50, and 0.66 mg Ra/cm radium source, were used
- The use of a specific pattern of distribution of radioactivity was recommended depending on the shape (linear, planar, and volume implant) and size of the implant
- Crossing needles are required to enhance dose at implant ends
- If the implants are not closed-ended or the shape of the implant is not square, the source strength should be adjusted
- The single-plane source arrangement implant is used to treat 1 cm thick slab of tissue, with the dose prescribed to a 0.5 cm away from the source plane
- For thicker slabs, two parallel planes are used to treat slabs of tissue with thickness up to 2.5 cm. The required total source strength is equally distributed between the two planes in proportion to their relative areas

Quimby System or Memorial System for Interstitial Implants

- Developed by Quimby in 1932 [8–11]
- A uniform distribution of source strength allows a higher dose in the center of the treatment volume than near the periphery
- Constant intensity (0.5 or 1.0 mg Ra/cm radium source) was used
- To deliver the prescription dose, a system of tables and rules has been generated to provide the total source strength for a uniform distribution of the source activity
- Dose value obtained from the Quimby tables represents the minimum dose within the target volume
- Typically, dose rates used in the Quimby System for patient treatments (60–70 cGy/h) are much higher than the Patterson–Parker (Manchester) system (40 cGy/h)

Paris System for Interstitial Implants

- This system was developed by Pierquin, Dutreix, and Chassagne for ^{192}Ir wire implants in 1960s and 1970s [12, 13]
- The Paris system is used for single and double plane implants
- The source strength (activity/cm) is uniform and identical for all sources in the implant
- Sources are linear and their placements are parallel
- Adjacent sources must be equidistant from each other. Source separation should be determined according to active implant length
- The prescription dose is made to the "central plane," which is perpendicular to the direction of the sources, at the midpoint of the implant
- Since crossing needles are not used, the active source length is 30–40 % longer than the target length
- In volume implants, cross-sectional source distribution forms a series of equilateral triangles or squares

- The reference isodose is 85 % of the average basal dose, which is defined by the minimum dose between the sources

Stockholm System for Intracavitary Implants

- Based on a fractionated course of radiation treatment using ^{226}Ra sources over a period of 1 month with two or three applications [14, 15]
- 60–80 mg radium sources were placed inside the vagina using an intravaginal applicator while 30–90 mg of radium was placed inside uterus using an intrauterine tube
- A total radiation dose of 6500–7100 mg-h was prescribed for the cervical cancer treatment

Manchester System for Intracavitary Implants

- It was published in 1938 by Tod and Meredith (updated in 1953) and remains in use today [16–18]
- Defines treatment in terms of dose to a point representative of the target, and which is anatomically comparable from patient to patient. The dose points should not be in a region of high-dose gradient (i.e., sensitive to small changes in applicator position)
- A "dose-limiting point" Point A was originally defined as 2 cm lateral to the center of the uterine canal and 2 cm superior to the mucosal membrane of the lateral fornix in the plane of the uterus
- Later Point A was redefined to be 2 cm superior to the external cervical os (or cervical end of the tandem) and 2 cm lateral to the cervical canal
- Manchester system can be characterized by the dose to four points;
  - Point A
  - Point B = 5 cm lateral to the mid pelvis. For example, this would be to Point A, when the central canal is not displaced . This could be further from Point A

if the tandem is favoring one side of the pelvis due to anatomy

- Bladder point - the most dependent portion of the foley balloon with 7 cc of contrast
- Rectum point defined as 0.5 cm posterior to the posterior vaginal mucosa at the lower end of the intruterine source or mid vaginal source
- Figure 2.2 shows definition of points A and B
- If the tandem displaced the central canal, Point A moves with the canal, but Point B remains fixed at 5 cm from midline
- 20, 15 – 10, and 15 – 10 – 10 mg of Ra was loaded in the short, medium, and long uterine tubes. 17.5, 20, and 22.5 mg of Ra was loaded in the small, medium, and large ovoids
- Designed such that:
  - Dose rate at Point A was approximately 0.53 Gy/h for all allowed applicator loadings
  - Vaginal contribution to Point A was limited to 40 % of the total dose

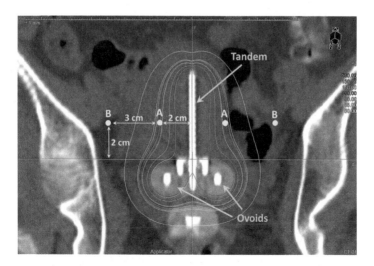

FIG. 2.2. Definition of points A and B for intracavitary implant according to the Manchester system

- The rectal dose should be 80 % or less of the dose to Point A
- In the absence of external beam, 80 Gy to Point A was prescribed in two applications with total of 144 h
- In 1938 Tod showed that toxicity to the pyramid shaped area, "paracervical triangle," in the medial edge of the broad ligament (where uterine vessels cross the ureter) was the main dose limiting factor in the treatment of the uterine cervix
- The validity of this point for this was illustrated in a study of over 500 cases, which showed a clear relationship between the tolerance of normal tissues and the dose received to this area

Paris System for Intracavitary Implants

- A single application of radium brachytherapy was prescribed for cervical cancer treatment [12, 13]
- Unlike the Stockholm system, almost an equal amount of radium was used in the uterus and the vagina in the Paris system
- The system used two cork colpostats in the form of a cylinder and an intrauterine tube
- The system was designed to deliver a dose of 7000–8000 mg-h of radium over a period of 5 days
- One intrauterine source contained three radium sources with source strengths in the ratio of 1:1:0.5. The source strength of the topmost uterine source was the same as the strengths in the colpostats

Problems with Older Dosimetric Systems

- Since both the Paris and the Stockholm Systems used intrauterine tubes, which were separate from the vaginal colpostats, these systems had a loose geometry
- With the use of external-beam radiotherapy which specified the prescription in terms of the absorbed

dose, the use of Milligram-hours of radium as a unit in brachytherapy was no longer acceptable
- In addition, dose prescription in this unit ignored the importance of tolerance of different critical organs to radiation. This was because the dose to important anatomical targets could not be quantified adequately with the use of this dose prescription method

Dose Optimization

- Optimization is shaping of the isodose line. Normalization is scaling of the isodose lines
- Goals of optimization:
  - Homogeneous dose distribution in the target
  - Coverage of the target with minimum prescription dose
  - Sparing dose to critical organs with high-dose gradient outside the target
- Optimization methods:
  - Manual dwell weights
  - Manual dwell times
  - Geometrical optimization (distance and volume optimization)
  - Graphical optimization
  - Inverse planning optimization (IPSA, HIPO, etc.)
- Optimization of dose distribution is usually achieved by weighting the relative spatial and temporal distribution of sources in order to achieve the required dose at prescription point/volume coverage
- Source dwell position and relative dwell times are analytically optimized in order to achieve the desired dose distribution
- Typical optimization algorithms initially assign dwell times for all source dwell positions based on their respective distances to each other
- To compensate for the reduced dose contribution from the other dwell positions, a dwell position at larger distance from any other dwell positions will be assigned larger dwell times

- A homogeneous dose distribution, as defined by the ratio of volume of high dose to volume of prescription dose (e.g., dose homogeneity index (DHI) = $1 - V150/V100$) will be the result of this initial optimization
- More advanced optimization techniques include graphic optimization and inverse planning optimization
- Graphic optimization allows graphical control over desired isodose lines, with the dwell locations and time updated accordingly
- Inverse planning is an anatomy-based dose distribution optimization approach [19]
- Similarly to IMRT, inverse planning in brachytherapy requires 3D-imaging (CT, MRI, Ultrasound, etc.) and the segmentation (contouring) of Volumes of Interest (VOI)
- Optimized dose distributions should be carefully reviewed to avoid unintended high-dose regions or gradients arising due to control of target/OAR dose distributions

Dose Calculation

Fundamental Problems with Old Dose Calculation Protocols

- Real brachytherapy source gives anisotropic distribution since it is not exactly equivalent to a point source.
- Old protocols calculate photon fluence in free space and do not take into account photon scattering in a scattering medium (tissue)
- For accurate dose calculation in clinical applications, dose distributions should be calculated in a scattering medium (water equivalent medium)

AAPM TG-43 Protocol

The AAPM recommended TG-43 dosimetry protocol to resolve the fundamental problems with the old dose calculation protocols [20, 21]. From the AAPM-TG 43 protocol, dose rate, $\dot{D}(r,\theta)$ at Point P with polar coordinate (r,θ) in a medium is

$$\dot{D}(r,\theta) = S_{\mathrm{K}} \cdot \Lambda \cdot \frac{G_{\mathrm{L}}(r,\theta)}{G_{\mathrm{L}}(r_0,\theta_0)} \cdot g_L(r) \cdot F(r,\theta)$$

- r: the distance (in centimeters) from the center of the active source to the point of interest
- θ: the angle specifying the point of interest relative to the source longitudinal axis
- r_0: the reference distance which is specified to be 1 cm in this protocol
- θ_0: the reference angle on the source transverse plane and is specified to be 90° or $\pi/2$ radians
- Figure 2.3 shows the geometry used in the dose calculation based on the AAPM-TG 43 protocol
- S_{K}: air-kerma strength
  - $S_{\mathrm{K}} = \dot{K}_\delta(d)d^2$

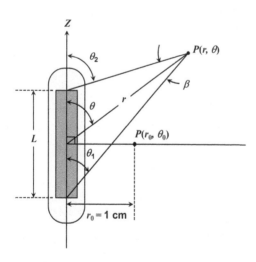

FIG. 2.3. Illustration of geometry used in the TG-43 dose calculation formalism

- air-kerma rate at the point along the transverse axis of the source in free space
- a measure of brachytherapy source strength
- units of $1\ U = 1\ \mu\ Gy\ m^2 h^{-1} = 1\ cGy\ cm^2 h^{-1}$
- measured in vacuo meaning that it must not include effects due to attenuation or scattering in a medium
- must be measured at a distance much larger than the source length (typically of the order of 1 m)
- include contributions from photons greater than δ (energy cutoff, typically 5 keV) to exclude low-energy or contaminant photons
- usually determined by an NIST wide angle free air chamber

- Λ: dose-rate constant

  - $$\Lambda = \frac{\dot{D}\left(r_0, \theta_0\right)}{S_K}$$

  - the dose rate to water as a distance of 1 cm on the transverse axis of a unit air kerma strength source in a water phantom
  - depends not only on the radioactive material type and quantity but also the source construction
  - $\Lambda = 0.686$ for ^{103}Pd, 0.965–1.036 for ^{125}I, 1.12 for ^{192}Ir.

- $G_L(r, \theta)$: geometry function
  - accounts for the variation of relative dose due to the spatial distribution of activity within the source
  - generalizes the inverse square correction
  - considering the fall-off of the photon fluence
  - ignoring photon attenuation and scattering in the source

  - $$G_L\left(r,\theta\right) = \begin{cases} \dfrac{\beta}{Lr\sin\theta} & if \quad \theta \neq 0° \\ \left(r^2 - L^2/4\right)^{-1} & if \quad \theta = 0° \end{cases}$$

  line-source approximation

  - $G_P\left(r,\theta\right) = r^{-2}$ point-source approximation

- $g_L(r)$: radial dose function

- $$G_L\left(r\right) = \frac{\dot{D}\left(r,\,\theta_0\right)}{\dot{D}\left(r_0,\,\theta_0\right)} \frac{G_L\left(r_0,\,\theta_0\right)}{G_L\left(r,\,\theta_0\right)}$$

- accounts for the effects of absorption and scatter in the medium along the transverse axis of the source
- Figure 2.4 shows the radial dose functions for the most commonly used brachytherapy sources

- $F(r, \theta)$: 2D anisotropy function

- $$F\left(r,\theta\right) = \frac{\dot{D}\left(r,\theta\right)}{\dot{D}\left(r,\,\theta_0\right)} \frac{G_L\left(r_0,\,\theta_0\right)}{G_L\left(r,\,\theta_0\right)}$$

- accounts for the anisotropy of dose distribution around the source
- including the effects of absorption and scatter in the medium
- Figure 2.5 shows anisotropy function for ^{192}Ir source

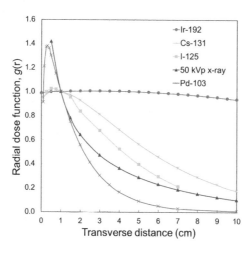

FIG. 2.4. Radial dose functions in water for [103]Pd, 50 kVp x-ray, ^{125}I, [131]Cs, and ^{192}Ir sources

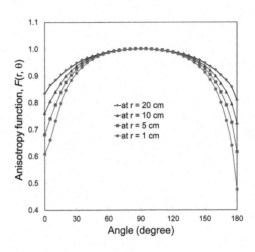

FIG. 2.5. Anisotropy function for ^{192}Ir Flexitron source

■ Dose rate at the implant:

$$\dot{D} = \dot{D}_0 e^{-\lambda t}$$

■ Cumulative dose:

$$D_{\text{cum}} = \dot{D}_0 \int_0^t e^{-\lambda t} dt = \frac{\dot{D}_0}{\lambda}\left(1 - e^{-\lambda t}\right)$$

■ Total delivered dose from short treatment time $\left(t \ll t_{1/2}\right)$:

$$D_{\text{cum}} = \dot{D}_0 \int_0^t e^{-\lambda t} dt \cong \frac{\dot{D}_0}{\lambda}\left\{1 - \left(1 - e^{-\lambda t}\right)\right\} = \dot{D}_0 t$$

■ Total delivered dose from permanent implant $\left(t \to \infty\right)$:

$$D_{\text{cum}} = \dot{D}_0 \int_0^\infty e^{-\lambda t} dt = \frac{\dot{D}_0}{\lambda} = \dot{D}_0 \tau$$

- $\dot{D}_0$: initial dose rate (Gy/h)
- $\lambda = \dfrac{\ln 2}{T_{1/2}}$: decay constant
- $T_{1/2}$: half-life of the radioisotope
- $\tau = \dfrac{1}{\lambda}$: mean lifetime of the radioisotope

Model-Based Dose Calculation (MBDCA, AAPM TG-186 Protocol)

- Monte Carlo simulations in brachytherapy geometries show errors incurred with the AAPM TG-43 approach [22]
- The significant dose differences in nonwater media (tissues, applicators, and air-tissue interfaces) were seen in the low energy region (<50 keV)
- For the dependence of scatter dose in the 3D geometry, either the radiation transport simulation in the actual media or multiple-dimensional scatter integration is used in the MBDCA approaches

Grid-Based Boltzmann Equation Solvers (GBBS)

- The linear Boltzmann transport equation (LBTE) is the governing equation for radiation transport
- The GBBS are deterministic methods for solving the true continuous LBTE by discretizing the phase-space variables (space, angle, and energy)
- The GBBS was commercially integrated into the Acuros® TPS by Varian Medical Systems

Monte Carlo Simulations (MC)

- In order to solve the LBTE, the MC simulations were used with random sampling

- The MC codes include PTRAN, EGSnrc, MCNP, GEANT4, etc
- In order to the LBTE by random sampling, the MC simulations were used
- The MC is the current state of the art in computational dosimetry, but not optimized for calculation speed
- Pre-calculated phase-space files were used to accelerate calculation speed
- Not commercially available for brachytherapy planning

Collapsed-Cone Superposition/Convolution Method (CCC)

- CC is a point kernel superposition method
- For calculation efficiency, the CCC algorithm uses angular discretization ("collapsed cones") of the kernels along a radiation transport grid
- The primary dose was calculated through a direct ray tracing of the primary photons using the kerma approximation
- The secondary dose from first scatter and multiple scatters was calculated separately with different kernels for heterogeneities
- The CCC algorithm has implemented in the Oncentra® BrachyTPS from Elekta (Veenendaal, The Netherlands)

References

1. International Commission on Radiation Units and Measurements (ICRU). 1985 dose and volume specification for reporting and recording intracavitary therapy in gynecology. Report 38 of ICRU. Bethesda: ICRU Publications.
2. Brenner DJ, Hall EJ, Randers-Pehrson G, Huang Y, Johnson GW, Miller RW, Wu B, Vazquez ME, Medvedovsky C, Worgul BV. Quantitative comparisons of continuous and pulsed low dose rate regimens in a model late-effect system. Int J Radiat Oncol Biol Phys. 1996;34:905–10.

3. Chen CZ, Huang Y, Hall EJ, Brenner DJ. Pulsed brachytherapy as a substitute for continuous low dose rate: an in vitro study with human carcinoma cells. Int J Radiat Oncol Biol Phys. 1997;37:137–43.
4. Visser AG, van den Aardweg GJ, Levendag PC. Pulsed dose rate and fractionated high dose rate brachytherapy: choice of brachytherapy schedules to replace low dose rate treatments. Int J Radiat Oncol Biol Phys. 1996;34:497–505.
5. Williamson JF. Clinical brachytherapy physics. In: Perez CA, Brady LW, editors. Principles and practice of radiation oncology. 3rd ed. Philadelphia: Lippincott Williams and Wilkins; 1998. p. 405–67.
6. Paterson R, Parker HMA. A dosage system for gamma ray therapy. Br J Radiol. 1934;7:592–612.
7. Paterson R, Parker HMA. A dosage system for interstitial radium therapy. Br J Radiol. 1952;25:505–16.
8. Quimby EH. The grouping of radium tubes in packs on plaques to produce the desired distribution of radiation. Am J Roentgenol. 1932;27:18.
9. Quimby EH. Dosage tables for linear radium sources. Radiology. 1944;43:572–7.
10. Quimby EH, Castro V. The calculation of dosage in interstitial radium therapy. Am J Roentgenol. 1953;70:739–49.
11. Glasser O, Quimby EH, Taylor LS, et al. Physical foundations of radiology. 3rd ed. New York: Harper & Row; 1961.
12. Pierquin B. Precis de Curietherapie. Endocurietherapie et Plesiocurietherapie. Paris: Masson; 1964.
13. Pierquin B, Dutreix A, Paine C, Chassagne D, Marinello G, Ash D. The Paris system in interstitial radiation therapy. Acta Radiol Oncol. 1978;17(1):33–48.
14. Heymann J. The so-called Stockholm method and the results of treatment of uterine cancer at Radiumhemmet. Acta Radiol. 1935;16:129–48.
15. Kottmeier HL. Surgical and radiation treatment of carcinoma of the uterine cervix. Experience by the current individualized Stockholm Technique. Acta Obstet Gynecol Scand. 1964;43(2):1–48.
16. Tod M, Meredith WJ. A dosage system for use in the treatment of cancer of the uterine cervix. Br J Radiol. 1938;11:809–24.
17. Tod M, Meredith WJ. Treatment of cancer of the cervix uteri – a revised Manchester method. Br J Radiol. 1953;26:252–7.
18. Meredith WJ. Radium dosage: the Manchester system. Edinburg: Livingston; 1967.

19. Lessard E, Pouliot J. Inverse planning anatomy-based dose opti-
    mization for HDR-brachytherapy of the prostate using fast
    simulated annealing algorithm and dedicated objective function.
    Med Phys. 2001;28(5):773–9.
20. Nath R, Anderson LL, Luxton G, Weaver KA, Williamson JF,
    Meigooni AS. Dosimetry of interstitial brachytherapy sources:
    recommendations of the AAPM Radiation Therapy Committee
    Task Group No.43. American Association of Physicists in
    Medicine. Med Phys. 1995;22(2):209–34.
21. Rivard MJ, Coursey BM, DeWerd LA, Hanson WF, Huq MS,
    Ibbott GS, Mitch MG, Nath R, Williamson JF. Update of AAPM
    Task Group No. 43 Report: a revised AAPM protocol for
    brachytherapy dose calculations. Med Phys. 2004;31(3):633–74.
22. Beaulieu L, Carlsson Tedgren A, Carrier JF, Davis SD, Mourtada
    F, Rivard MJ, Thomson RM, Verhaegen F, Wareing TA,
    Williamson JF. Report of the Task Group 186 on model-based
    dose calculation methods in brachytherapy beyond the TG-43
    formalism: current status and recommendations for clinical
    implementation. Med Phys. 2012;39(10):6208–36.

Chapter 3
Treatment Delivery Technology for Brachytherapy

J. Adam M. Cunha and Dae Yup Han

Introduction

Because of the wide range of applications and tumor sites treated with brachytherapy, delivery technology is extremely diverse. Brachytherapy is customizable and allows for personalized design of applicators and implants tailored to each patient. This chapter will summarize the most popular delivery techniques. We will cover a few helpful rules of thumb for the physics and planning of brachytherapy implants. Then, we will cover the most common types of brachytherapy procedures: permanent seed implants and afterloader-based temporary implants. Finally, we will discuss microsphere brachytherapy.

J.A.M. Cunha, PhD (✉) • D.Y. Han, PhD
Department of Radiation Oncology, University of California,
San Francisco, 1600 Divisadero St, Box 1708, Suite H1030,
San Francisco, CA 94115, USA
e-mail: Adam.Cunha@ucsf.edu; DaeYup.Han@ucsf.edu

© Springer International Publishing AG 2017
J. Mayadev et al. (eds.), *Handbook of Image-Guided Brachytherapy*, DOI 10.1007/978-3-319-44827-5_3

General Physics and Technology

- Inverse r-squared law results in quick fall off of dose
- As a rule of thumb, the 50 % isodose line is separated from the 100 % isodose line by a distance of approximately 1 cm. This is a useful point of reference when estimating expected dose to organs at risk
- As a rule of thumb, the half-life of the Ir-192 sources used most commonly for high dose rate (HDR) brachytherapy will cause a drop in activity of approximately 1 % per day
- Temporary implants result in no radiation being left in the patient when they leave the clinic/hospital. Permanent implants do leave radioactive material in the patient
- A vast database of information on brachytherapy sources can be found at the web site of the Imaging and Radiation Oncology Core (IROC) at M.D. Anderson Cancer Center (http://rpc.mdanderson.org). This database, the Joint AAPM/IROC Houston Registry of Brachytherapy Sources Meeting the AAPM Dosimetric Prerequisites, includes both currently available sources and older sources no longer available
- Forward-based planning, e.g., Point-A-based cervical brachytherapy has been a standard of brachytherapy for decades, but its use has been falling out of favor over the last decade due to the target dose coverage and normal tissue dose sparing techniques available with modern inverse planning techniques. Inverse planning uses anatomical information to inform the dose distribution. Inverse Planning Simulated Annealing (IPSA) was one of the first widely implemented inverse planning systems for brachytherapy [1–3]
- Specialized clinics may produce custom applicators for each patient and modern additive manufacturing (3D printing) techniques can be especially useful. If custom materials are used for patient-specific applicators; however, it is critical to understand the dosimetric properties of the fabrication materials for the photon energy range of the source being used [4, 5]

Permanent Implant Brachytherapy

General Facts

- Most common uses: Prostate, Brain
- Typical dose rate at time of implant: 0.4–2.0 Gy/h.
- Treatment dose delivered on a timescale of weeks/months.
- Radiation dose rate decays to background in approximately 5 half-lives
- No shielding required for implant room
- Exposure to physicists and physicians during preparation and implant is low but non-zero
- Seeds may be ordered loose or in preloaded needles
- Radiation sources are placed within or on the cancer volume and left in place indefinitely
- Because the radiation is left in the patient after discharge, security scans will pick up a signal above background for the first few months. UCSF gives each patient an identification card to provide to, e.g., airport security (Fig. 3.1).

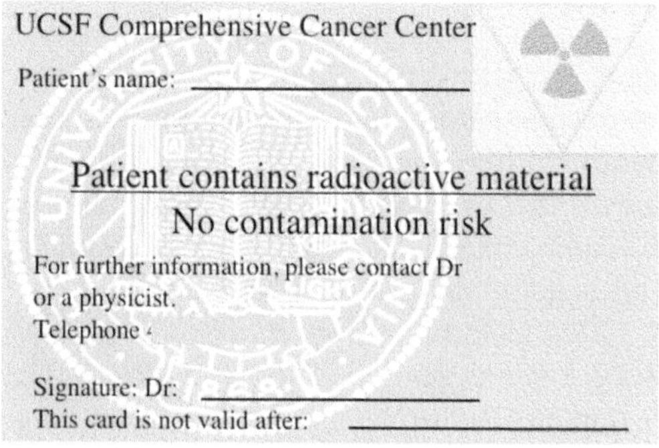

UCSF Comprehensive Cancer Center

Patient's name: _____

Patient contains radioactive material
No contamination risk

For further information, please contact Dr
or a physicist.
Telephone ⸱

Signature: Dr: _____
This card is not valid after: _____

FIG. 3.1. Radiation card. The identification card provided by UCSF for each patient after a procedure that places radioactive material in the body permanently. This card should be carried by patients to be shown, e.g., to airport security

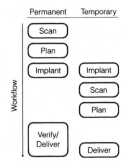

Fig. 3.2. Workflow. The implant workflow for the two most common sealed source brachytherapy delivery types: permanent seed implants and afterloader-based (temporary, HDR) implants. Permanent implants are commonly called low dose rate implants, while temporary implants can be either low dose rate or high dose rate. The main difference is the timing of the dose planning, which is done prior to the implant procedure for permanent case and after the catheter insertion procedure for the temporary implant case

Workflow

- The standard workflow for permanent prostate implants is: Scan, Plan, Implant, Verify (S-P-I-V). Figure 3.2 shows the difference between the workflow for permanent implants and temporary brachytherapy treatment like high dose rate brachytherapy
- *Scan*—The pre-implant scan is generally done under the same conditions as will be present for the implant. This is generally trans-rectal ultrasound
  - Often called a *volume study*
  - Performed several days to a few weeks prior to implant to allow time for dose planning and seed ordering/delivery
  - MR spectroscopy in prostate may be used to identify local lesions

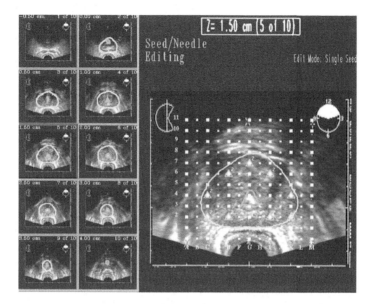

FIG. 3.3. Template. A pre-implant plan for a prostate permanent-seed implant. Note the *grid of white dots* corresponds to the needle insertion grid placed on the perineum of the patient. This is co-registered with the trans-rectal ultrasound used to obtain the image

■ *Plan*—Planning is done using the pre-implant scan and planning software specifically designed for the task. The template grid used for needle insertion is overlaid on the ultrasound image to provide a 3D matrix of seed placement locations typically 0.5 cm in the left-right and anterior-posterior directions, and 5 cm in the superior-inferior direction (Fig. 3.3)
 ■ Often referred to as the *preplan* since it is done prior to the implant (contrast with the afterloaded brachytherapy workflow)
 ■ Generate a dose plan based on the image set obtained.
 ■ Planning may be done manually or with inverse planning

- Seed order-to-delivery times are approximately 1 week
- Seeds my come preloaded in needles ready for implant or loose. If they are ordered loose, the medical physicist is responsible for loading each needle with the correct seed configuration
- *Implant*—The needle template used to guide the needle insertion is placed on the perineum and the current (live) ultrasound implant is aligned with the preplan scan. This co-registers the planned prostate volume with the position of the prostate at the time of the surgical procedure
  - Done under anesthesia in an operating room
  - Typical time: 1 h
  - After the procedure, the patient generally takes 1–3 h to recover from anesthesia at which point they are able to leave the hospital
- *Verify*—Post-implant dosimetry is required to verify the placement of the seeds and to record the dose delivered to the patient
  - Most commonly done using CT imaging
  - Up to 30 days after the implant but can be done on the day of the implant. If done on the day of the implant, edema needs to be accounted for since it will cause the dose coverage to appear cooler (Fig. 3.4) [6].
- The workflow for brain or other implants that do not incorporate pre-implant planning is simpler: Steps 1-Scan and 2-Implant are not performed. A number of seeds are ordered prior to the operation based on the expected size of the resection cavity. The implant immediately follows surgical resection of the bulky mass of the tumor in the operating room. After surgical resection of the tumor, the seeds are glued one-by-one to the inner surface of the resection cavity in an approximately 1 cm × 1 cm grid. A post-implant CT scan is obtained to perform the dosimetry of the implant and recorded in the patient's medical record

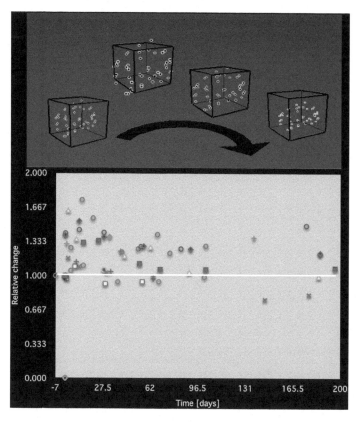

FIG. 3.4. Edema. Prostate edema as a function of time after a permanent implant for a sample of 10 randomly selected patients from our clinic. While edema doesn't have a significant effect for all patients, it can cause an increase in the volume of the prostate by a factor of two. This can have a significant impact on the dose delivered to the gland

TABLE 3.1 Common PPI sources: the three most commonly used sealed brachytherapy sources for permanent implants

Radionuclide	Half-life (days)	Average energy (keV)	Year introduced	Typical monotherapy seed strength (mCi)	(U)
125-I	59.4	28.4	1965	0.3–0.6	0.4–0.8
103-Pd	17.0	20.7	1986	1.1–2.2	1.4–2.8
131-Cs	9.7	30.4	2004	2.5–3.9	1.6–2.5

Common Radionuclides

The three most common radionuclides for permanent implants are Iodine-125, Palladium-103, and Cesium-131 (Table 3.1).

- 125-I
  - Decay: γ-ray emitting, characteristic X-rays are produced by e^- capture
  - Average energy: 0.028 MeV
  - Half-life: 60 days
  - Half value layer (lead): 0.02 mm
  - Commonly used in clinic with hot loading
- 103-Pd
  - Decay: e^- capture with emission of characteristic X-rays, γ ray emitting
  - Average energy: 0.021 MeV
  - Half-life: 17 days
  - Half value layer (lead): 0.01 mm
  - Commonly used in clinic with hot loading
- 131-Cs
  - Decay: Electron capture with emission of characteristic X-rays and electrons. Electrons are absorbed in seed wall.
  - Average energy: 0.029 MeV
  - Half-life: 9.7 days
  - Half value layer (lead): 0.03 mm

- Source models: Sources are manufactured by a number of different vendors. The design of each source is different for each vendor as can be seen in Fig. 3.5a, b.

Afterloader-Based Brachytherapy

General Facts

- The main advantage of afterloader-based brachytherapy is that is simple utilize time as a treatment planning variable
- Minimum dwell times are generally 0.1 s with typical dwell times ranging from 0.1 to 60 s or longer
- Typical dose rate: 12 Gy/h or more [7]
- Typical treatment times are on the order of 10 min
- Shielding:
  - Linac vault design is sufficient for HDR brachytherapy;
  - CT room design is NOT sufficient for HDR brachytherapy
- Cancer site use:
  - Common: prostate, gynecologic, breast, skin
  - Less common: oral cavity, base of tongue, nasopharynx, bronchial, kidney, keloids
  - No sites are explicitly contraindicated
  - Main restriction on site use is accessibility via intracavitary applicator or interstitial needle

Workflow

The standard workflow for afterloader-based brachytherapy is: Implant, Scan, Plan, Deliver (I-S-P-D). The procedure is described in detail in the report of AAPM Task Group 59 [8] and is illustrated in Fig. 3.6.

- *Implant*—Applicators are chosen depending on the tumor site being treated. Figure 3.7a–h shows some of

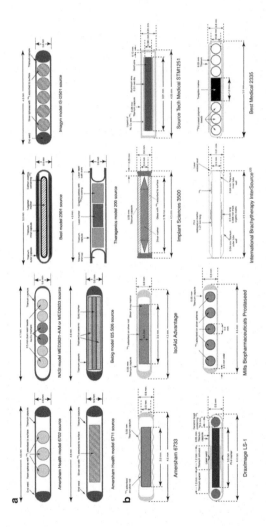

Fig. 3.5. (a, b) LDR sources. The internal structure of several sealed radiation sources used for seed implant brachytherapy (a) TG-43 [4] and (b) TG-43 update [5]. ((a): Used with permission from ICRU, International Commission on Radiation Units and Measurements. Dose and volume specification for reporting intracavitary therapy in gynecology. ICRU Report 38 1985; Bethesda, Maryland, USA; (b): Used with permission from Han DY, Webster MJ, Scanderbeg DJ, Yashar C, Choi D, Song B, Devic S, Ravi A, Song WY. Direction-Modulated Brachytherapy for High-Dose-Rate Treatment of Cervical Cancer. I: Theoretical Design, International Journal of Radiation Oncology, Biology, Physics 2014; 89(3): 666–673)

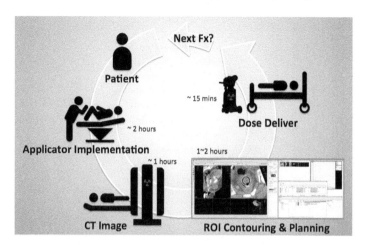

F<small>IG.</small> 3.6. HDR workflow. The typical afterloader-based brachytherapy workflow starts with applicator placement. This is followed by imaging of the applicator in place in the anatomy, structure delineation, and finally dose delivery. Fractioned treatments can have a different plan for each fraction if desired. In this case, care should be taken when reporting doses since contoured structures are not necessarily the same physical volumes for each fraction and aggregate doses to hotspots will be strictly less than a simple addition of the D1cc, D2cc, etc., values

the more common applicators. The following is not exclusive to the sites listed but are the most commonly used

- Intracavitary applicators come in various designs depending on the cavity shape and location. They are most commonly metal (non-CT, -MR compatible) or plastic (CT and MR compatible) though other materials can be used as long as the photon attenuation properties are known and biocompatibility is established
  - Types: Vaginal cylinder, tandem and ring, tandem and ovoids (Fletcher), breast balloon-type (SAVI®) (Cianna Medical, Aliso Viego, CA, USA,

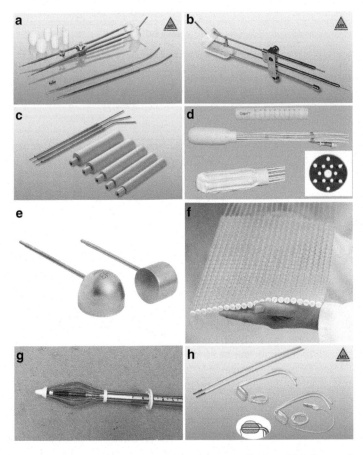

FIG. 3.7. (**a–h**) Applicators. Intracavitary applicators: Tandem and ovoids (**a**) and tandem and ring (**b**) with rectum retractor for cervical cancer; (**c**) tandem and cylinder for vaginal cancer; (**d**) Capri applicator for vagina and rectum cancer; flap-style applicator (**e**) and collimated-style applicator (**f**) for skin cancer; (**g**) SAVI applicator for breast cancer; (**h**) nasopharyngeal cancer applicator. Note that the thin plastic cover in (**f**) is critical for the absorption of secondary electrons produced in the Tungsten walls of the applicators. (Images used with permission of Varian (**a–d, h**), Elekta (**e, f**), and Cianna Medical)

and Contoura®, Hologic, Bedfor, MA, USA), naso-pharynx (Rotterdam), rectal cylinder, bronchial catheters, etc

■ Common uses: rectum wall, virginal wall, cervix, lumpectomy cavity, bronchus and esophagus, nasopharynx, etc

■ Interstitial applications generally make use of plastic catheters with a metal stylet that provides stiffness for puncture

■ Common uses: prostate, breast, cervix, vaginal wall, lips, tongue, penis, etc

■ Skin applicators have several types depending on the size and location of the tumor. There are a few main types:

■ Surface flaps can be used for large treatment areas and provide uniform spacing for the source dwell positions;

■ Collimated surface applicators (Leipzig, etc.) provide a narrow beam of dose and can include a flattening filter. It is critical that these tungsten applicators are used with a thin plastic cap in place between the applicator and the skin otherwise electron contamination from the high-Z material will result higher than planned superficial dose

■ *Scan (Imaging)*—Each of the four main imaging modalities can play a role in this step of the afterloader-based brachytherapy workflow

■ X-ray

■ Pros: 2D image, low soft tissue contrast
■ Cons: fast imaging time, cheap

■ CT

■ Pros: 3D image, fast imaging time, tissue density information
■ Cons: low soft tissue contrast, metal artifacts (e.g., hip, dental implants) make organ segmentation and catheter digitization difficult

- **MR**
  - Pros: 3D image, high soft tissue contrast
  - Cons: longer imaging time, cannot use metal applicators, no tissue density information, interstitial catheter definition can be difficult because the air inside the catheters is not well visualized
- **Ultrasound**
  - Pros: 2D/3D image, live image (used for image guided intestinal applicator implementation), high soft tissue contrast, Doppler imaging can help avoid vessels during interstitial insertion, cheap
  - Cons: Field of view can be shallower than extent of dose cloud, speed of sound can affect image co-registration with stereotactic needles, high density material (bone, needles) shadow and artifacts (mirror image artifact, speed displacement artifact, ring-down artifact)
- *Plan*—Key factors in planning mimic those in the previous step; however, a few unique points to keep in mind are:
  - Conventional X-ray-based planning
    - Hard to define target and organs due to no soft tissue contrast
    - Historic empirical plans (e.g., "point A" for cervical cancer)
  - 3D volumetric planning
    - Use 3D image modalities
    - Can delineate organs
    - Computer-based dose calculation (AAPM TG-43, AAPM TG-43U, and AAPM TG-168)
    - Computer-based plan optimization (IPSA, HIPO, etc.)
- *Deliver* (*Afterloaders*)—The afterloader allows the radioactive material to be positioned in the patient for delivery *after* the placement/insertion of the delivery applicator/interstitial needles (Fig. 3.8a–c)

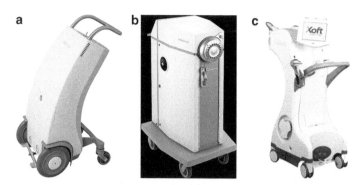

Fig. 3.8. (a–c) Afterloaders. Two of the most popular Ir-192 high dose rate (HDR) brachytherapy afterloaders: (a) MicroSelectron (Nucletron®/Elekta, Stockholm, Sweden); (b) VeriSource™ iX (Varian, Palo Alto, CA, USA); (c) The Xoft Axxent® electronic brachytherapy afterloader system (iCAD, Nashua, NH, USA). ((a): Used with permission of Elekta, Stockholm, Sweden; (b): Used with Permission of Varian, Palo Alto, CA, USA; (c): Used with permission of iCAD, Nashua, NH, USA)

- Source
  - 192-Ir source is encapsulated and attached on nitinol wire
  - Overall diameter ≤ 1 mm (MicroSelectron® (Elekta, Stockholm, Sweden) = 1.1 m, VariSource® (Varian, Paolo Alto, CA, USA) = 0.59 mm)
  - The source is stored built-in shielding with typical dose rates at 5 cm from the surface of the afterloader < 0.1 mR/h
  - Conventional activity is 10 Ci (370 GBq) for HDR and 1 Ci (37 GBq) for pulsed dose rate (PDR)
- Two servomotors are used for determining source position and deciding channel
- A dummy source (nonactivated source) is used to verify the accessibility of each dwell position before beginning the treatment
- Source calibration and safety check need to be performed as recommended in TG-40 and TG-56

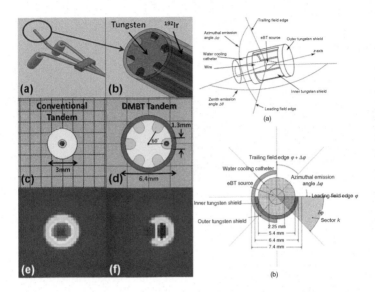

FIG. 3.9. New applicators. Direction-modulate brachytherapy (*left*) and rotate-shielding brachytherapy (*right*)

New Applicators/Concepts

Several new technologies for customized brachytherapy applicators have been explored in recent years; two of the most promising new technologies are mm-scale shielding and additive manufacturing (3D printing).

- mm-scale and dynamic shielding in cervical and uterine cancer applicators.
  - Figure 3.9 shows two designs of mm-scale shielded applicators, direction modulated brachytherapy (DMBT) [9, 10] and rotating-shield brachytherapy (RSBT) [11]
  - Both of these designs incorporate shielding into the tandem applicator that is placed through the cervix into the uterus
  - Care must be taking when performing dose planning with shielded applicators since the standard TG-43 dosimetry used for sealed-source brachytherapy

does not apply. TG-43 assumes an infinite water medium and is valid to acceptable uncertainties in traditional brachytherapy implants. However, shielding is explicitly not water and therefore Monte Carlo or model-based (TG-186) [12] dosimetry is required

- Additive manufacturing or 3D printing
  - This technology is posed to have a significant impact on the design of customized brachytherapy applicators because it allows for easy fabrication of designs incorporating internal substructure (i.e., catheter channels)
  - Biocompatibility must be verified to ensure placement in the body does not create adverse effects
  - Photon attenuation must be verified for any material used in the 3D printing of the custom applicator. Figure 3.10a, b shows a setup for testing a 3D printing material. PC-ISO showed almost identical attenuation properties to water and therefore standard TG-43-based treatment planning systems can be safely used for dose planning using applicators fabricated with PC-ISO

Sources for High Dose Rate Brachytherapy and Pulsed Dose Rate Brachytherapy

Source models for various afterloader models are shown in Fig. 3.11 [13].

- 192-Ir
  - Most commonly used source
  - Decay: β^-, γ, e^- capture
  - Average energy: 0.38 MeV (max 1.06 MeV)
  - Half-life: 74 days
  - Half value layer (lead): 3 mm
  - Typical activity at installation is 10 Ci (370 GBq)
  - Source exchanges typically occur every 2–4 months
- 60-Co
  - Decay: β^-, γ decay
  - Average energy: 1.25 MeV (max 1.33 MeV)

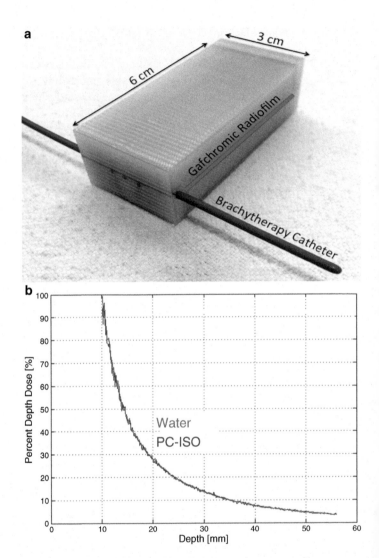

FIG. 3.10. (**a**, **b**). 3D printing. When introducing 3D printing to the brachytherapy clinic, it is imperative to understand both the photon attenuation and the biocompatibility of the materials being used. (**a**) An apparatus printed with the material PC-ISO to measure the attenuation properties of the material using film. (**b**) The depth dose curve in PC-ISO using an Ir-192 source compared to water; for this material the curves overlap almost exactly and therefore it is safe to use standard TG-43 dose calculations for treatment planning

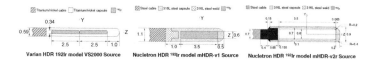

FIG. 3.11. HDR sources. The internal structure of several sealed radiation sources used for HDR brachytherapy

- Half-life: 5.3 years
- Half value layer (lead): 11 mm
- Typical activity is 0.5 Ci (18.5 GBq)
- 137-Cs
  - Decay: β⁻, γ ray emitting (β particles are absorbed by container)
  - Average energy: 0.66 MeV
  - Half-life: 30 years
  - Half value layer (lead): 6.5 mm
- Electronic radiation source brachytherapy—(Fig. 3.12a–c) Xoft® Axxent® System (iCAD, Inc, Nashua, NH, USA)
  - Isotope-free radiation allows medical professionals to remain in the room during treatment, with minimal shielding requirements
  - 50 kV X-ray source is low energy compared to the other afterloader type sources
    - This lower energy means shorter penetration distance, which can be beneficial for reducing dose to normal tissues in proximity to the tumor site
    - Also requires significantly more needles to provide an equal dose coverage to Ir-192
    - More surface dose compared to Ir-192 due to fast tissue attenuation
    - Primarily used for skin and surface-type applications but is approved for early-stage breast cancer, gynecological cancers, and non-melanoma skin cancer
  - Ability to turn on and off radiation at will makes regulation and radiation protection easier

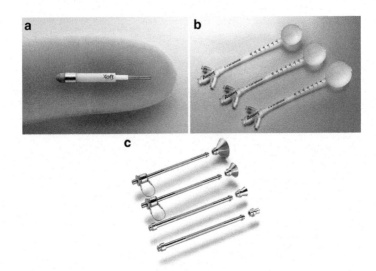

FIG. 3.12. (**a–c**) Xoft® (iCAD, Nashua, NH, USA). (**a**) The Xoft® electronic brachytherapy sources emits photons of energy 30–50 kVp. Being electronic, it does not emit any radiation when the source is not powered. The Xoft® applicators are very similar in design to traditional afterloader applicators; (**b**) The Xoft balloons for post-breast-lumpectomy brachytherapy; (**c**) The Xoft® skin applicator set. ((**a–c**): Used with permission of Used with permission of iCAD, Nashua, NH, USA)

Yttrium-90 Microsphere Brachytherapy

Microsphere brachytherapy using Yttrium-90 (90-Y) is a relatively new procedure that has been in practice since the mid 1980s. Its use originates with treatment of the liver, the vasculature of which makes it uniquely favored for a radiation treatment delivered via the blood. A comprehensive review of the development of the topic is available to the interested reader [14].

Clinical Uses

- Most often used to treat liver disease since EBRT is limited by normal tissue radiation tolerance (~35 Gy/fx in 1.8 Gy/day fractions) [15]

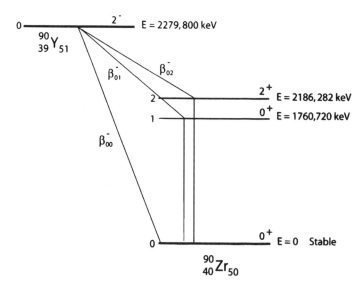

FIG. 3.13. Y90 decay. The radioactive decay scheme for Y-90

■ Interstitial brachytherapy for the liver is not generally considered an option due to the potential for bleeding from the interstitial needles

■ Portal vein (normal tissue) and hepatic artery (cancer tissue) circulatory system are used to controlling dose to organs with radiation imaging assessment

Physical Properties of 90-Y

■ See Fig. 3.13 [16]
■ Decay: 100 % β^- decay (90-Y → 90-Zr + e⁻ + antineutrino) (internal pair production emits β^+ decay)
■ Mean energy: 0.937 MeV and Max energy: 2.27 MeV
■ Half-life: 64.1 h
■ Half value layer: 50 mg/cm²
■ Mean-free path in tissue (tissue penetration depth): Max 11 mm (@2.28 MeV, Max energy) and mean 2.5 mm (@ 0.937 MeV, Mean energy)

- Particle maximum range [17]: 10,375 mm (air), 9.8 mm (plexiglass), 11.3 mm (water), 11.4 mm (tissue), 6.0 mm (glass), 1.63 mm (lead), 6.6–6.8 mm (bone)

Radiation Therapy Planning

- The treatment workflow is depicted in Fig. 3.14 with the main steps as follows [16]:
  - Radioembolization Brachytherapy Oncology Consortium (REBOC) Guidelines (1–2 weeks)
    - Consultation—Tumor board
    - Consensus for liver-directed therapy with 90-Y microspheres
  - Pretreatment screening evaluation (1–2 weeks)
    - Tumor mapping to delineate the extent of the disease
    - Vessel mapping to delineate the geometry of the treatment vector
  - Reviews imaging, dose, tumor volume, and catheter placement (1 week)
    - Delivery of 90-Y Microspheres to the planned treatment volume (few days)
  - Bremsstrahlung scan post-implant QA documentation
  - Lung dose assessment
    - Lung dose should considered to prevent pneumonitis
    - Total lung dose $< \sim 30$ Gy
    - Assessing lung shunt fraction using 99m-Tc MAA scans
    - Lung shunt (%) = (Lung Counts)/(Lung Counts + Liver Counts) × 100
  - Dose Limits
    - SIR Spheres® (Sirtex, Sydney, Australia)
      - SIR Spheres dose limit is based on activity: Max ~3.0 GBq (81.08 mCi)
      - Activity can be changed drawing microsphere solution by volume

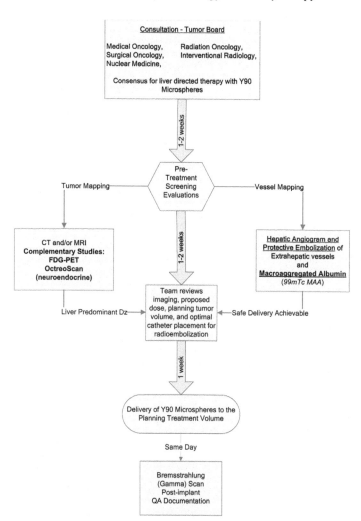

Fig. 3.14. Y90 workflow. A typical workflow for Y-90 microsphere brachytherapy of the liver

Table 3.2 SIR activity: SIR-Sphere® (Sirtex, Sydney, Australia) recommended activity (Empirical Method) and activity modification with lung shunt rate

90-Y Activity recommendation		Lung shunt modification		
Tumor fraction in liver (%)	Recommended activity	Lung shunt rate (%)	Reduction rate (%)	Total lung dose limit
>50	3.0 GBq (81.08 mCi)	<10	−0	<30 Gy
25–50	2.5 GBq (67.57 mCi)	10–15	−20	
<25	2.0 GBq (54.05 mCi)	15–20	−40	

Data from Dezarn WA, Cessna JT, DeWerd LA, Feng W, Gates VL, Halama J, Kennedy AS, Nag S, Sarfaraz M, Sehgal V, Selwyn R, Stabin MG, Thomadsen BR, Williams LE, Salem R. Recommendations of the American Association of Physicists in Medicine on dosimetry, imaging, and quality assurance procedures for 90Y microsphere brachytherapy in the treatment of hepatic malignancies. Medical Physics 2011;38:4824–4845, and from National Institute of Standards and Technology (http://www.nist.gov/pml/data/star/)

- ▨ Microsphere activity delivered as ~81 mCi in 5 mL water
- ▨ Dosimetry
  - ▪ Empirical method: Activity estimation based on tumor rate [%] of the total mass of the liver (Table 3.2)
  - ▪ Body Surface Area (BSA) method: Activity based on BSA and tumor involvement in liver

  $$\text{BSA (m}^2) = 0.20247 \times \text{height [m]}^{0.725} \times \text{weight (kg)}^{0.425}$$

  $$\text{Activity (GBq)} = (\text{BSA} - 0.2) + \text{Tumor Volume/Total Liver Volume}$$

  Lung shunt modification: no treatment for Lung Shunt >20 %

TABLE 3.3 SIR vs. Thera: Features of SIR Spheres® and TheraSphere®

SIR Spheres® (Sirtex, Sydney, Australia)	TheraSphere® (Theragenics, Atlanta, GA, USA)
– Material: Resin	– Material: Glass
– 90-Y is within the sphere	– 90-Y is integrated in the sphere
– Particle size: 20–60 µm	– Particle size: 20–30 µm
– 3 GBq = 40–80 × 10^6 spheres	– 3 GBq = 1.2 × 10^6 spheres
– Activity: 50 Bq/particle	– Activity: 2500 Bq/particle
– Specific gravity: Low (1.6 g/dL)	– Specific gravity: High (3.6 g/dL)

- TheraSphere® (Theragenics, Atlanta, GA, USA)
  - TheraSphere dose limit is based on target mass [kg]: 100–150 Gy [16]
  - Activity modification is prevented (TheraSphere should be ordered accounting Tx time)
  - Activity [GBq] = nominal target Dose [Gy] × liver Mass$_{PTV}$ [kg]/50 [Gy kg/GBq]
  - Max dose <30 Gy to prevent radiation pneumonitis
- Calculation of Absorbed Radiation Dose [16]
  - Dose$_{tissue}$ [Gy] = Activity$_{tissue}$ [GBq] × Lung Shunt Fraction × 49.38 [Gy kg/GBq]/M_{tissue} [Kg]
    - Tissue: Lung or liver
    - >90 % of 90-Y energy deposits in the first 5 mm of tissue (β^- decay)
    - 49.38 [Gy kg/GBq]: Total absorbed dose constant
    - Lung Shunt (LS) Fraction: to the lung LS, to the liver (1-LS)

Available Products

There are two main products available on the market for 90-Y brachytherapy, SIR Spheres, and TheraSphere. The features of each are listed in Table 3.3.

References

1. Pouliot J, Tremblay D, Roy J, Filice S. Optimization of permanent 125I prostate implants using fast simulated annealing. Int J Radiat Oncol Biol Phys. 1996;36(3):711–20.
2. Lessard E, Pouliot J. Anatomy-based dose optimization for HDR-brachytherapy of the prostate using fast simulated annealing algorithm. Med Phys. 2001;28(5):773–9.
3. Lessard E, Hsu I-C, Pouliot J. Inverse planning for interstitial gynecological template brachytherapy: truly anatomy based planning. Int J Radiat Oncol Biol Phys. 2002;54(4):1243–51.
4. Cunha JAM, Mellis K, Siauw T, Sudhyadhom A, Sethi R, Hsu I-C, Garg A, Goldberg K, Pouliot J. Evaluation of PC-ISO for customized, 3D printed, gynecologic 192Ir HDR brachytherapy applicators. J Appl Clin Med Phys. 2015;16(1):5168.
5. Sethi R, Cunha A, Mellis K, Siauw T, Diederich C, Pouliot J, Hsu I-C. Clinical applications of custom-made vaginal cylinders constructed using three-dimensional printing technology. J Contemp Brachyther. 2016;8(3):208–14.
6. Crehange G, Krishnamurthy D, Cunha JA, Pickett B, Kurhanewicz J, Hsu I-C, Gottschalk AR, Shinohara K, Roach III M, Pouliot J. Cold spot mapping inferred from MRI at time of failure predicts biopsy-proven local failure after permanent seed brachytherapy in prostate cancer patients: Implications for focal salvage brachytherapy. Radiother Oncol. 2013;109:246–50.
7. ICRU, International Commission on Radiation Units and Measurements. Dose and volume specification for reporting intracavitary therapy in gynecology. ICRU report 38, Bethesda; 1985.
8. Kubo HD, Glasgow GP, Pethel TD, Thomadsen BR, Williamson JF. High dose-rate brachytherapy treatment delivery: report of the AAPM Radiation Therapy Committee Task Group No. 59. Med Phys. 1998;25(4):375.
9. Han DY, Webster MJ, Scanderbeg DJ, Yashar C, Choi D, Song B, Devic S, Ravi A, Song WY. Direction-modulated brachytherapy for high-dose-rate treatment of cervical cancer. I: Theoretical design. Int J Radiat Oncol Biol Phys. 2014;89(3):666–73.
10. Han DY, Safigholi H, Soliman A, Ravi A, Leung E, Scanderbeg DJ, Liu Z, Owrangi A, Song WY. Direction modulated brachytherapy (DMBT) for treatment of cervical cancer. II: Comparative

Planning study with intracavitary and intracavitary-interstitial techniques. Int J Radiat Oncol Biol Phys. 2016;96(2):440–48.

11. Liu Y, Flynn RT, Kim Y, Yang W, Wu X. Dynamic rotating-shield brachytherapy. Med Phys. 2013;40(12):121703.

12. Beaulieu L, Tedgren ÅC, Carrier J-F, Davis SD, Mourtada F, Rivard MJ, Thomson RM, Verhaegen F, Wareing TA, Williamson JF. Report of the Task Group 186 on model-based dose calculation methods in brachytherapy beyond the TG-43 formalism: current status and recommendations for clinical implementation. Med Phys. 2012;39(10):6208.

13. Perez-Calatayud J, Ballester F, Das RK, DeWerd LA, Ibbott GS, Meigooni AS, Ouhib Z, Rivard MJ, Sloboda RS, Williamson JF. Dose calculation for photon-emitting brachytherapy sources with average energy higher than 50 keV: full report of the AAPM and ESTRO. American Association of Physicists in Medicine One Physics Ellipse, August 2012; also in Med Phys 2012;39:2904.

14. Kennedy AS, Nutting C, Coldwell D, Gaiser J, Drachenberg C. Pathologic response and microdosimetry of 90Y microspheres in man: review of four explanted whole livers. Int J Radiat Oncol Biol Phys. 2004;60:1552–63.

15. Dezarn WA, Cessna JT, DeWerd LA, Feng W, Gates VL, Halama J, Kennedy AS, Nag S, Sarfaraz M, Sehgal V, Selwyn R, Stabin MG, Thomadsen BR, Williams LE, Salem R. Recommendations of the American Association of Physicists in Medicine on dosimetry, imaging, and quality assurance procedures for 90Y microsphere brachytherapy in the treatment of hepatic malignancies. Med Phys. 2011;38:4824–45.

16. Kennedy A, Nag S, Salem R, Murthy R, McEwan AJ, Nutting C, Benson III A, Espat J, Bilbao JI, Sharma RA, Thomas JP, Coldwell D. Recommendations for radioembolization of hepatic malignancies using yttrium-90 microsphere brachytherapy: a consensus panel report from the radioembolization brachytherapy oncology consortium. Int J Radiat Oncol Biol Phys. 2007; 68(1):13–23.

17. National Institute of Standards and Technology. http://www.nist.gov/pml/data/star/.

Chapter 4
Image Guidance Systems for Brachytherapy

Laura Padilla and Dorin A. Todor

Introduction

- Image guidance is inextricably linked to the evolution of brachytherapy. This chapter will present an overview of the image guidance methods relevant for brachytherapy today or beginning to gain acceptance
- There are many perspectives one can have on imaging:
  - Applicator visualization vs. anatomy delineation vs. functional information
  - Single modality vs. multiple modalities
  - Contrast vs. depth vs. resolution vs. spatial accuracy
  - 2D vs. 3D vs. multidimensional
  - Ionizing vs. nonionizing radiation

L. Padilla, PhD (✉)
Department of Radiation Oncology, Virginia Commonwealth,
University Health System, 401 College Street, Box 980058,
Richmond, VA 23298, USA
e-mail: Laura.Padilla@vcuhealth.org

D.A. Todor, PhD
Department of Radiation Oncology, Virginia Commonwealth
University Health System, 401 College Street, PO Box 980058,
Richmond, VA 23298, USA
e-mail: Dorin.todor@vcuhealth.org

© Springer International Publishing AG 2017
J. Mayadev et al. (eds.), *Handbook of Image-Guided
Brachytherapy*, DOI 10.1007/978-3-319-44827-5_4

- With the advent of multiple imaging modalities, medical image registration has emerged as an active research field
- In brachytherapy, multiple applications are typically associated with multiple image datasets, each containing anatomy, applicators, and dose distributions in 3D, thus posing the difficult problem of adding dose to distorted targets and OARs for the purpose of evaluating plans
- Deformable registration and dose accumulations are not only difficult and interesting problems today but fields of research on their own
- The final goals of image guidance in brachytherapy are:
  - To reduce invasiveness by allowing minimally invasive procedures
  - Increase accuracy
  - Shorten procedure times and
  - Ultimately improve outcomes
- Without the claim for completeness and with the constraint of space, we hope that this chapter will give the reader a good overview of where image guidance is today in brachytherapy and where it might go tomorrow

2D

Planar Radiography

- Provides a 2D representation of the patient anatomy in a given orientation
- Has high resolution but low soft tissue contrast
  - Overlay of the anatomy makes it difficult to clearly distinguish individual soft tissue structures
  - Bones and areas of higher atomic number (i.e., metals, contrast-filled catheters/balloons) can be more easily differentiated

- Readily available but provides limited information which can impact treatment quality
- Used in brachytherapy as a tool for source localization in implants, treatment planning, and applicator insertion evaluation
- At least two images are necessary to obtain 3D information
- During source localization, the position and orientation of the sources is determined relative to the patient anatomy
  - Orthogonal images (images taken with a 90° separation) commonly used
    - It can prove difficult to relate the source on one orthogonal image to the other due to different appearance of anatomy in the two views
    - Poor image quality on the lateral film due to patient thickness in sites like the pelvis also increases the difficulty of associating sources on the two films
  - Non-orthogonal image pairs (isocentric images at angles <90°) can also be used
    - Advantage: Views are more similar (source position during image acquisition is closer between the two films)—Facilitates source identification
    - Disadvantage: The smaller the angle difference in the two images, the less accurate the 3D spatial localization becomes
  - Other 2D technique for source localization: "Stereo" films
    - Acquisition of two patient images with a linear displacement between the two
    - Done by moving either the patient or the X-ray source
    - Provides an easier mean of source localization in comparison to orthogonal film—the anatomy between the two films is easy to correspond
    - Has the worst depth reconstruction accuracy of the three [1]

- Source localization used in the past to calculate post-implant dosimetry of permanent implants
  - Since source positions cannot be accurately known within the patient anatomy, this technique is used to calculate the matched peripheral doses (contour volume dose equals the dose of the target) [1]
    - For prostate implants, this parameter is a poor indicator of the actual dose delivered to the gland [2]
  - Technique no longer routinely used in the clinic as Transrectal Ultrasound (TRUS) imaging is considered the standard for permanent prostate brachytherapy treatment planning [3]
- Treatment planning with radiographs:
  - Difficult to relate the dose distribution delivered to the dose received by the target and organs at risk
    - Target volume to be treated usually not visible due to lack of soft tissue contrast
    - Lack of true volumetric information
  - Limited visibility of soft tissue—plan based on dose prescription points and organs-at-risk points for dose specification
  - Example: Use of point A in the treatment of locally advanced cervical carcinoma using Tandem and Ovoid/Tandem and Ring applicators
    - Point A: Dose prescription point—Represents the crossing of the ureters with the uterine artery
    - Soft tissue is not visible on radiographs, a variety of surrogates used to localize this point on films = inconsistencies in the dose specifications due to lack of robustness of some of the surrogates
    - American Brachytherapy Society guidelines published in 2012 indicate that the point should be placed by tracing a line between the center of the ovoids (or most-lateral dwell positions in the ring), identifying the point at which it crosses the tandem, and moving superiorly along the tandem a length of 2 cm + the radius of the ovoids (or superior thickness of ring cap), as seen on the

lateral film. Then, the points should be placed laterally, 2 cm on each side, perpendicular to the tandem as seen on the AP film [4]

- Use of two orthogonal films is required
- Assumes a high quality applicator insertion — any deviation of the applicator geometry from the ideal (tandem and ovoids bisect on the AP film, ovoids are not displaced inferiorly to the flange, and they overlap each other on the lateral film) will affect the placement of the prescription point
- If films show poor applicator geometry, placement should be corrected before proceeding [4]
- Improper applicator geometry is detrimental to treatment outcomes

- Orthogonal radiographs are a good tool to evaluate brachytherapy applicator insertion quality (for tandem and ovoids/tandem and ring), even when volumetric treatment planning techniques are used [5, 6]

Fluoroscopy

- Continuous planar radiography to observe the patient's anatomy in real time
- Can be used during interstitial and permanent seed implants to monitor seed and needle positions
- This modality is complementary to ultrasound (US) during implants — sources cannot be easily seen on US but are readily seen in fluoroscopy [7]
- Registration of source positions from fluoroscopy on US images is being considered as means of real-time treatment planning for permanent prostate implants [7]

Ultrasound

- Uses sound waves to image the anatomy
- Nonionizing, inexpensive, and allows visualization of the anatomy in real time

- Quality of the image is highly dependent on the operator.
- Images can be difficult to interpret [8]
- Highly useful to guide applicator and needle insertions [2–4, 8, 9]
- During tandem insertion for gynecological procedures, the use of a transabdominal or transrectal probe as the tandem is placed helps reduce rate of uterine perforation [4]
    - Treatment with a tandem that has perforated the uterus can lead to significant irradiation and toxicity of adjacent organs at risk such as the bowel or bladder
- To maximize visualization of the pelvic anatomy when using US, there should be approximately 200 cm^3 of saline in the bladder [4]
- Work has been done to show the potential use of 2D US to plan brachytherapy treatments for gynecological cancers [10]
    - Images provide better soft tissue contrast than radiographs
    - Allows for more accurate visualization of organ boundaries and target volumes which can serve to create a more conformal plan even without a full 3D volumetric dataset [8, 10]
    - Figure 4.1a–d shows the ease of visualization of the soft tissue anatomy and applicator with newer US technology and it compares it to a sagittal MRI view
- US guidance during interstitial implants can help determine depth of insertion and avoid placement of sources outside the target volume = Reduced risk of bladder and bowel perforation, and better target implantation [4, 9]
- Transrectal US (TRUS) imaging commonly used for needle insertion guidance during transperineal prostate implants—recommended approach by ABS and GEC/ESTRO [3, 11]

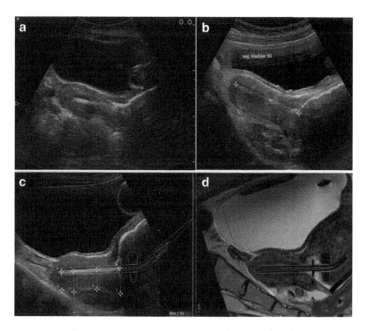

FIG. 4.1. Example of improvements in quality of ultrasound images with new ultrasound technology. (**a**) Sagittal view of applicator in uterus taken in 2008 with Falcon ultrasound unit (BK-Medical, Herlev, Denmark). (**b**) Sagittal view of applicator in uterus taken in 2010 with Flex focus 400 ultrasound unit (BK-Medical, Herlev, Denmark). (**c**) Sagittal view of applicator in uterus taken in 2012 with Flex focus 400 ultrasound unit (BK-Medical, Herlev, Denmark). (**d**) Sagittal view of applicator in uterus on MRI taken in 2012 same patient as in (**c**) (Used with permission of the Peter MacCallum Cancer Center and Elsevier from van Dyk S et al. Ultrasound use in gynecologic brachytherapy: Time to focus the beam. Brachytherapy. 2015 May–Jun;14(3):390–400)

3D

- Use of volumetric imaging for treatment planning of brachytherapy procedures has improved treatment outcomes and reduced toxicities
- 3D anatomical information during treatment planning allows for
  - Better target volume definition and organ at risk visualization
  - Improved dose optimization
- Several 3D imaging modalities are available for use—strengths and weaknesses vary and their validity for brachytherapy use depends on the anatomical site of interest

Computed Tomography (CT)

- Provides cross-sectional images of the anatomy = better soft-tissue definition than planar imaging
- Physicians can delineate the tumor volumes and organs at risk to allow for dose optimization of the treatment plan
- Better soft tissue contrast than planar imaging, but still inferior to Magnetic Resonance Imaging (MRI)
- Use is a lot more prevalent than MR because it is not as resource intensive and a large portion of departments have a CT scanner on site [8, 12]
- Excellent choice for source localization (within the limits of slice thickness and partial volume effects of the scanner), and it is preferred over radiographs [1]
  - Uncertainty of proper source identification no longer a concern, sources can be easily distinguished from the surrounding soft tissue
  - Dose distribution calculated from the sources can be directly evaluated with respect to the patient's anatomy depicted on the CT scan

- When utilizing CT for interstitial treatment planning, the choice of needles is essential to the image quality
- Titanium or flexible plastic needles produce fewer artifacts than stainless steel needles = better volume definition [4, 9]
- CT imaging is not the optimal imaging modality for prostate delineation
  - Gland not clearly visible
    - Posterior portion of prostate and anterior wall of rectum cannot be easily differentiated in non-contrast CT
    - Apex of prostate blends with anterior portion of the levator ani muscles and adjacent neurovascular bundles are not distinguishable — often get contoured as prostate [2]
  - Subjective delineation, yields inter/intraobserver variability = overestimation of the prostate volume in comparison to US or MR [7, 13]
  - Dosimetric parameters calculated from post-implant CT contours yield inter- and intraobserver variability in dose reporting [2, 7]
  - Despite these issues, CT often used for post-implant dosimetry due to ease of availability at most centers and clear visibility of the implanted sources
  - Contouring issues are well known, physicians can try to minimize them as they draw the volumes. Figure 4.2 illustrates differences in prostate shape and size when contoured with 3D TRUS, MR, and CT [13]
- CT can also be used to evaluate the potential pubic arch interference in prostate implants
  - Largest axial dimensions of prostate can be projected onto slice displaying the pubic arch to check for potential issues [2]
  - Important: If CT scan is not performed in the same position as needle insertion, differences in expected versus actual clearance may arise

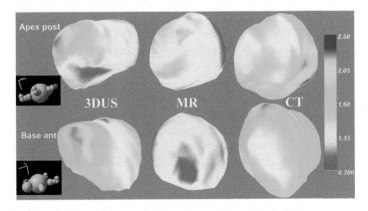

FIG. 4.2. Standard deviation (in mm, see color bar at right) in radial distance to contour vertices for 14 observations, averaged for all patients. The difference in apparent size reflects the differences between modalities. *CT* computed tomography, *MR* magnetic resonance, *3DUS* three-dimensional ultrasound (Used with permission from Smith WL et al. Prostate volume contouring: A 3D analysis of segmentation using 3DTRUS, CT, and MR. Int J Radiat Oncol Biol Phys. 2007 Mar 15;67(4):1238–47)

■ CT scans are used for treatment planning of HDR prostate treatments after TRUS-guided needle insertions
  ■ Due to the time elapsed between planning and treatment delivery, caudal needle retraction has been observed and should be corrected and verified [14]
■ Cone Beam CT (CBCT) imaging can be utilized to check needle positions
  ■ Study by Holly et al. showed a mean internal displacement of catheters of 11 mm during pre-treatment CBCT, which was corrected before dose delivery [14]
  ■ Alternative workflows are being investigated to alleviate treatment uncertainties stemming from prolonged time between insertion and delivery [15, 16]

- Use of TRUS for treatment planning is being considered, but needle reconstruction on TRUS is challenging and too inaccurate
- Combination of TRUS for soft tissue delineation and CBCT for needle reconstruction can lead to acceptable real-time dosimetry [16, 17]
- CBCT has also been used as an alternative to orthogonal film planning for gynecological diseases [18]

- Use of CT images for gynecologic treatment plans more common than MR despite its soft tissue contrast inferiority [12]
  - Due to the difficulties in assessing the target volume in CT, CT contouring guidelines specific to treatment planning of cervical brachytherapy are available [19]
  - Use of applicators that do not cause severe image artifacts is important and should be considered to maximize image quality

Ultrasound

- Transrectal Ultrasound (TRUS): Standard treatment planning modality for permanent perianal prostate seed implants [3], technique first used in 1983 by Holm et al. [20]
- Prostate clearly visible in the images and patient position between pre-implant scan and insertion can be closely replicated—TRUS used to guide needle insertion in the operating room
- When using TRUS, patient is positioned in the lithotomy position and a transrectal probe is used
  - Probe attached to stepping device that stabilizes it and allows for precise superior-inferior movement in set intervals. Figure 4.3 shows an illustration of the apparatus [21]

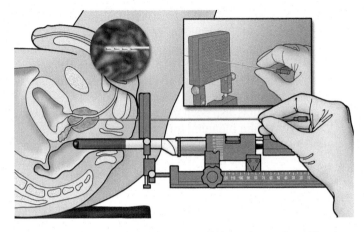

FIG. 4.3. Illustration depicting the needle insertion and seed implantation during a permanent prostate implant procedure with transrectal ultrasound guidance (Used with permission of Analogic Corporation from "Transrectal ultrasound guided prostate brachytherapy," by Brendan Carey MD, ebook)

- TRUS pre-implant volume study for treatment planning:
  - Axial slices of prostate, 5 mm apart, coverage at least from base to apex [2]
  - Overlay of insertion template placed on images to facilitate treatment planning
  - Patient should be in same position for pre-implant planning US scan and needle insertion
- Pre-implant planning with TRUS is preferred although MR can also be used [3]
- CT alone is not recommended over TRUS or MR because it is less reproducible, and the prostate volume is better identified using TRUS [7]
- Urethra visible on US—planner can avoid seed placement in or near it to limit its dose and minimize treatment-related complications
  - Aerated gel can be inserted into urethra to increase contrast and facilitate visualization [2]

- TRUS equipment with the capability of displaying both axial and sagittal slices:
  - Aids in proper seed placement in superior capsule of prostate
  - Helps visualize gland movement during needle insertion
- TRUS can also be used to check pubic arch interference during pre-implant scan [2]
  - Hard to identify the pubic arch on TRUS, but bone-soft tissue interface can be visualized and marked on the US screen
  - Probe can then be moved to visualize prostate on consecutive axial slices to check for clearance
- US inadequate for post-implant dosimetry: Prostate can be clearly visualized but the seeds cannot [7]
  - Image registration between TRUS and CT could alleviate this issue, but tissue distortion due to the probe in the rectum makes it a challenging problem. Effects of TRUS probe on prostate shape are visible in Fig. 4.2 [13]
- 3D US currently not used in planning of gynecological malignancies, but there is interest because it is a more readily available technology in developing countries [8]
- Use of robotic systems for image-guided brachytherapy is under development—Most currently geared towards prostate implants
  - Compilation of available systems through January 2012 has been published by AAPM in conjunction with GEC-ESTRO [22]
  - Systems use either TRUS or MR for image guidance and some even allow for automatic needle insertion and seed delivery without a physical template
- Doppler ultrasound imaging identifies areas with measurable blood flow signal
  - Can identify foci of growing tumor in the prostate by imaging increased microvessel density areas [23]—identification of intraprostatic lesions could be applied to tailor dose distribution to specific disease location

- Other applications of Doppler in brachytherapy include the detection of major vessels during interstitial implants to avoid injury [24]

MRI

- MRI is a noninvasive imaging technique that provides:
  - Volumetric information on the density of the certain atomic nuclei
  - Information on the structure, dynamics, and chemical environment of molecules
- Nuclear magnetic resonance (NMR), first observed in 1945, relies on the interaction of nuclei of certain magnetic isotopes with a static magnetic field
  - While nearly every element has at least one NMR active isotope, the common NMR active nuclei are H-1, C-13, P-31, and N-15
  - The easiest to observe nuclei have spin $I = 1/2$ and very high ($\approx 100\,\%$) abundance. Hydrogen (H-1) is particularly interesting because of the abundance of water in the human body, a low precession frequency at a 2 T field (~90 MHz), and relaxation times that make fast acquisitions of many FID (free induction decay) signals possible in times of the order of minutes
  - While NMR on heavier elements like P-31 or Na-23 (naturally abundant in the body) can reveal very interesting information (e.g., energy metabolism in various disease sites), multinuclear imaging is currently only a research tool
- MR spectroscopy (MRS) allows measurements of tissue metabolites levels. For example, in prostate the metabolites commonly measured and correlated with Gleason score are choline, spermine, and creatine
- In MRI, besides the density of protons, contrast can be obtained to demonstrate different anatomical structures or pathologies

- The return to equilibrium state of the nuclear spins after excitation is governed by the independent processes of T1 (spin-lattice) and T2 (spin-spin) relaxation. T1 and T2 are tissue specific
  - T1 is useful for identifying fatty tissue and in general for obtaining morphological information of soft tissues
  - T2 image weighting is useful for detecting edema and inflammation and assessing zonal anatomy for sites like prostate, cervix, and uterus
- While imaging anatomical structures or blood flow (typically associated with functional MRI) does not require contrast agents, such agents (gadolinium is a very common one) are sometimes used intravenously before or during the MRI to increase the speed at which protons are realigning with the magnetic field.
  - The shorter the relaxation time, the brighter the image
- Another parameter that can provide very interesting information is diffusion
  - Unlike in an isotropic medium, where water molecules are moving randomly, in biological tissues water motion is constrained by the morphology of the tissue
- Diffusion weighted imaging (DWI), for example, can image swelling due to changing (increase) of barriers to water diffusion. While most MRI imaging protocols take minutes or longer, a real-time MRI is possible due to new imaging pulse-sequences (FLASH) and fast iterative image reconstruction, leading to speeds of 50 frames per second at a resolution of 1–2 mm
- Being a nonionizing radiation imaging method, MRI has the advantage that can be done as many times as necessary
- From the general perspective of radiotherapy, MRI has two major limitations:
  - Spatial image distortions
  - Missing electron density information

- For brachytherapy, both these limitations are mild, since a small field will likely have smaller distortions and for HDR energy, the water world of TG-43 is a reasonable approximation at least for pelvic treatment sites (cervix, prostate). In the newer paradigm for dose computation, the Model Based Dose Computation Algorithms (MBDCA), electron density, and other material properties (interaction cross sections, tissue mass density, atomic number distribution) need to be assigned on a voxel-by-voxel basis. A CT to MRI co-registration, normally sufficient for EBRT dose computation, is needed but not sufficient for brachytherapy if dose is to be computed using MBDCA
- Field strength of the MRI scanner is important:
  - Lower fields (0.2–0.5 T) allow for larger bores or open magnets reducing patient claustrophobia. The price to pay is poor image quality
  - In order to increase quality and resolution, one has to consider fields in the range 1.5–3 T, but here the price is an increased image distortion
- MR compatibility:
  - Applicators used in brachytherapy, when MRI is used for imaging, have to be MR compatible. If MRI is used in an interventional mode, so have to be all the instruments, probes, needles, etc
  - When dummy markers are needed to outline the path of the radioactive source within applicators, catheters filled with $CuSO_4$ solution can be used to insure visibility on MR images
- While MRI for permanent seed implants evaluation is not as common as the CT-based one, it is a safe procedure at fields less than 3 T. Eddy currents induced in the titanium shells produce very little heating and artifacts during routine imaging. Detecting seeds in MR images is nontrivial as they look like voids, and they can compete with needle tracks (also voids). While MRI presents a clear advantage for delineating anatomy, when it comes to identifying seeds, a reason-

able solution is fusing MRI and CT and retrieving the seed positions from the CT dataset

■ MRI, MRS, and mpMR (multi-parametric MR, a combination of T2, ADC, DWI, DCE, and proton magnetic resonance spectroscopy imaging) are beginning to be commonly used for detecting and staging prostate cancer [25], as well as planning the biopsy and the treatment plans for both LDR and HDR

■ Whether in the setting of initial treatment or salvage after a recurrence, MR images of various flavors are typically co-registered with US (Ultrasound) or CT, which are primary imaging and real-time guidance methods (US) for these types of treatments. MRI allows for delineating of foci of disease and usually an MR-based or -augmented plan involves boosting these foci at higher doses

■ In 2005, the Groupe Europeen de Curietherapie-European Society for Therapeutic Radiology and Oncology (GEC-ESTRO) published recommendations on contouring of tumor target and organs at risk and reporting of dose volume parameters for image-guided brachytherapy (IGBT) for locally advanced cervix cancer [26], thus creating an impetus towards increased use of MRI

■ For cervical cancer, the obvious benefit of improved tumor detection and delineation is somehow diminished by the difficulty of integrating MRI into a HDR intracavitary brachytherapy workflow

■ A number of scenarios can be envisioned in order to take advantage of information contained in MRI images, but the main difficulty to overcome is the registration on MRI depicted anatomy without applicators to the CT anatomy with applicators, given the significant changes in anatomy produced by applicators. One elegant way to solve this problem is to place a Smit sleeve during the first CT-planned fraction, acquire an MRI scan with no applicator in place, and then co-register subsequent CT datasets to the MRI scan using the Smit sleeve visible in both CT and MRI [27]

PET

- Positron Emission Tomography is a nuclear medicine imaging method producing a 3D image of functional processes in a body
- A short-lived positron emitting radionuclide (F-18, O-15, N-13, Ga-68) is transported to the site to be imaged by an organic molecule (radiotracer), usually injected in the blood stream. After a wait period (~1 h), needed to increase concentration in the tissue of interest, the acquisition process starts
- The radioisotope decays through positron emission, and the positron emitted travels a short distance until it is annihilated by interaction with an electron. In the process, a pair of opposite photons is produced and it is this pair, detected in coincidence, which locates the site of the initial decay
- The most used radiotracer is fluorine-18 (F-18) fluoro-deoxyglucose (FDG), thus making FDG-PET almost synonym with PET. Since FDG is an analog of glucose (a sugar), high uptake areas will indicate high metabolic activity and glycolysis of cancer cells and depict metabolic abnormalities before morphological alterations occur
- 18F-FDG PET/CT has been primarily used as a diagnosis, staging, and restaging tool essential for an optimal management of cancer patients
- It has also been used to distinguish responders from nonresponders before any reduction in tumor size occurs. 18F-FDG PET/CT acquires PET and CT data in the same imaging session and allows accurate anatomical localization of the lesions detected on the 18F-FDG PET scan
- The combined acquisition of PET and CT has synergistic advantages over its isolated constituents and minimizes their limitations while enhancing each technique's advantages

- In the management of cervical cancer, lymph node metastasis is one of the poor prognostic factors, and PET-CT is more sensitive than other techniques (CT, MRI) for detecting pelvic and para-aortic lymph node metastasis [28]
- Thus, PET, by virtue of its lymph node detection, can upstage the clinical stage, modify treatment decision-making, and allow the radiation oncologist to extend the radiotherapy volume for inclusion of the metastatic lymph nodes. In brachytherapy, success is predicated on our ability to accurately define a high risk clinical target volume (HR-CTV) [26]
- FDG-PET/CT not only has the advantage that allows a good delineation of the tumor, but unlike MRI, does not require special applicators. Evaluating the utility of sequential 18F-fluorodeoxyglucose positron emission tomography (FDG-PET) imaging for brachytherapy treatment planning in patients with carcinoma of the cervix, the investigators found that 9 of 11 patients had decreasing tumor volume, and 3 patients had complete remission before treatment was completed [29]
- In prostate cancer, there is no established role for 18F-FDG PET/CT in the assessment of disease, since it has a low accuracy owing to the relatively low metabolic rate of the tumor as well as the interfering adjacent urinary excretion of the tracer. However, other new PET radiotracers such as 11C-choline and 18F-fluorocholine have shown promising results in the management of prostate cancer. In a recent study [30], it was shown that combining MRI and 18F-fluorocholine (FCH) PET/CT for patients with a biochemical relapse (BR) after prostate radiotherapy or brachytherapy, the site of relapse was identified in about 70 % of patients, thus facilitating the selection of the patients for local salvage treatment. A high detection rate by 11C-choline PET/CT of extracapsular disease might become a clinically useful tool in management of prostate cancer patients

- Breast is another disease site in which 18F-FDG-PET/ MR is used for preoperative cancer staging, with MRI having a higher sensitivity for primary tumors and PET for nodal metastases. In restaging, a major advantage of FDG PET imaging compared with conventional imaging is that it screens the entire patient for local recurrence, lymph node metastases, and distant metastases during a single whole-body examination using a single injection of activity, with a reported average sensitivity and specificity of 96 % and 77 %, respectively [31]

Challenges in the 2D to 3D Transition (Going from Points to 3D Geometry to Functional Structures)

- Traditionally, brachytherapy treatment planning performed using 2D films, with dose prescription and calculations to reference points
  - Poor soft tissue visualization in planar films — treatment plans could not be adapted to patient-specific anatomy
  - Organ dose reference points (defined by the International Commission on Radiation Units (ICRU) report 38 [32]) used to estimate the maximum dose received to these tissues. Figure 4.4a–c shows images from orthogonal films, CT and MR
- Use of 3D imaging much more time consuming and resource intensive, especially when using MRI, but superior visualization of anatomical structures yields more patient-specific, higher quality treatment plans
- For some brachytherapy procedures, such as prostate implants (TRUS with stepping devices), 3D imaging is commonplace and volumetric treatment planning is widely practiced
- More hesitation for gynecological treatments — doubts about necessity/value of 3D imaging for planning since

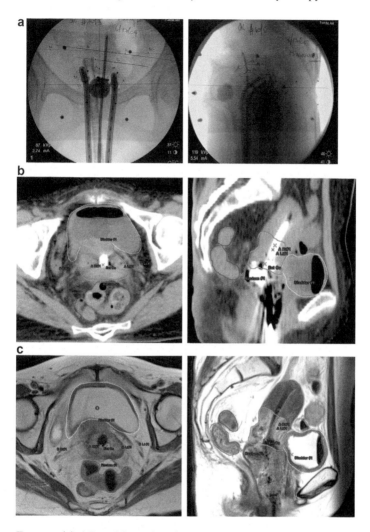

FIG. 4.4. (**a**) AP and lateral radiographs showing point A, point B, bladder and rectal and vaginal surface points. (**b**) CT images with point A, point B, HR-CTV (*orange*), bladder (*yellow*), rectum (*brown*), and sigmoid colon (*blue*). (**c**) MRI images with HR-CTV, bladder, rectum, and sigmoid colon. *CT* computed tomography, *HR-CTV* high-risk clinical target volume, *MRI* magnetic resonance imaging (Used with permission from Harkenrider MM et al. Image-Based Brachytherapy for the Treatment of Cervical Cancer. Int J Radiat Oncol Biol Phys. 2015 Jul 15;92(4):921–34)

historical 2D outcomes for cervical cancer management
are good

■ 2D planning achieved good tumor control and
infrequent major complications were seen for treatments of cervical cancer, but visualization of 3D
anatomy, using either CT or MR, has significantly
improved the tumor control probability and mini-
mized the normal tissue toxicity [33–35]

■ Point A defined based on applicator, not tumor

  ▪ Always a fixed distance away from applicator-
  does not account for the actual target volume to
  be treated

  ▪ Might lead to a prescription lower than necessary for bulky disease or higher for small target
  volumes [36]

  ▪ 2D planning based on point doses = oversimplifi-
  cation of the dose distribution of brachytherapy
  treatments and its effects on the anatomy of
  interest

  ▪ Volumetric dose parameters used to evaluate
  3D treatment plans include the D90 %, D100 %,
  and V100 % for the target volume (along with
  the V150 % and V200 % for interstitial plans)

■ Several publications highlight the discrepancies
between ICRU 38 organ point doses and volumetric dose parameters calculated based on 3D planning, especially for the bladder [5, 33, 34, 37–39]

  ▪ Volumetric parameters used to evaluate organs
  at risk (OARs): D2cc, D0.1cc [4]

  ▪ The ICRU reference bladder point has been
  reported to underestimate the D2cc by as much
  as 3.5 times [5]

  ▪ The rectal reference point has shown better correlation with the D2cc of the rectum, studies
  in the literature have reported the ICRU rectal
  reference dose point results in doses that are
  1–2.5 times lower than the maximal dose received
  by the rectum [5, 37]

- Underestimates of the actual dose delivered to the OARs are likely the reason why higher rate of toxicity is seen in patients treated with 2D versus 3D planning [5, 33]
- 3D imaging found to be a cost-effective option over traditionally 2D treatment plans for sites such as cervical cancer [40]
  - Use of CT imaging for cervical cancer implants has been reported to be about 55 % in the United States [4]
  - Inspection of the implant with 3D scans also allows identification of applicator or needles that have perforated organs and should be repositioned, or not loaded during treatment = minimizes toxicity [4, 9]
- Use of 3D image-based planning has improved the outcomes of many brachytherapy procedures from permanent prostate seed implants to intracavitary treatments for gynecological diseases
- Better and more consistent definition of treatment volumes and dose prescriptions yield better plans and better dose reporting for treatment outcome evaluations

Other Imaging Methods Specific to Brachytherapy

- Anatomy is delineated in various imaging modalities and while model-based methods have been around for a while, it still requires a significant effort from physicians. Similarly, despite recent supervised detection algorithms and library of solid applicators, a planner will spend considerable time outlining applicators in the body
- An elegant solution, which requires a different type of imaging, involves the use of a tracking device. Tracking devices, despite not being common in brachytherapy, are an essential component of image-guided surgery systems

- Since optical trackers are difficult to use in a crowded clinical environment because of their unobstructed markers-to-cameras line-of-sight stringent requirement, electromagnetic trackers were developed and they are relatively new for clinical applications
- These systems localize small electromagnetic field sensors in an electromagnetic field of known geometry
  - Their main advantage is that they have no line-of-sight limitation, but their disadvantages include susceptibility to distortion from nearby metal sources and limited accuracy compared to optical tracking
- A number of research groups have developed solutions for automatic catheter reconstruction using electromagnetic tracking in brachytherapy environments.
  - The EM-tracked catheter representations were found to have an accuracy of <1 mm when compared with TRUS- and CT-user-delineated catheters, in the laboratory environment as in the brachytherapy operating room [41]. Reconstruction times are of the order of seconds, thus making automatic catheter reconstruction faster and more precise than the manual one
- Another interesting application is the real-time tracking of a HDR source. Two groups have developed similar methods essentially using a flat panel detector in conjunction with a matrix of markers in a known geometry relative to the panel [42]. The exit dose from a patient is enough to produce images of the markers; each image is paired with its marker and ray back tracing can provide information about the 3D position of the source. Bondal et al. have further developed the method by comparing, in real-time, the planned dwell position of the source with the actual position as retrieved by the intersection of all rays; if the distance becomes greater than a predefined threshold (by the source being placed in the wrong catheter, for example), the treatment automatically stops

Tools for Multi-Modality Imaging

- Brachytherapy, as the rest of radiation therapy, has made the leap from 2D to 3D, from planning based on single modality imaging—traditionally fluoroscopy, US or CT—to multi-modality imaging, verification, and assessment

- Unlike EBRT, where large variations in anatomy are not expected to occur from fraction to fraction, brachytherapy poses specific and challenging problems by placement of applicators which do produce major changes in anatomy (e.g., T&O HDR cervical cancer brachytherapy) as well as major patient posture changes (e.g., from lithotomy to supine)

- In the fall of 2012, Medical Physics hosted an interesting point counterpoint debate on the subject whether "it is not appropriate to 'deform' dose along with deformable image registration [DIR] in adaptive radiotherapy" [43]

- Even when restricting the image sets to H&N patients imaged in the same position with very similar modalities (CT and CBCT), the conclusion is that "in spite of all methods resulting in comparable geometrical matching, the choice of DIR implementation leads to uncertainties in dose warped, particularly in regions of high gradient and/or poor imaging quality" [44]

- In brachytherapy, image registration involves the combination of several image sets/modalities at one time point or multiple image sets from several time points.

  - The most common version of "registration" is reconstruction of applicators (from a library or a previous fraction) followed by propagation of contours from different image modalities and/or time points

  - Dose accumulation is used mostly in relation to OARs and commonly employs "parameter addition" rather than dose warping. Deformable registration in OARs (bladder, rectum, sigmoid) is not used on a regular basis due to large uncertainties and unreliable deformations

- Intra- and inter-fraction movements of the tumor relative to the applicator is limited in cervix intracavitary applications, and therefore registration between image series should always be performed in reference to the applicator, and registration on bone is strongly discouraged
- In prostate permanent seed implant brachytherapy, ultrasound and fluoroscopy have been traditionally used in conjunction: one has good ability to visualize anatomy using a rectal probe but poor resolution in determining seed position, the other allows for very clear visualization of the seeds and needles but has essentially no ability to see soft tissues or interfaces
    - Most often these two modalities are used for qualitative guidance during the procedure and CT is used at a later time to assess the quality of the implant by retrieving the geometry of the implant and segmenting the anatomy
    - Many investigators have worked to refine the quantitative use of the fluoroscopy + ultrasound combination, the main idea being "fusing" or registering, using a system of fiducial markers or the seeds themselves, the ultrasound volumetric dataset with 3D seed positions retrieved from fluoroscopy acquired in multiple poses. With complete information about the anatomy and seed positions, one would be able to retrieve the dosimetry of the implant in near real time

References

1. Nath R, et al. Code of practice for brachytherapy physics: report of the AAPM Radiation Therapy Committee Task Group No. 56. Med Phys. 1997;24(10):1557–98.
2. Yu Y, et al. Permanent prostate seed implant brachytherapy: report of the American Association of Physicists in Medicine Task Group No. 64. Med Phys. 1999;26(10):2054–76.

3. Davis BJ, et al. American Brachytherapy Society consensus guidelines for transrectal ultrasound-guided permanent prostate brachytherapy. Brachytherapy. 2012;11(1):6–19.
4. Viswanathan AN, Thomadsen B, A.B.S.C.C.R. Committee. American Brachytherapy Society consensus guidelines for locally advanced carcinoma of the cervix. Part I: general principles. Brachytherapy. 2012;11(1):33–46.
5. Pelloski CE, et al. Comparison between CT-based volumetric calculations and ICRU reference-point estimates of radiation doses delivered to bladder and rectum during intracavitary radiotherapy for cervical cancer. Int J Radiat Oncol Biol Phys. 2005;62(1):131–7.
6. Viswanathan AN, et al. The quality of cervical cancer brachytherapy implantation and the impact on local recurrence and disease-free survival in RTOG Prospective Trials 0116 and 0128. Int J Gynecol Cancer. 2012;22(1):123.
7. Nath R, et al. AAPM recommendations on dose prescription and reporting methods for permanent interstitial brachytherapy for prostate cancer: report of Task Group 137. Med Phys. 2009; 36(11):5310–22.
8. van Dyk S, et al. Ultrasound use in gynecologic brachytherapy: time to focus the beam. Brachytherapy. 2015;14(3):390–400.
9. Beriwal S, et al. American Brachytherapy Society consensus guidelines for interstitial brachytherapy for vaginal cancer. Brachytherapy. 2012;11(1):68–75.
10. Van Dyk S, et al. Conformal brachytherapy planning for cervical cancer using transabdominal ultrasound. Int J Radiat Oncol Biol Phys. 2009;75(1):64–70.
11. Hoskin PJ, et al. GEC/ESTRO recommendations on high dose rate afterloading brachytherapy for localised prostate cancer: an update. Radiother Oncol. 2013;107(3):325–32.
12. Viswanathan AN, et al. International brachytherapy practice patterns: a survey of the Gynecologic Cancer Intergroup (GCIG). Int J Radiat Oncol Biol Phys. 2012;82(1):250–5.
13. Smith WL, et al. Prostate volume contouring: a 3D analysis of segmentation using 3DTRUS, CT, and MR. Int J Radiat Oncol Biol Phys. 2007;67(4):1238–47.
14. Holly R, et al. Use of cone-beam imaging to correct for catheter displacement in high dose-rate prostate brachytherapy. Brachytherapy. 2011;10(4):299–305.

15. Batchelar D, et al. Validation study of ultrasound-based high-dose-rate prostate brachytherapy planning compared with CT-based planning. Brachytherapy. 2014;13(1):75–9.
16. Even AJ, et al. High-dose-rate prostate brachytherapy based on registered transrectal ultrasound and in-room cone-beam CT images. Brachytherapy. 2014;13(2):128–36.
17. Ng A, et al. A dual modality phantom for cone beam CT and ultrasound image fusion in prostate implant. Med Phys. 2008; 35(5):2062–71.
18. Reniers B, Verhaegen F. Technical note: cone beam CT imaging for 3D image guided brachytherapy for gynecological HDR brachytherapy. Med Phys. 2011;38(5):2762–7.
19. Hegazy N, et al. High-risk clinical target volume delineation in CT-guided cervical cancer brachytherapy: impact of information from FIGO stage with or without systematic inclusion of 3D documentation of clinical gynecological examination. Acta Oncol. 2013;52(7):1345–52.
20. Holm HH, et al. Transperineal 125iodine seed implantation in prostatic cancer guided by transrectal ultrasonography. J Urol. 1983;130(2):283–6.
21. Brendan Carey M. Transrectal ultrasound-guided prostate brachytherapy. Analogic Ultrasound.
22. Podder TK, et al. AAPM and GEC-ESTRO guidelines for image-guided robotic brachytherapy: report of Task Group 192. Med Phys. 2014;41(10):101501.
23. Polo A. Feasibility of functional imaging for brachytherapy. J Contemp Brachyther. 2009;1:45–9.
24. Yoshida K, et al. Interstitial brachytherapy using virtual planning and Doppler transrectal ultrasonography guidance for internal iliac lymph node metastasis. J Radiat Res. 2012;53(1):154–8.
25. Aydin H, et al. Detection of prostate cancer with magnetic resonance imaging: optimization of T1-weighted, T2-weighted, dynamic-enhanced T1-weighted, diffusion-weighted imaging apparent diffusion coefficient mapping sequences and MR spectroscopy, correlated with biopsy and histopathological findings. J Comput Assist Tomogr. 2012;36(1):30–45.
26. Haie-Meder C, et al. Recommendations from Gynaecological (GYN) GEC-ESTRO Working Group (I): concepts and terms in 3D image based 3D treatment planning in cervix cancer brachytherapy with emphasis on MRI assessment of GTV and CTV. Radiother Oncol. 2005;74(3):235–45.

27. Trifiletti DM, et al. Implementing MRI-based target delineation for cervical cancer treatment within a rapid workflow environment for image-guided brachytherapy: a practical approach for centers without in-room MRI. Brachytherapy. 2015;14(6):905–9.

28. Jover R, et al. Role of PET/CT in the evaluation of cervical cancer. Gynecol Oncol. 2008;110(3 Suppl 2):S55–9.

29. Lin LL, et al. Sequential FDG-PET brachytherapy treatment planning in carcinoma of the cervix. Int J Radiat Oncol Biol Phys. 2005;63(5):1494–501.

30. Quero L, et al. 18F-Choline PET/CT and prostate MRI for staging patients with biochemical relapse after irradiation for prostate cancer. Clin Nucl Med. 2015;40(11):e492–5.

31. Lind P, et al. Advantages and limitations of FDG PET in the follow-up of breast cancer. Eur J Nucl Med Mol Imaging. 2004;31 Suppl 1:S125–34.

32. ICRUM. Dose and volume specification for reporting intracavitary therapy in gynecology. Bethesda, MD: International Commission on Radiation Units and Measurements; 1985.

33. Viswanathan AN, Erickson B. Seeing is saving: the benefit of 3D imaging in gynecologic brachytherapy. Gynecol Oncol. 2015; 138(1):207–15.

34. Harkenrider MM, et al. Image-based brachytherapy for the treatment of cervical cancer. Int J Radiat Oncol Biol Phys. 2015;92(4):921–34.

35. Rijkmans EC, et al. Improved survival of patients with cervical cancer treated with image-guided brachytherapy compared with conventional brachytherapy. Gynecol Oncol. 2014;135(2):231–8.

36. Narayan K, et al. Comparative study of LDR (Manchester system) and HDR image-guided conformal brachytherapy of cervical cancer: patterns of failure, late complications, and survival. Int J Radiat Oncol Biol Phys. 2009;74(5):1529–35.

37. Ling CC, et al. CT-assisted assessment of bladder and rectum dose in gynecological implants. Int J Radiat Oncol Biol Phys. 1987;13(10):1577–82.

38. Kim RY, Shen S, Duan J. Image-based three-dimensional treatment planning of intracavitary brachytherapy for cancer of the cervix: dose-volume histograms of the bladder, rectum, sigmoid colon, and small bowel. Brachytherapy. 2007;6(3):187–94.

39. Schoeppel SL, et al. Three-dimensional treatment planning of intracavitary gynecologic implants: analysis of ten cases and implications for dose specification. Int J Radiat Oncol Biol Phys. 1994;28(1):277–83.

40. Kim H, et al. Cost-effectiveness analysis of 3D image-guided brachytherapy compared with 2D brachytherapy in the treatment of locally advanced cervical cancer. Brachytherapy. 2015; 14(1):29–36.
41. Bharat S, et al. Electromagnetic tracking for catheter reconstruction in ultrasound-guided high-dose-rate brachytherapy of the prostate. Brachytherapy. 2014;13(6):640–50.
42. Song H, et al. Tracking brachytherapy sources using emission imaging with one flat panel detector. Med Phys. 2009;36(4): 1109–11.
43. Schultheiss TE, Tome WA, Orton CG. Point/counterpoint: it is not appropriate to "deform" dose along with deformable image registration in adaptive radiotherapy. Med Phys. 2012;39(11): 6531–3.
44. Veiga C, et al. Toward adaptive radiotherapy for head and neck patients: Feasibility study on using CT-to-CBCT deformable registration for "dose of the day" calculations. Med Phys. 2014; 41(3):031703.

Chapter 5
Quality Assurance
in Brachytherapy

Bruce Libby and Taeho Kim

Introduction

- This chapter will discuss brachytherapy quality assurance (QA), references from AAPM Task Groups, periodic QA, periodic QA, brachytherapy workflow, brachytherapy audit, and implementation.

Brachytherapy QA

- Quality Assurance (QA)
  - Complete set of procedures that are undertaken to ensure that the treatment is delivered according to the intent of the radiation oncologist [1, 2].

B. Libby, PhD (✉)
Department of Radiation Oncology,
University of Virginia Health System, 1335 Lee Street,
Box 800375, Charlottesville, VA 22908, USA
e-mail: bl8b@virginia.edu

T. Kim, PhD
Department of Radiation Oncology, Massey Cancer Center,
Virginia Commonwealth University, Richmond, VA, USA
e-mail: Taeho.kim@vcuhealth.org

© Springer International Publishing AG 2017   99
J. Mayadev et al. (eds.), *Handbook of Image-Guided
Brachytherapy*, DOI 10.1007/978-3-319-44827-5_5

- Brachytherapy QA
  - All of the tests performed prior to patient treatment
  - Range from ensuring that the radioactive source within the treatment planning system to ensuring that the source strength used
  - Treatment hardware and auxiliary systems, such as ultrasound or computer tomography (CT) systems [1, 3–5]
  - Codified within federal regulations, which are then adopted into state regulations of agreement states [2]
    - Periodic (treatment day) QA need not be performed by an authorized medical physicist (AMP), but needs to be reviewed by an AMP within 15 days [2].
    - Source calibration for high dose rate (HDR) afterloader systems must be performed by an AMP.
    - Requirements are stricter than for external beam systems [6].

References from AAPM Task Groups

- The state or federal regulations for brachytherapy
- American Association of Physicists in Medicine (AAPM) Task Group (TG) reports [3, 4, 7, 8]
  - TG-43: dose calculation in the treatment planning system
  - TG-53: QA for the treatment planning system
  - TG-59: safety aspects of brachytherapy treatment
  - TG-186: [9] advanced dose calculations

Periodic QA

- A complete QA program must account for the entire treatment process. Brachytherapy is a complex treatment that requires expert users performing sometimes mundane tasks in a method that ensures the patient is treated properly [1, 3, 7, 10, 11].

- Periodic QA in 10CFR35
- QA performed prior to each use, usually daily, of the HDR equipment [1, 2].
- Minimum tests
- State regulations incorporated with the federal regulations
- Required tests with 10CFR35:
  - Door interlocks (functional)
  - Source exposure indicator lights (functional)
  - Audio and visual monitoring of the patient (functional)
  - Emergency response equipment availability
  - Radiation monitors used to indicate the source position (functional)
  - Timer accuracy
  - Clock
  - Correct source activity
- Additional period tests specified and performed prior to each treatment day
- Implementation of the Periodic QA
  - Quality Assurance Daily Check on HDR Unit in Fig. 5.1
    - Checklist
    - All of the tests performed prior to each treatment day
    - QA performed in an identical fashion independent of the person performing the procedures
    - System hardware issues will be discovered prior to any patient treatment
    - These tests need not be performed by an AMP, but an AMP is required to review the performance of the tests within 15 days.
    - Any daily test failure should be reported to the AMP immediately.
      - Those failures can either be resolved prior to treatment, or treatments are cancelled until proper repairs are made.
  - An example of a failed test in Fig. 5.2a, b

Quality Assurance Daily Check on HDR Unit
Varisource iX S/N _____
Source S/N _____

No:	DATE [mm/dd/yy]: Location						
1.	Current Date & Time on HDR Unit [Correct]						
2.	Decayed Activity on HDR Unit [Correct ±1%]						
3.	Turret/Indexer locked [Interlocked]						
4.	Key off at Afterloader [Interlocked]						
5.	Key off at Console [Interlocked]						
6.	Door open [Interlocked]						
7.	Position Verification Test [±1 mm]						
8.	Applicator Inspection/length [121.4±2 mm]						
9.	A/V System [Operable]						
10.	Source Indicator on Afterloader [Operable]						
11.	Source Indicators at Console [Operable]						
12.	Interrupt Button @ Console [Operable]						
13.	Door Radiation Indicator [Operable]						
14.	Door Interrupt Button [Operable]						
15.	Door opening [Operable]						
16.	Timer Accuracy [30±1 sec]						
17.	Primalert +Backup Power Unit [Operable]						
18.	Survey Meter in range [Range on unit]						
19.	Emergency Response Kit: pig, lid, forceps, suture removal kit, syringe [Present]						
20.	Emergency Procedures Posted						
21.	Printer paper [Present]						
	Performed by (initials)						
	Reviewed by Authorized Physicist (signature)						
Comments:							

FIG. 5.1. Periodic QA checklist. The document shows all of the tests that are performed prior to each treatment day. The checklist provides the QA procedures in an identical fashion including ensuring the time and date at the treatment console and the treatment console printer

- Result of the Position Verification Test (PVT):
  - Performed with the Varisource® system (Varian Inc, Palo Alto, CA, USA)
  - Internal ruler and digital camera

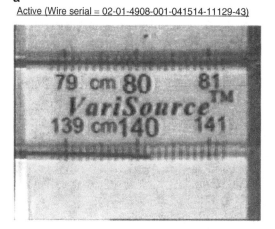

a

Active (Wire serial = 02-01-4908-001-041514-11129-43)

Planned (cm): 140.0   Actual (cm): 140.20

b

FIG. 5.2. (**a, b**) Position Verification Test (PVT) performed with the Varisource® system (Varian Inc, Palo Alto, CA, USA). (**a**) The result of PVT using an internal ruler and digital camera shows the true source position differs from the required source position by 2 mm. (**b**) The film test shows that the source position is within 1 mm, indicating an issue with the PVT test catheter

- Source position differs from the required source position by 2 mm, which is larger than the required 1 mm source position accuracy in Fig. 5.2a.
- Film of the source position: the source position is within 1 mm in Fig. 5.2b.
- This figure shows that there was an issue with the PVT test catheter, and the vendor was contacted to correct this issue.
- Additional Periodic QA
  - Quarterly (Procedure shown in Fig. 5.3)
  - Or at the time the radioactive source replaced
  - Regulations specify
  - AMP must perform the quarterly QA
  - Tests include:

Department of Radiation Oncology
Source Exchange QA Procedure

Date: _____

Note: All shipping and receiving of the HDR source is performed by Radiation Safety Office
Records are kept in that office.

x	Well-chamber placed in room to acclimate.
x	Thermometer
x	Barometer
x	Electrometer fully charging and warming up.
x	EBT film for PermaDoc
x	Vendor source calibration paper data entered into Source Calibration spreadsheet.
x	Radiation detection and survey meters available.
x	Radiation Safety office delivers new source and picks up old source
x	Shipping papers accurately reflect source received.
x	Radiation detection survey indicates both old and new source are in proper locations.
x	PermaDoc source placement films indicate positioning within 1 mm. (EBT film)
x	All covers secure on the unit, and the service work is complete.
x	Radiation levels 10 cm from the surface are < 1 mR/hr.
	Actual Value: mR/hr
x	Radiation levels at 1 m from the shipping container are < 1 mR/hr.
x	Service Engineer's radiation surveys approved.
x	Source Calibration performed and Starting Factor entered into console.
x	Source decay spreadsheet printed (2). (Source File and DailyQA notebook)
x	Old source packaged, labelled and picked up by EHS

[x] **AREA SURVEY (source out)**

Area	Actual Reading in mR/hr	Expected Value in mR/hr	Maximum Allowable Reading*
Treatment door			2
Second vault			2
Hallway			2

*Based on a workload of 2 hrs/wk and ALARA 0.1

[x] **Survey Meter:**
Model, Serial Number Calibration due date: _____

[ ] _____
AMP

FIG. 5.3. Quarterly QA procedure

- Verification of the source activity (shown in Fig. 5.4)
- Timer linearity
- Source position accuracy
- Source retraction with backup battery
- Function of the source transfer tubes
- Applicators and transfer tube-applicator interfaces
- Annual HDR Emergency Response Training (shown in Fig. 5.5)

HDR Source Calibration

| Date: | | | | Source Number: | |

Well Chamber Model and Serial Number
Chamber Calibration Factor: 0.1186 xe9 Cl/A Calibration Due Date
Electrometer Model and Serial Number   1.000 nA/"nA" Calibration Due Date

= Temperature C.
= Pressure (mm of Hg)
= TPC

Setup:	Dwell Distance (cm)	Dwell	Electrometer Reading ("nA")
		1	
Lung catheter		2	
ORIGIN = 136		3	
Step length = 2 mm		4	
15 D.P at 10 sec each		5	
-300V bias		6	
		7	
		8	
		9	
		10	
		11	
		12	
		13	
		14	
		15	
	Maximum		

Measured Activity = (Max)(Elec.Cal.Fact.)(Chamber CalFact)(TPC)

| Measured Activity: | Ci |

Time of Calibration:		
Decimal part of day:		
Meas. Act. at Noon (Ci)		on

Vendor Activity (Ci)	
Vendor Date	
Vendor Time (CST)	
Vendor Time (EST)..(add 1 h)	
Vendor Time Decimal Days	
Activity at Noon EST	
Elapsed Days	
Vendor Act. at Noon TODAY	
% Diff. = (Vendor/Meas. - 1) x 100	
Console Displayed Activity	
%Diff. Console Act.vs. Meas.Act.	

Physicist

FIG. 5.4. HDR source calibration. Verification of the source activity

■ Brachytherapy Treatment Planning System QA
  ■ Quality assurance for the brachytherapy treatment planning system (RTP)
  ■ Verification of dose calculation [4]

Annual HDR Emergency Response Training (paraphrased from Varisource iX User Guide, Varian Inc.)

Emergency Equipment:

-long handled forceps

- lead pig

-suture removal kit

-survey meter

-stop watch

Emergency Response Procedures:

The in room radiation monitor (Primalert) should be observed at all times through the AV system. A survey meter should be used to confirm that the source is retracted into the safe. A stop watch should be used to estimate the time that the patient and personnel were exposed to the source.

1) Press the **stop** button on the treatment console
2) Press the **stop** button on the Door Display Panel
3) Open the treatment room door, which is interlocked into the source retraction system. Observe both the Primalert and the survey meter.
4) Press the **stop** button on the Afterloader.
5) Use the hand crank on the afterloader to return the source to the shielded position
6) Remove the transfer guide tube and/or applicator from the patient and place the applicator/transfer guide tube in the lead pig. Move the patient to the treatment room entrance and survey the patient to ensure the source is not in the patient. Remove the patient from the treatment room.
7) Close the treatment room door and notify emergency contacts as soon as possible.

-

FIG. 5.5. Annual HDR emergency response training. (Adapted with permission from Varisource iX User Guide; Varian Inc. Palo Alto, CA, USA)

- Acceptance testing of the software includes:
  - Vendor-specific tests to ensure that the software functioning.
  - New versions of the software must be accepted prior to clinical use.
- Dose calculation verification for each type of brachytherapy source used.

- Test plan for brachytherapy dose calculation commissioning
- Tests include:
  - Source entry into the RTP system
  - Source library
  - Source strength and decay
  - Single source/multiple source dose calculations
- Imaging Equipment QA
  - QA program for any imaging equipment in the brachytherapy program [5].
  - Imaging equipment needs proper QA prior to each use.
  - Dedicated CT, MR, or cone-beam CT scanners become more common [12–15].
  - In 10CFR35.10.a.3, interlocks must be present to prevent dual operation of more than one radiation producing device.
  - In Task Group 66, "does not address CT-scanning and related QA procedures for special procedures like....brachytherapy," [5] a QA program for the imaging equipment needs to be established.
    - Periodic (daily), monthly, and annual QA for these scanners may be much simpler to perform.
    - CT unit
      - CT units dedicated to brachytherapy without the external lasers so no QA of the laser system.
      - Exposure controls used to limit scanning dose for pediatric patients not necessary for a brachytherapy CT scanner.
      - However, the implementation of heterogeneity calculations in brachytherapy (TG-186) requires the accurate determination of Hounsfield numbers to properly calculate the patient dose [9].
      - QA for determination of CT number to density for a range of material densities required.

- Ultrasound systems
  - Planning low dose rate brachytherapy, such as prostate seed implants, for many years [16]
  - Recently, more common in HDR treatments
  - In TG-128, QA for ultrasound systems clinically used for brachytherapy [17]
- Second Dose Check
  - Independent dose check [7]
    - Second dose check consists of the constancy of Curie-seconds for the plan (in the case of a library plan that is used for standard cases).
    - Commercial second check software such as RadCalc® (Lifeline Software, Inc., Austin, TX, USA) or IMSure™ (Standard Imaging, Middleton, WI, USA)
- Major Source of Errors
  - A review of brachytherapy treatment errors published by the Nuclear Regulatory Commission
  - Mundane tasks lead to treatment errors [18]
  - One of the most common errors:
    - Incorrect measurement of the treatment catheter length [10].
    - For simple treatments (i.e., single catheter), a standard length may be used.
    - Length may not be correctly used in the treatment planning system.
      - In the Nucletron® system (Elekta, Stockholm, Sweden), there are two standard catheter lengths-1000 and 1500 mm.
      - Use of the incorrect standard length will lead to an incorrect treatment.
      - All catheter lengths should be measured prior to treatment to ensure proper treatment [7].
    - An example of a method to measure the treatment lengths in Fig. 5.6.
      - Simulation sheet shows the measured length for each catheter.
      - Subtraction of 1.4 cm from the length of each catheter to ensure that the lengths inputted into

Multi-Catheter Simulation Sheet

Patient Name:
MR #:
Treatment Site:

Catheter Number	Length -1.4cm =total	Catheter Number	Length -1.4cm =total
1		11	
2		12	
3		13	
4		14	
5		15	
6		16	
7		17	
8		18	
9		19	
10		20	

Treatment Diagram

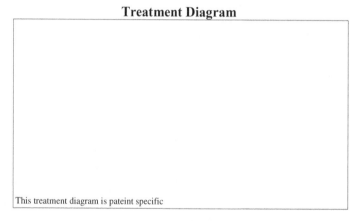

This treatment diagram is pateint specific

FIG. 5.6. Example of the applicator length check chart is shown. The length of each applicator with a transfer tube should be measured prior to treatment. The 1.4 cm difference between the measured and used length is due to a feature in the Varisource® platform (Varian Inc, Palo Alto, CA, USA), as published in Varian technical note

the treatment planning system comply with the Varian technical report on catheter length [19].
■ Simulation sheet also includes space for a treatment diagram to ensure that the transfer guide tubes are attached to the correct catheter.

- Prior to initiation of treatment, a second physicist, dosimetrist, or other trained personnel must review the connection of the afterloader to the patient to ensure that catheters are connected properly [10, 11].
- Labeling of catheters within the treatment planning system must be reviewed to ensure that the treatment plan corresponds to the physical connection at the machine [20].
- Another major source of errors:
  - Improper placement of the treatment applicator [10, 18].
  - If not placed properly, it is impossible to treat the patient in compliance with the written directive.
  - For example, a vaginal cylinder misplaced in the patient's rectum instead of the vagina [18].
    - While the user was able to argue that the dose to the vaginal cuff was within the regulatory limit for that single fraction (and within the regulatory limit for the course of the treatment), the improper placement could have been discovered if a proper QA program had been in place at that facility.
  - Two examples of the discovery of the improper placement of the applicator in Fig. 5.7a–d [11].
    - Placement of a tandem and ovoid (T&O) applicator, followed by a CT scan used for treatment planning.
    - In Fig. 5.7a, the tandem is placed properly into the Smit sleeve, but the sleeve had become dislodged from the patient's cervix.
    - In Fig. 5.7c, the tandem is not placed completely into the Smit sleeve in the patient's cervix.
    - The applicator is removed and properly placed in Fig. 5.7b, d.

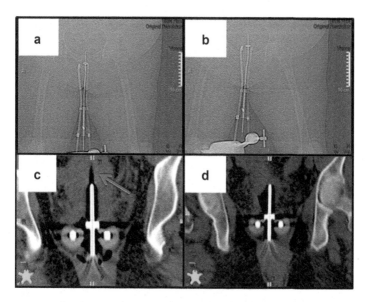

FIG. 5.7. (**a–d**) Tandem and ovoid misplacements. (**a**) The applicator is improperly positioned in the proximal vagina after the Smit sleeve was unknowingly dislodged. (**b**) Proper placement of applicator after identification. (**c**) Tandem was not inserted to proper depth. *Arrow* indicates air gap in Smit sleeve. (**d**) Tandem placed in the Smit sleeve at proper depth. (Used with permission from Kim T, Showalter TN, Watkins WT, Trifiletti DM, Libby B. Parallelized patient-specific quality assurance for high-dose-rate image-guided brachytherapy in an integrated computed tomography–on-rails brachytherapy suite. Brachytherapy 2015 Nov-Dec;14(6):834-9)

Brachytherapy Workflow

- ■ A flow chart of the brachytherapy process
  - ■ AAPM TG-59 [7]
  - ■ Illustrating the steps
  - ■ Workflow for a simple vaginal cylinder treatment may not be as complex as that for a prostate treatment in which ultrasound guidance and CT are used.
  - ■ Following the flow chart for each patient treatment ensures that the treatment itself, not just the treatment hardware, has been properly vetted for possible errors prior to treatment.

112   B. Libby and T. Kim

- Several publications that have modified the work-flow presented in TG-59.
    - Account for advances in brachytherapy treatments and performance of brachytherapy treatments within a rapid workflow environment [10, 11, 21–23]
    - QA in parallel steps in Fig. 5.8 by Kim et al.
        - Additional QA steps to TG-59 QA steps
        - Catheter length measurement, as specified in a Varian Technical Note [19] performed by

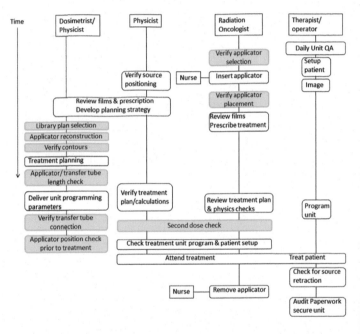

FIG. 5.8. Parallelized patient-specific QA procedures based on one medical physicist model of TG-59. The steps in *block boxes* indicate the routine procedure in TG-59 and the steps with *green* indicate our novel workflow. (Used with permission from Kim T, Showalter TN, Watkins WT, Trifiletti DM, Libby B. Parallelized patient-specific quality assurance for high-dose-rate image-guided brachytherapy in an integrated computed tomography–on-rails brachytherapy suite. Brachytherapy 2015 Nov-Dec;14(6):834-9)

dosimetrist, physics resident, or second physicist, while the primary physicist and radiation oncologist are preparing the treatment plan
- Similar modification to the TG59 flow chart [23] by Damato et al.

Brachytherapy Audit

- Departmental audit of a brachytherapy program
  - Guidance on areas that need to be addressed within a department's brachytherapy program
  - To identify any problem areas within the brachytherapy program
  - To prepare the brachytherapy program for inspections by regulatory agencies
  - To prepare for accreditation, and as a tool for internal audits
    - Can be performed by personnel within the department
    - Can be included in an external review of either the brachytherapy program or a complete review of the radiation oncology department
  - List of 83 items reviewed [24]

Implementation

Development of QA Program

- Development of a proper QA program for brachytherapy
  - Implementation of all relevant state and federal regulations
  - Relevant AAPM Task Group reports along with recent publications to ensure that the best practices of the field are included in the QA program.
  - Different program based on the size of the department

- For example, implementation of parallel workflow in Fig. 5.8 may be difficult in a small department [11].
- Modification of the flow chart for serial workflow can be easily accomplished.

Development of Audit Program

- Brachytherapy program requires a dedicated team.
  - Authorized user, authorized medical physicist, nurse, and possibly radiation therapist or dosimetrist
  - To ensure that all treatments comply with the legal requirements as well as the published best practices within the field
  - Brachytherapy audit program
    - Performed on a regular basis
    - Modified based on changes within the brachytherapy program [24]
    - Pretreatment audit of the program
      - All members of the brachytherapy team are comfortable with the treatment process.
      - All members of the brachytherapy team are aware of any pitfalls that may occur during the initiation of the new program.

References

1. Kutcher GJ, Coia L, Gillin M, Hanson WF, Leibel S, Morton RJ, Palta JR, Purdy JA, Reinstein LE, Svensson GK. Comprehensive QA for radiation oncology: report of AAPM radiation therapy committee task group 40. Med Phys. 1994;21:581.
2. USNRC. Medical use of byproduct material. 10CFR Part 35. Washington, DC: USNRC; 2007.
3. Nath R, Anderson LL, Meli JA, Olch AJ, Stitt JA, Williamson JF. Code of practice for brachytherapy physics: report of the AAPM Radiation Therapy Committee Task Group No. 56. Med Phys. 1997;24:1557–98.

4. Fraass B, Doppke K, Hunt M, Kutcher G, Starkschall G, Stern R, Van Dyke J. American Association of Physicists in Medicine Radiation Therapy Committee Task Group 53: quality assurance for clinical radiotherapy treatment planning. Med Phys. 1998;25:1773–829.

5. Mutic S, Palta JR, Butker EK, Das IJ, Huq MS, Loo LND, Salter BJ, McCollough CH, Van Dyk J. Quality assurance for computed-tomography simulators and the computed-tomography-simulation process: report of the AAPM Radiation Therapy Committee Task Group No. 66. Med Phys. 2003;30:2762–92.

6. Klein EE, Hanley J, Bayouth J, Yin FF, Simon W, Dresser S, Serago C, Aguirre F, Ma L, Arjomandy B. Task Group 142 report: quality assurance of medical accelerators. Med Phys. 2009;36:4197–212.

7. Kubo HD, Glasgow GP, Pethel TD, Thomadsen BR, Williamson JF. High dose-rate brachytherapy treatment delivery: report of the AAPM Radiation Therapy Committee Task Group No. 59. Med Phys. 1998;25:375–403.

8. Nath R, Anderson LL, Luxton G, Weaver K, Williamson JF, Meigooni AS. Dosimetry of interstitial brachytherapy sources: recommendations of the AAPM Radiation Therapy Committee Task Group No. 43. Med Phys. 1995;22:209.

9. Beaulieu L, Tedgren ÅC, Carrier JF, Davis SD, Mourtada F, Rivard MJ, Thomson RM, Verhaegen F, Wareing TA, Williamson JF. Report of the Task Group 186 on model-based dose calculation methods in brachytherapy beyond the TG-43 formalism: current status and recommendations for clinical implementation. Med Phys. 2012;39:6208–36.

10. Thomadsen BR, Erickson BA, Eifel PJ, Hsu IC, Patel RR, Petereit DG, Fraass BA, Rivard MJ. A review of safety, quality management, and practice guidelines for high-dose-rate brachytherapy: executive summary. Pract Radiat Oncol. 2014;4:65–70.

11. Kim T, Showalter TN, Watkins WT, Trifiletti DM, Libby B. Parallelized patient-specific quality assurance for high-dose-rate image-guided brachytherapy in an integrated computed tomography–on-rails brachytherapy suite. Brachytherapy. 2015;14(6):834–9.

12. Orcutt KP, Libby B, Handsfield LL, Moyer G, Showalter TN. CT-on-rails-guided HDR brachytherapy: single-room, rapid-workflow treatment delivery with integrated image guidance. Future Oncol. 2014;10:569–75.

13. Ménard C, Susil RC, Choyke P, Gustafson GS, Kammerer W, Ning H, Miller RW, Ullman KL, Crouse NS, Smith S. MRI-

guided HDR prostate brachytherapy in standard 1.5 T scanner. Int J Radiat Oncol Biol Phys. 2004;59:1414–23.

14. Trifiletti DM, Showalter TN. Image-guided brachytherapy in cervical cancer: past, present and future. Future Oncol. 2015;7. [Epub ahead of print].

15. Trifiletti DM, Libby B, Feuerlein S, Kim T, Garda A, Watkins WT, Erickson S, Ornan A, Showalter TN. Implementing MRI-based target delineation for cervical cancer treatment within a rapid workflow environment for image-guided brachytherapy: a practical approach for centers without in-room. MRI Brachyther. 2015;14(6):905–9.

16. Yu Y, Anderson LL, Li Z, Mellenberg DE, Nath R, Schell M, Waterman FM, Wu A, Blasko JC. Permanent prostate seed implant brachytherapy: report of the American Association of Physicists in Medicine Task Group No. 64. Med Phys. 1999;26:2054–76.

17. Pfeiffer D, Sutlief S, Feng W, Pierce H, Kofler J. AAPM Task Group 128: quality assurance tests for prostate brachytherapy ultrasound systems. Med Phys. 2008;35:5471–89.

18. G.N.R.C. (NRC), NRC information notice 2013-16 – State of Illinois.

19. Channel Length Measurement with the VariSource series afterloader product line. Varian Customer Technical Bulletin-Brachytherapy. 2008; 1–8.

20. Damato AL, Devlin PM, Bhagwat MS, Buzurovic I, Friesen S, Hansen JL, Lee LJ, Molodowitch C, Nguyen PL, O'Farrell DA. Independent brachytherapy plan verification software: improving efficacy and efficiency. Radiother Oncol. 2014;113:420–4.

21. Mayadev J, Qi L, Lentz S, Benedict S, Courquin J, Dieterich S, Mathai M, Stern R, Valicenti R. Implant time and process efficiency for CT-guided high-dose-rate brachytherapy for cervical cancer. Brachytherapy. 2014;13:233–9.

22. Wilkinson DA, Kolar MD. Failure modes and effects analysis applied to high-dose-rate brachytherapy treatment planning. Brachytherapy. 2013;12:382–6.

23. Damato AL, Lee LJ, Bhagwat MS, Buzurovic I, Cormack RA, Finucane S, Hansen JL, O'Farrell DA, Offiong A, Randall U. Redesign of process map to increase efficiency: reducing procedure time in cervical cancer brachytherapy. Brachytherapy. 2015;14(4):471–80.

24. Prisciandaro J, Hadley S, Jolly S, Lee C, Roberson P, Roberts D, Ritter T. Development of a brachytherapy audit checklist tool. Brachytherapy. 2015;14(6):963–9.

Part II
Clinical Applications
of Image-Guided Brachytherapy

Chapter 6
Anesthesia and Procedural Care for Brachytherapy

Brandon A. Dyer, Alison Nielsen, Mitchell Kamrava, and Jyoti Mayadev

Key Concepts

- The cornerstone to providing safe, effective anesthesia during brachytherapy—be it local, conscious sedation, deep sedation, neuraxial, or general anesthesia—is a thorough pre-procedural evaluation including a history and physical which allows the practitioner to better understand the patient's medical comorbidities,

B.A. Dyer, MD • J. Mayadev, MD (✉)
Department of Radiation Oncology, University of California
Davis Medical Center, Comprehensive Cancer Center,
4501 X Street, G0140, Sacramento, CA 95817, USA
e-mail: bdyer@ucdavis.edu; jmayadev@ucdavis.edu

A. Nielsen, MD
Department of Anesthesiology and Pain Medicine, University of
California, Davis Medical Center, 4150 V Street, Suite 1200 PSSB,
Sacramento, CA 95817, USA
e-mail: aanielsen@ucdavis.edu

M. Kamrava, MD
Department of Radiation Oncology, University of California,
Los Angeles, 200 UCLA Medical Plaza, Suite B265, Los Angeles,
CA 90095, USA
e-mail: mkamrava@mednet.ucla.edu

© Springer International Publishing AG 2017   119
J. Mayadev et al. (eds.), *Handbook of Image-Guided
Brachytherapy*, DOI 10.1007/978-3-319-44827-5_6

current medications, pertinent drug and contact allergies and response, and review of pertinent laboratory results to prior anesthetics

■ An individualized anesthesia plan should be developed well in advance of any foreseen procedure to mitigate patient risk and allow ample time for changes in the anesthetic plan

■ In general, the indications and risks to patients receiving anesthesia for brachytherapy are similar to other procedures. A thorough pre-procedural anesthesia evaluation should be completed by an experienced practitioner to help minimize patient risk and develop a peri-procedural anesthetic plan

■ In patients deemed at high risk for thrombosis (e.g., certain cardiac dysrhythmias, prosthetic heart valve, history of deep vein thrombosis or prior thromboembolism) warfarin should be bridged with enoxaparin or low molecular weight heparin to minimize peri-procedural risk of bleeding

■ Premedication may be given to the patient for anxiolytics or post-procedural nausea and vomiting prophylaxis

■ Example cases and anesthesia techniques are provided

Rationale for Anesthesia Care During Brachytherapy

■ Brachytherapy, whether intracavitary or interstitial, involves instrumentation and placement of applicators or catheters into cavities or tissues throughout the body; the creation of a safe and effective anesthetic is paramount to procedural success

■ In addition to improving peri-procedural patient comfort, poorly controlled pain has been shown to delay healing [1], decrease appetite, and contribute to mortality [2–4]

■ Poor pain control will likely create a more difficult procedural environment (e.g., unwanted patient movement). Suboptimal initial pain management has been shown to prolong the need for pain medications, increase the required dose of medications and decrease the effectiveness response to these medications [1, 5]

■ There are many options for providing anesthesia for brachytherapy. The optimal plan is the one that takes into account patient comorbidities and preferences, while minimizing anesthetic risk

Anesthetic Options for Brachytherapy

■ Include local, conscious sedation, deep sedation/ Monitored Anesthesia Care (MAC), regional (spinal, epidural, or combined spinal epidural), or general anesthesia

■ Ultimately, anesthesia in brachytherapy allows for patient comfort during and following the procedure and allows the provider to safely and efficiently place the necessary procedural devices

■ There are multiple types of anesthesia available which can be used individually or jointly to tailor the degree of anesthesia required, depending on individual patient factors and procedural requirements

Examples of Anesthesia in Brachytherapy

Pre-procedural Brachytherapy Optimization

■ Prior to brachytherapy intervention, all patients expected to receive peri-procedural anesthesia using local sedation, or conscious sedation are usually evaluated in the radiation oncology clinic. Those patients needing deep, neuraxial, or general sedation with an anesthesiologist are evaluated in the pre-procedural anesthesia clinic at least 3 days prior to the procedure

■ The pre-procedural anesthesia evaluation considers the patient's medical comorbidities including:

- Pulmonary conditions, cardiovascular conditions including EKG review, neurologic or psychiatric conditions, gastrointestinal issues, hepatic or renal conditions, endocrine and hematological conditions as well as physical exam of the airway, heart and lungs and assignment of an ASA score, and patients Mallampati airway assessment.[1]
- Pre-procedural evaluation also involves review of important laboratory studies, including CBC with differential, BMP + Mg, and PT/INR, aPTT (for patients expected to receive epidural or spinal anesthetics) to be completed no more than 48 h prior to the procedure
- An example anesthesia checklist is provided in Table 6.1. Additional workup and potential delay of brachytherapy treatment may occur for unstable diseases (e.g., unstable angina or a current respiratory tract infection)

Standards/Guidelines for Monitoring Patient During Anesthesia

- The American Society of Anesthesiologist (ASA) has defined standards and guidelines for patient monitoring during anesthesia (e.g., continuous pulse oximetry, frequent blood pressure readings, continuous EKG monitoring and qualitative and quantitative measurements of ventilation depending on the type of anesthesia used)

---

[1]American Society of Anesthesiologists (ASA) score is a subjective assessment of a patient's overall health that is based on five classes (I–V). I—Patient is a completely healthy fit patient. II—Patient has mild systemic disease. III—Patient has severe systemic disease that is not incapacitating. IV—Incapacitating systemic disease threatening to life. V—Moribund patient not expected to survive 24 h.

TABLE 6.1 Pre-procedural
anesthesia evaluation

ASA score
Anesthesia plan
Informed consent
Use of blood products
Jehovah's witness
Hx of anesthetic complications
Pulmonary
Pneumonia
COPD
Asthma
Shortness of breath
Dyspnea on exertion
Recent URI
Sleep apnea
Cardiovascular
Pacemaker/AICD
HTN
Valvular problems/murmur
Myocardial infarction
CAD
CABG/stent
Dysrhythmias
Angina
CHF
Orthopnea
PND
EKG reviewed

(continued)

TABLE 6.1 (continued)

Neurologic/Psych
Seizures
Neuromuscular disease
TIA
CVA
Headache
Psychiatric history
GI/hepatic/renal
Hiatal hernia
GERD
PUD
Hepatitis
Liver disease
Renal disease
Bowel prep
Endocrine/other
Diabetes mellitus
Hypothyroidism
Hyperthyroidism
Blood dyscrasia
Arthritis
Autoimmune disorder

Post-anesthesia Patient Monitoring

- In addition, most institutions have defined patient monitoring protocols for post-anesthesia care units (PACU) and criteria requirements for home discharge

Anesthesia Instructions for Patients

■ Patients should be given adequate pre-procedural and post-procedural written and verbal instructions, including instructions about food, drink, OTC medications, anticoagulants, and bowel prep (if required)
■ Example instructions:
  ■ Days before your procedure do not take any of the following: ibuprofen (Advil® [Pfizer, New York, NY, USA], Motrin® [Johnson & Johnson, New Brunswick, NJ, USA]), naprosyn (Aleve®, Bayer, Leverkusen, Germany), aspirin (Ecotrin® [Prestige Brands, Tarrytown, NY, USA], Bayer® [Bayer, Leverkusen, Germany], Excedrine® [Novartis, Basel, Switzerland], Bufferin® [Novartis, Basel, Switzerland], Alka-Seltzer® [Bayer, Leverkusen, Germany], or any product containing aspirin-check the label), Echinacea, garlic capsules, ginko, ginseng, kava, St. John's Wart, Valarian, or Vitamin E, warfarin, coumadin
    ■ NOTE: If the anesthetic plan includes a spinal, epidural, or combined spinal epidural, more conservative anticoagulant restrictions may be required because of the risk for epidural or spinal hematoma with neuraxial technique [6]
  ■ Do not take Lovenox® (Sanofi, Paris, France) or fragmin the day before your procedure
  ■ Take Tylenol® (Johnson & Johnson, New Brunswick, NJ, USA) (Acetaminophen) for pain
  ■ Continue to take regular medications until 2 h before your procedure with a small sip of water
  ■ Avoid eating for 8 h prior to the procedure—this includes chewing gum or hard candy

■ Failure to follow fasting guidelines may result in the delay or cancelation of the scheduled procedure [7]

■ Take a bath or shower on the morning of your procedure and wear clean casual, loose clothing to your procedure

■ You must have a responsible adult to provide a ride home from discharge

Sample Bowel Prep Regimen

■ Typically used for patients receiving brachytherapy implants where the patient will be immobilized for more than 4 h, where having an empty rectum will affect dosimetry or help limit radiation-attributable toxicity, i.e., prostate or interstitial gynecologic procedures

■ Example bowel prep:
  ■ Start a clear liquid diet at noon the day prior to the procedure. Clears include: water, tea, coffee (without milk products), apple juice, cranberry juice, 7-up, broth (chicken, beef, vegetable), jello without fruit
  ■ Do not drink any juice with pulp and do not drink alcohol, no red jello
  ■ At noon the day before the procedure, take two 5 mg bisacodyl delayed-release tablets
  ■ At 4 PM the evening prior to the procedure, begin drinking polyethylene glycol solution. Drink 250 mL (8 oz) every 10 min to a total volume of 500 mL (or in some cases, 1000 mL)
    ■ TIP: Bowel prep goes bad so it needs to be ordered prior to every implantation
  ■ For patients who will be hospitalized overnight, or with retained applicators you need to induce constipation to prevent bowel movements:
    ■ Following completion of the initial brachytherapy procedure, take Imodium 4 mg tablet sched-

uled BID for induced constipation prior to next treatment, not to exceed 16 mg/day. Give an additional 4 mg after each bowel movement

■ After the procedure, the patient can advance their diet as tolerated

Pre-procedural Workflow

■ A peripheral IV is established for all patients
■ An immediate pre-procedural note is documented, including any changes since the anesthesia evaluation, day of procedure vitals, day of procedure limited physical exam of heart, lungs and airway, documentation of medications and NPO status, and assignment of ASA score
■ Pre-procedure CBC, BMP, PT/INR, aPTT, and UA results are reviewed and supplemental blood products or electrolyte are administered
■ Initiate 0.9 % normal saline IV infusion
■ Provide 1–2 mg oral/IV lorazepam for pre-procedural anxiolytics and appropriate oral/IV pain medications depending on the case and expectations of pain. Additional pre-procedural oral/IV medication can be given based on individual patient factors. Ondansetron (an antiemetic) is available, but not always given
■ Is taken to the procedural room/operating room and monitoring and supplemental oxygen is begun prior to initiation of further anesthetic
■ Oxygen therapy can include a nasal cannula at 2–3 L/min or a simple face mask at 6–8 L/min. It is suggested to also monitor continuous end-tidal carbon dioxide during sedation procedures
    ■ Consideration of pre-procedural administration of pre-procedural antibiotics prior to the initiation of a brachytherapy procedure. If there is an allergy, alternative agents may be used

Monitored Anesthesia Care (MAC)

Careful selection and administration of medications and diligent monitoring of the patient is required for optimal patient outcome and the desired procedural and post-procedural anesthetic outcome. Monitored anesthesia care (MAC) is anesthesia administered by an anesthesia provider and often includes sedative doses of induction agents of infusions of short-acting narcotics (such as propofol or remifentanil).

- Careful monitoring of spontaneous patient respirations and titration of medications to desired effect and required
- The most common drug combination is midazolam for sedation (highly potent and inducing temporary amnesia) and fentanyl for analgesia
  - Remifentanil can be added and used in conjunction with fentanyl, especially for patients who are especially sensitive and require brief additional analgesia coverage
- The American Society of Anesthesiologist definition of the continuum of sedation is defined in Table 6.2.

Local Anesthesia

- Involves anesthetic infiltration at the procedural site, including nerve blocks and tumescent techniques
- Useful for breast, vulvar, vaginal, cervix, and prostate cases
- Typical local anesthetic agents used in brachytherapy:
  - Vary in potency, onset of action and duration, Table 6.3. In addition to providing local anesthesia, these agents are also bacteriostatic and may help decrease the risk of infections [8]. Lidocaine, bupivacaine, prilocaine, mepivacaine, and etidocaine
- 1 % lidocaine infiltration is often preferred
  - The addition of 1:100,000 or 1:200,000 epinephrine to the anesthetic agent will prolong the anesthetic

TABLE 6.2 Continuum of depth of sedation

	Minimal sedation	Moderate sedation	Deep sedation	General anesthesia
Responsiveness	Normal to verbal and tactile stimulus	Purposeful response to verbal or tactile stimulus	Purposeful to repeated or painful stimulus	Unarousable, even to repeated painful stimulus
Cardiovascular function	Unaffected	Usually maintained	Usually maintained	Potentially impaired
Airway	Unaffected	No intervention required	Potential intervention required	Intervention required
Ventilation	Unaffected	Adequate	Potentially inadequate	Intervention required

Used with permission from American Society of Anesthesiologists (ASA). Committee of Origin: Quality Management and Departmental Administration. Continuum of Depth of Sedation; Definition of General Anesthesia and Levels of Sedation/Analgesia. 2009. Amended 2014. A copy of the full text can be obtained from ASA, 1061 American Lane, Schaumburg, IL 60173-4973 or online at www.asahq.org

Table 6.3 Anesthetic agent

	Maximum dose	Duration of action
Lidocaine	7.0 mg/kg with EPI	30–60 min
	4.5 mg/kg without EPI	
Bupivacaine	225 mg with EPI	30–90 min
	175 mg without EPI	
Prilocaine	600 mg with EPI	30–90 min
	500 mg without EPI	
Mepivacaine	7.0 mg/kg with EPI	45–90 min
Etidocaine	8.0 mg/kg with EPI	120–180 min
	6.0 mg/kg without EPI	
*EPI	Epinephrine	

effect as a result of the vasoconstrictive properties of epinephrine
- If more prolonged anesthesia is desired, lidocaine can also be mixed with other agents listed in Table 6.3.
- Lidocaine toxicity at 4 mg/kg of body weight
- Use the smallest gauge needle that is still feasible and practical for anesthetic injection
  - For easily visualized tissue, such as the breast, vulva, labia majora or perineum, apply topical anesthetic (EMLA cream or lidocaine jelly) before syringe injection to improve patient comfort, then anesthetic infiltration into the deeper cutaneous and subcutaneous tissues
    - 1 % lidocaine jelly can be applied to mucosal surfaces prior to infiltration of anesthesia; EMLA cream can be applied to non-mucosal tissues

Local Anesthesia for Interstitial Breast Brachytherapy

- Apply an entire tube of EMLA cream to the breast at least 2 h prior to arrival to clinic on the day of the procedure
- Application should be 2 mm thick and cover the whole breast
    - *TIP: Instruct patients to wrap breast with plastic food wrap after application to keep their clothes clean*
- Infiltrate anesthetic nearing the point of tumescence, then gently massage the area to better distribute the anesthetic agent
- For tissues with difficult or partial visualization (cervix, prostate) a single, superficial infiltration of anesthetic to allow for subsequent needle repositioning and anesthetic infiltration with minimal patient discomfort is recommended

Example: Lidocaine for Interstitial Breast Brachytherapy (APBI)

- 1 % Lidocaine with epinephrine 1:100,000 = 10 mg lidocaine/mL with 10 μg/mL of epinephrine
- Aim for a 10 % mixture of lidocaine to sterile saline
- Give 1 mL 8.4 % bicarbonate per 10 mL of mixture of lidocaine and sterile saline to decrease the sting of the lidocaine
    - 80 kg patient
    - Likely use 100 mL of total mixture depending on cavity size and projected brachytherapy volume, so 10 mL of lidocaine 10 mg/1 mL = 100 mg of lidocaine
    - 10 mL of 8.4 % sodium bicarbonate
    - 80 mL of sterile saline

Example: SAVI Insertion

- 10 mL 1 % lidocaine with epinephrine 1:100,000, as above
- Inject a 1 mL wheal of the lidocaine mixture into the superficial skin using a 23-27G needle and allow time for analgesia to take effect
- Using the remaining 9 mL of lidocaine mixture and an 18G needle, inject the remaining anesthetic into the lumpectomy cavity using ultrasound guidance

Example: Cervical Intracavitary or Interstitial Insertion to Use a Cervical Local Anesthesia Block

- Apply 1 % lidocaine jelly to all mucosal surfaces of the vagina, allow several minutes for full effect
- Use 10–15 mL 1 % lidocaine with epinephrine 1:100,000 (no dilution required)
- Using a 21G spinal needle, infiltrate 10–15 cm^3 lidocaine in a clock face pattern around the cervix, avoiding 9 and 3 o'clock due to the cervical vessels
- Inject the remaining mixture into/through the cervical os, or expected tandem tract. Allow time for analgesia to take effect

Conscious Sedation

- Also known as procedural sedation where IV anxiolysis, sedatives or dissociative agents and analgesics are provided
- Requires frequent or continuous monitoring of cardiopulmonary status (electrocardiography, pulse oximetry, capnography, blood pressure, heart rate) during a

procedure in the absence of securing the patients airway with an endotracheal tube

- Allows for purposeful patient response to verbal or tactile stimulus and can be particularly beneficial in large patients, in assisting with positioning and peri-procedural feedback
- Conscious sedation is provided by nurses who have additional training to administer limited IV medications (such as midazolam and fentanyl)
- In conscious sedation, the patient should still be responsive to verbal or tactile stimulation, require no airway intervention, and have adequate spontaneous ventilation and usually well-maintained cardiovascular function. MAC may advance to deep sedation and analgesia, such that the patient may only respond to repetitive painful stimuli, may require some airway interventions (such as chin lift and jaw thrusts). Spontaneous ventilation may be inadequate; however, cardiovascular function is still usually maintained
- Typically used agents include versed and fentanyl. Example dosing schedules are outlined in Table 6.4. Nurses certified in conscious sedation typically use fentanyl and versed in a conscious sedation protocol. Anesthesiologists may use propofol or remifentanil during MAC. Propofol is unreversible and has a high risk of apnea, remifentanil has a high risk of apnea and would need to be administered by an anesthesiologist or nurse certified in anesthesiology
- An approach for the co-administration of midazolam and fentanyl is as follows:
  - In general, use smaller doses for patients with impaired hepatic or renal function
    - Give midazolam first at 0.02 mg/kg (2 mg recommended maximal dose)
    - Wait 2–5 min for effect, redose if necessary
    - Give fentanyl at 0.5 µg/kg

TABLE 6.4 Sedative/dissociative agent

	Dose	Effect of duration
Propofol	0.5–1.0 mg/kg IV bolus followed by 0.5 mg/kg q3-5m as needed to achieve appropriate sedation	3–10 min, unchanged with impaired renal or hepatic function
Ketamine	1–2 mg/kg IV bolus followed by 0.25–0.5 mg/kg q5-10m as needed to achieve appropriate sedation	10–20 min, unchanged with impaired renal or hepatic function
Midazolam	0.5–2 mg administered over ≥2 min (smaller doses may be used in the elderly); titrate to effect by repeating doses every 2–3 min if needed; usual total dose 2.5–5 mg [9]	30–60 min [10, 11], no dose adjustment for renal impairment unless on dialysis; longer duration of action in patients with hepatic dysfunction
Analgesic agent		
Fentanyl	0.5–1 µg/kg every 2 min until adequate sedation and analgesia achieved [11]; max dose 5 µg/kg or 250 µg total	30–60 min [11], unchanged with impaired renal or hepatic function
Remifentanyl	Bolus 0.5–1.0 µg/kg over 30–60 s; if continuous infusion ± midazolam then 0.025–2 µg/kg/min	3–10 min, unchanged with impaired renal or hepatic function
Morphine	2–3 mg q5m as needed to achieve appropriate sedation [12, 13]	3–6 h, caution with hepatic or renal dysfunction; metabolized in liver with renal excretion

- ▦ Wait 2 min for effect, redose every 2 min to effect, titrate to effect
- ▦ NOTE: Reversal agents (narcan and flumazenil) should be readily available and the provider should be training in basic rescue airway skills and moderate sedation procedures

General Anesthesia

- ■ Most cases can be conducted with conscious sedation or monitored anesthesia care
- ■ However, in some situations patients may require a general anesthetic. General anesthesia is only administered by a qualified anesthesia provider and renders the patient unconscious and insensate where airway intervention is often required (e.g., intubation) and hemodynamics may be impaired
- ■ Often outpatient departments are not equipped or coded to safely accommodate a general anesthetic. Should the treating physician feel that deep sedation is required, a formal evaluation by an anesthesiologist should be performed and procedural anesthesia and patient monitoring should be overseen by the evaluating anesthesiologist, or other qualified provider

Neuraxial Anesthetic — Spinal

- ■ Spinal anesthetic provides neuraxial anesthesia by anesthetizing nerves exiting the spinal cord. Depending on the dose, spinal anesthesia can provide analgesia superiorly to the T4 dermatome
- ■ Can help to eliminate or decrease total systemic pain medications that may suppress the respiratory drive and cause side effects such as nausea and vomiting

- Particularly useful in patients receiving interstitial brachytherapy implantation who benefit from a 2–3 h window of anesthesia control
- During spinal anesthesia for a procedure, additional medications are given for anxiolysis or sedation
- A combined spinal epidural (CSE) can be used to prolong analgesia with use of a continuous epidural infusion, well beyond the actual procedure
- Spinal anesthesia often provides a dense sensory and motor block. Once the spinal resolves, a PCA or PRN IV or PO narcotic medications can be given for analgesia
- Spinal anesthesia is typically accomplished with 0.75 % preservative-free bupivacaine to a total dose of 10–12 mg. Analgesia usually sets up within 8–10 min and last for 210–240 min
- Introduction of spinal anesthesia is a procedure performed by an anesthesia provider at the mid-to-low lumbar level using a spinal needle
- Both sympathetic and parasympathetic nerves are blocked in addition to sensory and motor nerves. The extent of the block depends on the spinal dose, patient positioning, baricity of the solution, and technique influence the final dermatomal level
- Patients receiving spinal or epidural anesthesia may have to adhere to more strict anticoagulation guidelines because of the risk of spinal or epidural hematoma [7]
- There are data to suggest that spinal or epidural anesthesia during bacteremia is a risk for infection of the central neuraxis [14]. Pre-procedural bacteremia or sepsis is a general contraindication for neuraxial anesthesia
- Some patients may require light sedation with spinal anesthetic placement—spinals are not placed in adult patients who are deeply sedated or under general anesthesia because of the increased risk of nerve injury.
- Patients are usually positioned in the sitting position for spinal anesthetic placement; however, the lateral

decubitus position is possible. Prone needle placement is rare without fluoroscopy guidance

■ Aseptic technique should be used for the placement of spinal anesthesia

■ As part of spinal anesthesia management, all patients will require hemodynamic monitoring including blood pressure, heart rate, and oxygen saturation (pulse oximeter plethysmography)

■ Once spinal anesthesia is discontinued patients should be monitored for several hours, or as long as is safe and reasonable given the anesthetic agent used

Common Side Effects and Complications of Spinal Anesthesia

■ Side effects: Hypotension and urinary retention

■ Complications include post-dural puncture headache, nerve damage, spinal/epidural hematoma, or infection (which is rare)

Neuraxial Anesthetics — Epidural

■ Epidural anesthesia is another neuraxial technique which often allows for procedural and post-procedural analgesia by use of a continuous epidural catheter infusion

■ Epidurals can be employed in conjunction with the use of oral pain medications as a way to eliminate or dose de-escalate other systemic pain medications

■ Placement is performed by an anesthesiologist, or other qualified provider from mid thorax to low lumbar level

■ A needle is placed within the epidural space using aseptic technique and a catheter is introduced so manual intermittent epidural bolus dosing (patient or physician controlled) or continuous infusion of a lower dose anesthetic can be administered

■ Patient-controlled epidural analgesia (PCEA) allows patients to dose their epidural similarly to how a PCA is used. In the author's practice, only a PCA is used routinely

- ■ Has been shown to decrease the time required to achieve pain relief, provide psychological comfort to the patient by being able to control their own care, decrease the total dose and need for other systemic medications, and reduce the incidence of motor blockade [15]
- ■ It is possible to use a continuous background infusion with superimposed PCA or either approach alone; however, in practice only use the patient-controlled approach with morphine (2 mg with a 10 min interval lockout) or hydromorphone (0.2 mg with a 10 min interval lockout). In general, do not use a basal continuous rate with the hydromorphone PCA due to medication half-life and the risk of respiratory depression
- ■ Patient monitoring is required with administration of neuraxial anesthesia. However, if a low-dose infusion is used for post-procedural analgesia (e.g., 0.1 % bupivacaine 6–10 mL/h) typical inpatient monitoring is all that is required. Patients may have motor weakness during an epidural infusion so typically they cannot ambulate without assistance. Also patients require a foley catheter during epidural infusion because of the urinary retention
- ■ After the epidural is discontinued, the patient needs to achieve adequate pain control, be able to urinate and ambulate prior to discharge
- ■ Dangers of epidural are the same as with spinal anesthesia in the above section

Post-procedural Care

- ■ At the completion of the brachytherapy procedure, the patient continues to be monitored to achieve post-procedural milestones, and as long as is safe and reasonable given the anesthetic agents used. Often

TABLE 6.5 Aldrete score

	Score
Activity	
Able to move four extremities voluntarily or on command	4
Able to move two extremities voluntarily or on command	2
Able to move 0 extremities voluntarily or on command	0
Respiration	
Able to breathe deeply and cough freely	2
Dyspnea or limited breathing	1
Apneic	0
Consciousness	
Fully awake	2
Arousable on calling	1
Not responding	0
Circulation	
Blood pressure ± 20 % of pre-anesthetic level	2
Blood pressure ± 20–50 % of pre-anesthetic level	1
Blood pressure ± 50 % of pre-anesthetic level	0
Color	
Normal	2
Pale, dusky, blotchy, jaundiced, other cyanotic	1
Cyanotic	0

A score of ≥9 is required for discharge
Used with permission from Aldrete JA. The post-anesthesia recovery score revisited. J Clin Anesth. 1995;7(1):89–91

post-procedural criteria for discharge include the use of Aldrete's original scoring system [16], Table 6.5, or another validated post-anesthesia discharge scoring system. Patients who had a spinal or epidural must be

able to void before discharge and have full recovery of sensory and motor block prior to discharge home
- Discuss foreseeable anesthesia complications and provide discharge instructions
- Sample discharge instructions
  - For breast brachytherapy patients:
    - Apply a combination of Nystatin (Mycostatin) cream mixed with 20 % zinc oxide to the breast for 7 days to help prevent bacterial and fungal infections and aid in the healing process
    - Consideration of oral antibiotics for 7–10 days
    - Avoid submerging the breast when the catheters are in the breast
    - Tape plastic food wrap over breast while showering. If breast becomes wet, pat dry with a clean towel
    - No baths, swimming pools, jacuzzis, or saunas when the catheters are in the breast
    - Use oral pain medications as needed
    - Indirectly apply ice packs to the breast/chest wall for symptomatic relief and swelling
  - For GYN/GU patients:
    - Encourage patients to perform sitz baths twice daily for 5 days after the implant
    - Use a combination of Nystatin (Mycostatin) cream mixed with 20 % zinc oxide to be applied to the perineal region TID for 7 days to help prevent bacterial and fungal infections and aid in the healing process
    - Use oral pain medications as needed
    - Indirectly apply a perineal ice pack BID for 3 days to help decrease labial swelling
    - For GYN/GU patients, it is common to experience mild urinary burning for 2–3 days post-implantation, have loose or frequent bowel movements, vaginal discharge, cramping, tenderness or itching, sore perineum or labia, and fatigue

- ▨ If developing severe bleeding or dysthesias, for GYN/GU patients, also if developing severe burning with urination, sharp lower pelvic or abdominal pain contact the medical office immediately
- ■ For all patients:
  - ▨ Contact the treating provider immediately if:
    - ▪ Temperature greater than 100.5 °F
    - ▪ Streaking erythema at the site of brachytherapy implantation
    - ▪ If developing severe bleeding or dysthesias, for GYN/GU patients, also if developing severe burning with urination, sharp lower pelvic or abdominal pain contact the medical office immediately
- ▨ Sexual activity may be resumed as soon as the patient feels comfortable, usually after a period of pelvic rest

Conclusion

- ▨ Adequate pre-procedural patient evaluation is necessary to identify any potential anesthesia contraindications and establish a safe and feasible anesthesia plan
- ▨ Proper patient selection and type of anesthesia care is essential
- ▨ Peri-procedural patient monitoring, including: blood pressure, heart rate, and oxygen saturation (pulse oximeter plethysmography) are required for conscious sedation and monitored anesthesia care. General anesthesia also requires continuous end-tidal carbon dioxide and temperature monitoring
- ▨ If the use of spinal or epidural anesthesia is anticipated, establishing a relationship with an anesthesia provider should be pursued well in advance of the anticipated procedure so anticoagulation status and lab work can be reviewed

■ Post-procedure, established patient care instructions covering expected symptoms and red-flags should be covered, as well as providing medications for symptomatic control

■ There is a great degree of flexibility for brachytherapy anesthesia and even very sick patients can safely receive brachytherapy with relative ease with good procedural comfort

References

1. Gouin JP, Kiecolt-Glaser JK. The impact of psychological stress on wound healing: methods and mechanisms. Crit Care Nurs Clin North Am. 2012;24(2):201–13.

2. Smith D, Wilkie R, Uthman O, Jordan JL, McBeth J. Chronic pain and mortality: a systematic review. PLoS One. 2014;9(6): e99048.

3. Katz J, Jackson M, Kavanagh BP, Sandler AN. Acute pain after thoracic surgery predicts long-term post-thoracotomy pain. Clin J Pain. 1996;12(1):50–5.

4. Sharrock NE, Cazan MG, Hargett MJ, Williams-Russo P, Wilson Jr PD. Changes in mortality after total hip and knee arthroplasty over a ten-year period. Anesth Analg. 1995;80(2):242–8.

5. Indelli PF, Grant SA, Nielsen K, Vail TP. Regional anesthesia in hip surgery. Clin Orthop Relat Res. 2005;441:250–5.

6. Horlocker TT, Wedel DJ, Rowlingson JC, et al. Regional anesthesia in the patient receiving antithrombotic or thrombolytic therapy: American Society of Regional Anesthesia and Pain Medicine Evidence-Based Guidelines (Third Edition). Reg Anesth Pain Med. 2010;35(1):64–101.

7. Anesthesiologists ASo. Practice guidelines for preoperative fasting and the use of pharmacologic agents to reduce the risk of pulmonary aspiration: application to healthy patients undergoing elective procedures. Anesthesiology. 2011;114(3):495–511.

8. Johnson SM, Saint John BE, Dine AP. Local anesthetics as antimicrobial agents: a review. Surg Infect (Larchmt). 2008;9(2): 205–13.

9. Waring JP, Baron TH, Hirota WK, et al. Guidelines for conscious sedation and monitoring during gastrointestinal endoscopy. Gastrointest Endosc. 2003;58(3):317–22.

10. Horn E, Nesbit SA. Pharmacology and pharmacokinetics of sedatives and analgesics. Gastrointest Endosc Clin N Am. 2004; 14(2):247–68.
11. Bahn EL, Holt KR. Procedural sedation and analgesia: a review and new concepts. Emerg Med Clin North Am. 2005;23(2): 503–17.
12. Aubrun F, Mazoit JX, Riou B. Postoperative intravenous morphine titration. Br J Anaesth. 2012;108(2):193–201.
13. Lvovschi V, Aubrun F, Bonnet P, et al. Intravenous morphine titration to treat severe pain in the ED. Am J Emerg Med. 2008;26(6):676–82.
14. Horlocker TT, McGregor DG, Matsushige DK, Schroeder DR, Besse JA. A retrospective review of 4767 consecutive spinal anesthetics: central nervous system complications. Perioperative Outcomes Group. Anesth Analg. 1997;84(3):578–84.
15. van der Vyver M, Halpern S, Joseph G. Patient-controlled epidural analgesia versus continuous infusion for labour analgesia: a meta-analysis. Br J Anaesth. 2002;89(3):459–65.
16. Aldrete JA. The post-anesthesia recovery score revisited. J Clin Anesth. 1995;7(1):89–91.

Chapter 7
Breast Brachytherapy and Clinical Appendix

Kara D. Romano, Daniel M. Trifiletti, Bruce Libby, and Timothy N. Showalter

Introduction

Rationale for Brachytherapy

- Brachytherapy developed primarily as form of partial breast irradiation
- Partial breast irradiation aims to reduce volume of treated breast and adjacent organ and to shorten treatment duration
- Supported by rationale that the majority recurrences after breast-conserving surgery (BCS) develop near the tumor bed within the index quadrant [1]
- Brachytherapy has potential advantages over external beam radiation therapy (RT) for partial breast irradiation, including smaller volume of normal tissue treated, fewer challenges due to setup variations and respiratory motion

K.D. Romano, MD (✉) • D.M. Trifiletti, MD • B. Libby, PhD
T.N. Showalter, MD, MPH
Department of Radiation Oncology, University of Virginia Health System, PO 800393, Charlottesville, VA 22908, USA
e-mail: kara.e.downs@gmail.com; daniel.trifiletti@gmail.com; BL8B@hscmail.mcc.virginia.edu; tns3b@hscmail.mcc.virginia.edu

© Springer International Publishing AG 2017   145
J. Mayadev et al. (eds.), *Handbook of Image-Guided Brachytherapy*, DOI 10.1007/978-3-319-44827-5_7

Goal of Brachytherapy

- Brachytherapy usually delivered as postoperative accelerated partial breast irradiation (APBI) after curative-intent BCS, with goals of reducing risk of local recurrence while sparing normal tissue
- Compared to traditional external beam whole breast irradiation (WBI), the goal of breast brachytherapy is to give a high radiation dose to smaller breast tissue volume over a shorter period of time
- Breast brachytherapy has also been delivered as re-irradiation following BCS for ipsilateral breast tumor recurrence

Timing

- RT is most often delivered as adjuvant therapy after BCS in breast cancer
- Brachytherapy can be used as monotherapy APBI or to boost the tumor bed after whole breast irradiation (WBI)
- APBI allows delivery of adjuvant radiation after breast conservation surgery with ≤1 week duration of treatment
- Brachytherapy boost can be delivered following standard WBI, which may improve lumpectomy cavity dosimetry over other techniques such as electron therapy [2]
- Brachytherapy under evaluation for delivery as intra-operative RT [3]

Pertinent Anatomy for Brachytherapy

- The target is typically defined as the lumpectomy cavity, which can be identified on imaging by a seroma or surgical clips and guided by surgical incisions on the skin

- Organs at risk include:
  - Skin: Balloon surface to skin distance a primary factor limiting initial use of balloon brachytherapy applicators. A 5 mm distance required in NSABP B-39 trial [4]
  - Chest wall and pectoralis muscles: Excluded from the planning target volume for evaluation (PTV_EVAL)
  - Heart: Cardiac sparing is an increasingly emphasized focus of breast RT
  - Uninvolved normal breast tissue: This represents the ipsilateral breast tissue not included in the PTV_EVAL
- CT image (Fig. 7.1) shows a brachytherapy balloon applicator in place with the PTV_EVAL sculpted away from ribs and 5 mm from skin. Target coverage is ≥90 % of the dose delivered to ≥90 % of the PTV_

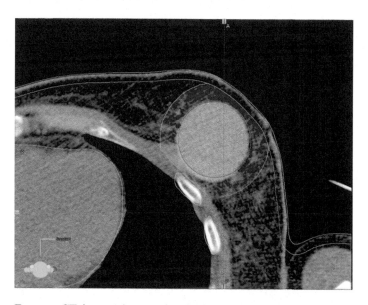

Fɪɢ. 7.ɪ. CT image shows a brachytherapy balloon applicator in place with the PTV_EVAL sculpted away from ribs and 5 mm from skin

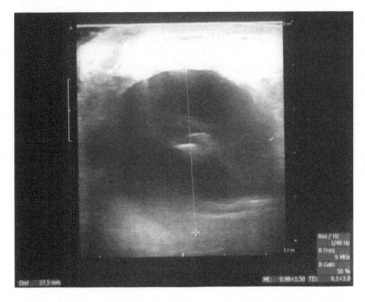

FIG. 7.2. Ultrasound image shows a seroma with the balloon applicator and catheters centered appropriately. Image guidance prior to each fraction confirms this position

EVAL target volume. Skin and rib maximum point doses ≤145 % prescription dose and ideally ≤125 %
- Ultrasound image (Fig. 7.2) shows a seroma with the balloon applicator and catheters centered appropriately. Image guidance prior to each fraction confirms this position
- CT image (Fig. 7.3) of a left breast applicator placement, which demonstrates that the dose to the heart is ≤30 % of the prescription dose

Pathology

Typical Pathology

- Ductal histology [5]

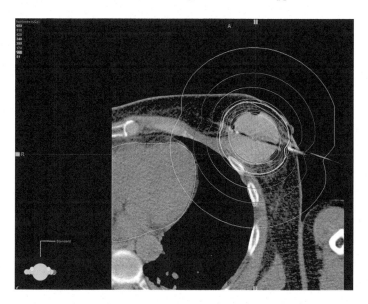

FIG. 7.3. CT image of a left breast applicator placement, which demonstrates that the dose to the heart is ≤30 % of the prescription dose

- Ductal carcinoma in situ (DCIS), 15–20 % of newly diagnosed cases
- Invasive ductal carcinoma (IDC), ~85 % of newly diagnosed cases
- Lobular histology [6–9]
  - Lobular carcinoma in situ (LCIS)
  - Invasive lobular carcinoma (ILC), 4–15 % of newly diagnosed cases
  - LCIS has been associated with increased risk of bilateral, invasive breast cancer [6]

Foundation of Rationale for Brachytherapy

- Majority of ipsilateral breast tumor recurrences occur within or near the tumor bed [10]

- Majority of ipsilateral breast tumor recurrences are in the index quadrant [1, 11–13]
- Some women opt out of breast conservation due to the logistical burden of whole breast irradiation over 3–6 weeks [14–16], so accelerated courses may improve compliance with adjuvant RT after BCS
- Twenty percent of women treated with BCS never receive radiation [17]
- Brachytherapy provides a highly conformal dose to the highest risk area
- Spares unnecessary risk of treatment to normal tissue in low risk patients
- Disease free survival acceptably low after brachytherapy in patients who would have been treated with WBI

Local Recurrence

- Available evidence demonstrates low ipsilateral breast tumor recurrence rates after brachytherapy
- Evidence summarized in Table 7.1

Disease Free Survival

- Evidence summarized in Table 7.1

Selection Criteria

Selecting Candidates for Implantation

- Select patients with early stage breast cancer at risk for local failure who would benefit from adjuvant RT
- Select patients at sufficiently low risk for recurrence in distant portions of the ipsilateral breast (>1 cm from the lumpectomy cavity), nodal failure, and distant failure

TABLE 7.1 Clinical outcomes of whole and partial breast irradiation in published literature

	Design	Pts	Year	Inclusion	Technique	Follow up	Local Recurrence	Disease-Free Survival
Whole breast irradiation								
NSABP B-17 [31]	Randomized	818	2001	DCIS	BCS vs. BCS+WBI	10 years	31 % vs. 15 %	NR
NSABP B-06 [32]	Randomized	1851	2002	Invasive	TM vs. BCS vs. BCS+WBI	20 years	39 % vs. 14 %	36 % vs. 35 % vs. 35 %
EBCTCG Group meta-analysis [33]	Meta-analysis	10,801	2011	Invasive	BCS vs. BCS+WBI	10 years	35 % vs. 19 %[a]	NR
Partial breast irradiation								
Polgar et al. APBI [34]	Randomized	258	2007	Invasive	WBI vs. PBI (HDR interstitial or electron beam)	5 years	3.4 % vs. 4.7 %	90 % vs. 88 %
Polgar et al. APBI Interstitial [35]	Prospective, nonrandomized	45	2010	Invasive	HDR multicatheter interstitial	12 years	9.3 %	75 %
Shah et al. Interstitial [36]	Matched-pair analysis	398	2011	Invasive	WBI vs. PBI (LDR or HDR interstitial)	12 years	3.8 % vs. 5.0 %	87 % vs. 91 %

(continued)

Table 7.1 (continued)

	Design	Pts	Year	Inclusion	Technique	Follow up	Local Recurrence	Disease-Free Survival
Pooled ASBS and WBH analysis [37]	Pooled analysis	1961	2012	Invasive DCIS	APBI (LDR/HDR interstitial, balloon, 3D-CRT partial breast)	5 years	3.2 %	89 %
Shah et al. Mammosite Registry Trial [38]	Prospective, nonrandomized	1449	2013	Invasive DCIS	HDR Mammosite Balloon brachytherapy	5 years	3.8 %	NR
Kamrava et al. PROMIS Study [39]	Pooled analysis	1356	2015	Invasive DCIS	APBI (LDR or HDR multicatheter interstitial)	10 years	7.6 %	NR
Strnad et al. APBI Interstitial [40]	Randomized	1184	2016	Invasive DCIS	WBI vs. APBI (HDR multicatheter interstitial)	5 years	0.92 % vs. 1.44 %	94.45 % vs. 95.03 %
NSABP B-39 [4]	Randomized	4000	Pending	Invasive DCIS	WBI vs. APBI (HDR interstitial, balloon, 3D-CRT partial breast)	–	–	–

Pts patients, DCIS ductal carcinoma in situ, BCS breast conservation surgery, WBI whole breast irradiation, NR not reported, TM total mastectomy, PBI partial breast irradiation, HDR high dose rate, LDR low dose rate, APBI accelerated partial breast irradiation, 3D-CRT three-dimensional conformal radiation therapy
[a]Includes any recurrence (locoregional or distant)

- Multiple groups have published consensus statements to guide clinicians on the appropriate selection of patients for APBI [5, 10, 18, 19]
- Selection criteria varies amongst the consensus guidelines with some conflicting recommendations
  - ASTRO considers patients as "suitable," "cautionary," and "unsuitable" based on specified risk factors for recurrence including factors such as age, tumor size, margin status, hormonal receptor status, and histology, original statement in 2009, with an update in 2016
  - ABS guidelines incorporated more recent data on APBI into a simpler classification
  - Theoretic risk of increased local recurrence with lobular histology due to multicentric nature of this histology; however, several clinical series have demonstrated that APBI with brachytherapy is safe in patients with ILC [7–9]
  - Guidelines summarized in Table 7.2
- As data from APBI mature, we expect these groups to be updated as several recent studies demonstrate that the current groups overlap in the risk of local recurrence [20–25]

Choice of Brachytherapy Applicator

- If cavity is small (less than 15 cm^3), irregular, closed, after adjuvant chemotherapy that has markers, or not well localized cavity, consider interstitial implantation If an oncoplastic tissue rearrangement has been performed, consider interstitial multicatheter implantation
- Spherical cavities—consider a balloon based applicator such as the multi-lumen Mammosite, Contura
- Elongated, irregular cavities—consider SAVI strut-based implantation

TABLE 7.2 Selection criteria for accelerated partial breast irradiation by consensus statement or clinical trial

	ASTRO "suitable" [18]	ASTRO "cautionary" [18]	ABS "acceptable" [5]	NSABP B39 Protocol [4]	ASTRO "unsuitable" [18]
Year published	2016	2016	2013	2011	2016
Age (yo)	≥50	40–49[b]	≥50	≥18	<40
Tumor size (cm)	≤2	2.1–3.0	≤3	≤3	>3
Margin	≥2 mm	Close (<2mm)	Negative	Negative	Positive
Hormonal status	Positive	Negative	Any	Any	–
Histology	Ductal	Lobular	Any	Any	–
LVSI	None	Limited	None	Yes	Extensive
Pure DCIS	Yes, <2.5 cm, low grade	Yes	Yes	Yes	If >3 cm in size
Multifocal	Clinically unifocal, ≤2 cm total	Clinically unifocal, ≤3 cm total	–	Microscopic, <3 cm total	If microscopically multifocal >3 cm in total size or if clinically multifocal
Multicentric	Unicentric	Unicentric	–	Unicentric	Present
Nodal status	pN0	pN0	pN0	pN0-1[a] No ECE	pN1, pN2, pN3

ASTRO American Society for Therapeutic Radiology and Oncology, *ABS* American Brachytherapy, *yo* years old, *LVSI* lymphovascular space invasion, *DCIS* ductal carcinoma in situ, *pN* pathologic nodal status, *ECE* extracapsular extension
[a]At least size axillary lymph nodes must be pathologically evaluated if pN1
[b]ASTRO cautionary is ≥50 with at least 1 feature of size 2.1–3 cm, LVSI, ER−, T2, close <2 mm margins, lobular, EIC <3 cm

When to Implant

- Most commonly, APBI implantation occurs within 1–4 weeks of BCS
- APBI intra-cavitary balloon implants: placed within 1–4 weeks after surgical resection and prior to chemotherapy
- APBI interstitial implants: a clear lumpectomy cavity is required, thus implantation can occur prior to surgical resection or after (if clips or seroma define the cavity)
- Boost brachytherapy: following completion of traditional WBI
- If chemotherapy is indicated, wait >2 weeks after completion of APBI before initiating
- For noninvasive image-guided boost brachytherapy (Accuboost), can be delivered as APBI 1–4 weeks after BCS or as boost either interdigitated with or immediately following external beam RT

Clinical Guidelines to Judge Readiness for Implantation

- Applicator placement may occur at the time of the breast-conserving surgery procedure or as a delayed separate procedure
- Surgical incisions must be adequately approximated
- No postoperative wound healing complications
- Seroma cavity must be visualized. Since seromas resolve several weeks after BCS, this is a reason to avoid delays

Medical Operability: Anesthesia Consent, Guidelines for CBC, Anticoagulation

- Obtain perioperative pre-anesthesia evaluation, depending on your institutional requirements. Procedure may be performed with local anesthesia

- Complete blood count (CBC)
- Prothrombin time/International normalized ratio (PT/INR) and Partial thromboplastin time (PTT)

Image Guidance Utilization

- Use of image guidance pre-procedure

  - Ultrasound (US), Mammography, Computed Tomography (CT), and Magnetic Resonance Imaging (MRI) are all useful to define pre-lumpectomy tumor characteristics and lumpectomy cavity
  - Delineate lumpectomy cavity based on clips, radiopaque markers, seroma, and soft tissue changes

- Types of image guidance to potentially use and pros/cons

  - Imaging with Ultrasound (US)
    - Lumpectomy cavity is visible on ultrasound using surface probe
    - Potential inter-user variability in image quality and the ability to clearly discern the lumpectomy cavity
    - Appealing due to low cost, ease of setup, mobility of units, and lack of additional exposure to ionizing radiation
    - Widely available
  - Imaging with computed tomography (CT) and CT on rails
    - CT provides three-dimensional confirmation of applicator placement and may complement ultrasound for evaluation if available
    - 3D treatment planning and optimization work to improve dose conformality
    - Customized dose distributions with CT-based planning can be tailored to match each patient's anatomy and lumpectomy cavity volume using multichannel applicators

- ▦ Not always readily available during implantation but may be used at time of simulation to permit adjustment of applicator
- ■ Emerging imaging considerations
  - ■ Magnetic Resonance Imaging (MRI)
    - ▦ Superior soft tissue delineation to CT
    - ▦ Complicated logistics including available equipment and cost
  - ■ Accuboost/mammography
    - ▦ Immobilization with mammogram paddles
    - ▦ Avoids target delineation issues, respiratory motion, and movement
    - ▦ kV image obtained to target the tumor bed and to select appropriate applicator
    - ▦ Breast is compressed and treated in parallel opposed fields in two orthogonal axes
- ■ Use of image guidance during procedure
  - ■ Confirm applicator placement, measure distance to skin and other pertinent structures, develop a customized plan for each patient with a unique dose distribution
  - ■ Mammogram images used for Accuboost, permit localization of lumpectomy cavity based on surgical clips
- ■ Transverse ultrasound image (Fig. 7.4a, b) shows visualization of the lumpectomy cavity by ultrasound guidance (A) and needle placement for interstitial brachytherapy is guided by real-time ultrasonography (B)

Guidelines for Implantation

Pre-procedure Advice

- ■ Review preoperative imaging, surgical report, and pathology report prior to implant

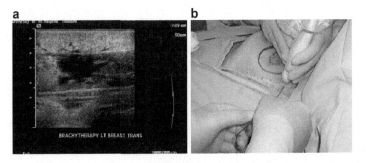

Fig. 7.4. Transverse ultrasound image shows visualization of the lumpectomy cavity by ultrasound guidance (**a**) and needle placement for interstitial brachytherapy is guided by real-time ultrasonography (**b**) (Used with permission of Elsevier from Patel RR, Das RK. Image-guided breast brachytherapy: an alternative to whole-breast radiotherapy. The Lancet Oncology 2006 May;7(5):407–415)

- Physical exam can define location of seroma relative to lumpectomy incision
- Plan catheter insertion angle with consideration of anticipated location and direction of catheter tubing. Consider patient comfort for catheter tubing location (catheter aimed lateral and caudal is preferred)
- Position patient supine with ipsilateral arm raised and ready access to ultrasound unit and/or CT
- Prior to the day of implant, advise patients to wear a soft, loose fitting bra without under wiring and to wear a button-up shirt for comfort
- Consider pre-procedural antibiotics, especially in the interstitial cases, with a post-procedure course of 7–10 days

Procedure Tips

- Closed-cavity techniques are preferred over placement through lumpectomy incision
- Radio-opaque surface marker can be placed on breast prior to CT imaging to help physician plan needle direction for insertion

- Use local anesthetic and consider mild sedation with oral medication (e.g., lorazepam). See additional recommendations in Chap. 6 on anesthesia
- Initial ultrasound or CT visualization of the lumpectomy cavity is important, and permits determining size of seroma as well as proximity to skin and chest wall
- The needle track can be first visualized and confirmed with needle prior to trochar insertion
- A small 1–1.5 cm stab incision is made prior to insertion of the trochar and applicator
- Expand the applicator after first confirming position of the device in the lumpectomy cavity. Expand until the device fits snug against the cavity
- Applicator sutured into position using drain stitch technique
- Apply dressings over the applicator insertion site prior to sending patient home
- The applicator tubing can be tucked within a soft bra between treatments
- Use magic marker or sticker to make skin mark that orients proper rotation of the applicator at time of CT simulation, which serves as landmark during treatment

Verification of Brachytherapy with Visual and Imaging

- CT scan is acquired for treatment planning, and the implant procedure and treatment planning can be done up to 3 days before the start of treatment
- Proper applicator fit confirmed on CT, and any necessary adjustments made, prior to treatment planning
- Rotation of applicator verified based on visual inspection of applicator and skin marks, aim for rotation less than 10°, or you may need to replan
- Prior to each treatment, applicator positioning verified with ultrasound or CT imaging

Evaluation of Implantation

Distribution of Implant

- Appropriate placement is confirmed via cross-sectional imaging
- Confirm location and configuration of applicator in the tumor cavity
- Tissue-balloon/device conformance: the surface of the device should be in contact with the lumpectomy cavity surface. In the B-39 trial, conformance was considered adequate when the volume of trapped air or fluid was <10 % of the PTV_EVAL volume
- Balloon/device symmetry: In the B-39 trial, no more than 2 mm deviation from expected dimensions was permitted for single-lumen balloon applicators
- Device surface to skin distance: Although multi-lumen devices permit sculpting of dose distributions, a distance of 5 mm is favored to deliver safe maximum skin dose

Review Imaging Real Time or When a Change Is Needed

- Ultrasound and CT imaging are useful for reviewing implant
- Applicator manipulation options include suctioning of air or fluid through a vacuum port, altering the fill volume, advancing or retracting the applicator, or changing devices
- Additional imaging is performed to evaluate implant
- A final CT is required after applicator adjustment for treatment planning
- Adjustments and replans may require additional CT and/or ultrasound imaging during the treatment course
- Sagittal CT images (Fig. 7.5) demonstrating an applicator that needed adjustment. Image on the left demonstrates a large air cavity posterior to the balloon. The applicator was adjusted and air suctioned through

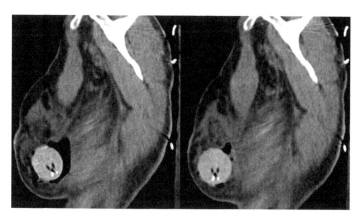

FIG. 7.5. Sagittal CT images demonstrating an applicator that needed adjustment. Image on the *left* demonstrates a large air cavity posterior to the balloon. The applicator was adjusted and air suctioned through the vacuum port of the applicator. Repeat CT scan (image on *right*) confirmed placement and decreased size of the air cavity deep to the applicator. Permission credit statement (Used with permission of Elsevier from Trifiletti DM, Shoalter TN, Libby B, Brenin DR, Schroen AT, Reardon KA, Showalter SL. Intraoperative breast radiation therapy with image guidance: Findings from CT images obtained in a prospective trial of intraoperative high-dose-rate brachytherapy with CT on rails. Brachytherapy 2015 Nov–Dec;14(6):919–24)

the vacuum port of the applicator. Repeat CT scan (image on right) confirmed placement and decreased size of the air cavity deep to the applicator

Treatment Planning Considerations [2]

Optimal Brachytherapy Doses

■ HDR Iridium-192

  ■ Primary treatment: 34 Gy in 10 fractions over 5 treatment days; 32 Gy in 8 fractions over 4 treatment days has also been reported

- Boost treatment: 10 Gy in 2 fractions over 1–2 treatment days

- LDR Iridium-192

  - Primary treatment: 45–50 Gy/0.50 Gy per hour
  - Boost treatment: 15–20 Gy/0.50 Gy per hour

- Use of image guidance for target volume delineation [26, 27] prior to breast-conserving surgery, identify tumor location in the breast by physical exam and preoperative imaging (mammogram/MRI) to delineate an imaging-related target volume
- Obtain detailed knowledge of the surgical procedure (type, number and location of clips, and position of skin scar) and surgical resection margins in six directions
- Obtain post-implant imaging to confirm placement and allow for individualized treatment planning
- Contour lumpectomy cavity guided by architectural distortion, surgical clips, seroma, scar and imaging-related target volume
- CTV = lumpectomy cavity + at least 1–2 cm margin
- Consider non-isotropic geometrical extension of the lumpectomy cavity based on pathologic information of margin status
- Typically, CTV = PTV
- However, if there are uncertainties, add an additional 5–10 mm to CTV
- PTV_EVAL = PTV – 5 mm from skin and pulled away from chest wall
- PTV_EVAL allows for dosimetric planning and evaluation with regard to nearby critical structures

Optimization of Target Volume: Point Based, Volume Based [28]

- Target coverage:

  - ≥95 % of the PTV_EVAL target volume to receive ≥90 % of the dose

- V150% $\leq$50 cm^3, V200 $\leq$20 cm^3

- Dose homogeneity index (DHI) for interstitial implants should be $\geq$0.75 and is calculated as: $(1-V150)/V100$

- Air/Seroma $\leq$10 % PTV_EVAL

- <60 % of the whole breast to receive $\geq$50 % of the dose

- Skin and rib maximum point doses $\leq$145 % prescription dose and ideally $\leq$100 %

- Dose should be sculpted away from heart, skin, ribs/chest wall

- Newer multicatheter applicators should allow for improved sparring of the skin and chest wall with improved volume coverage

Optimal Dose Distribution with Isodose Curves

- Multi-dwell, multichannel balloon applicators provide superior dose coverage to single-channel applicators by reducing anisotropy at the individual catheter tips

- If air is present between applicator and normal tissue, this pushes the target outside the normal isodose distribution and target coverage is calculated as:

$$\% \, PTV\_EVAL \, coverage - 100\left[volume \, of \, air \, / \, volume \, of \, PTV\_EVAL\right] \Rightarrow 90\%$$

- CT images (Fig. 7.6a–c) of breast interstitial implant showing how target coverage and irradiation to organs at risk changes with the number and position of catheters place

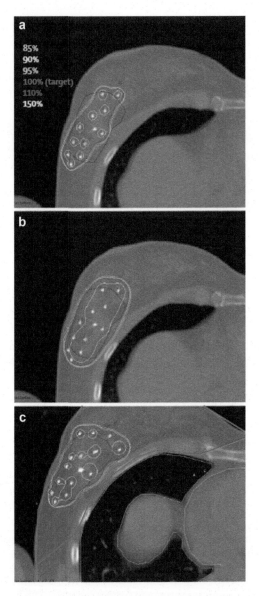

FIG. 7.6. (**a–c**) CT images of breast interstitial implant showing how target coverage and irradiation to organs at risk changes with the number and position of catheters place (Used with permission of Elsevier from Patel RR, Das RK. Image-guided breast brachytherapy: an alternative to whole-breast radiotherapy. The Lancet Oncology 2006 May;7(5):407–415)

Toxicity (Table 7.3)

Toxicity Side Effect Review: Common, Rare

- Common: dermatitis (acute), seroma, (acute), skin dimpling-indentation (late), telangiectasia (late), hyperpigmentation (late) fibrosis (late)
- Rare: bleeding (acute), infection (acute), delayed wound healing or complications (subacute), pneumonitis (subacute), fat necrosis (late), rib fracture (late), neuropathic pain (late)
- Potentially lower toxicity than external beam whole breast, as less normal tissue is irradiated
- Two most important factors in cosmesis: tumor size and skin spacing [29]
- Good-to-excellent cosmesis and high treatment-related satisfaction has been reported [30]
- NSABP B-39/RTOG 0413 will allow for comparison of treatment-related toxicity and cosmesis between APBI and WBI

Management of Brachytherapy Toxicity

- Grade 1 and 2 dermatitis: wash with soap and water to prevent bacterial superinfection, use non-scented cream to prevent moist desquamation, wear loose-fitting cotton clothing
- Itching and irritation: use topical corticosteroids
- Grade 3 dermatitis: apply nonadhesive dressings to regions of moist desquamation

Table 7.3 Toxicity and cosmetic outcomes following breast brachytherapy in current literature

	Treatment technique	Dose	Toxicity	Cosmesis "good/excellent"
Polgar et al. APBI interstitial [35]	HDR multicatheter interstitial	$7 \times 4.3 - 5.2$ Gy (HDR)	2.2 % Fibrosis 2.2 % Fat necrosis 0 % Telangiectasia	78 %
Polgar et al. APBI vs. WBI [34]	HDR multicatheter interstitial or EB	7×5.2 Gy (HDR) or 50 Gy (EB)	NR	78 % (81 % HDR, 70 % EB) vs. 63 % (WBI)
Strnad et al. APBI vs. WBI [40]	HDR multicatheter interstitial	8×4.0 Gy (HDR) or 7×4.3 Gy (HDR) or 50 Gy at 0.60– 0.80 Gy/h (PDR)	3.23 % Grade 2–3 late skin toxicity 0 % Grade 3 fibrosis	NR
Benitez et al. HDR Mammosite balloon [41]	HDR Mammosite balloon	10×3.4 Gy (HDR)	9.3 % Infection 21 % Seroma, asymptomatic 12 % Seroma, symptomatic requiring aspiration	83 %

Yashar et al. SAVI for APBI [42]	HDR SAVI	10×3.4 Gy (HDR)	1.9 % Telangiectasia 9.8 % Hyperpigmentation 1.9 % Fibrosis 1.9 % Fat necrosis, asymptomatic 1.9 % Seroma, symptomatic	NR
Vicini et al. ASBS Mammosite Registry [43]	HDR Mammosite balloon	10×3.4 Gy (HDR)	13 % Seroma, symptomatic 2.3 % Fat necrosis	91 %
Cuttino et al. Contura Balloon Phase 4 Registry [44]	HDR Contura multi-lumen balloon	10×3.4 Gy (HDR)	8.5 % Infection 4.4 % Seroma, symptomatic	88 %
Kamrava et al. PROMIS Study [39]	HDR or LDR multicatheter interstitial	50 Gy at 52 cGy/h×96 h (LDR) 8–10×3.2–3.4 Gy (HDR)	NR	91 % between 1 and 5 years 84 % with >5 years

EB electron beam, *HDR* high dose rate, *Gy* Gray, *cGy* Centigray, *PDR* pulsed dose rate, *SAVI* strut adjusted volume implant, *NR* not reported, *h* hour

Appendix A

Jyoti Mayadev, Timothy Showalter

Breast Case Study 7.1

Description of the Stage, Case

- Sixty-five-year-old female with a biopsy-proven invasive ductal carcinoma of the right breast upper outer quadrant clinically measuring 1.1 cm diagnosed by screening mammogram and confirmed by an US-guided core biopsy
- She chooses breast conservation therapy and undergoes lumpectomy and sentinel lymph node biopsy
- Final pathology confirms a 1.5 cm invasive ductal carcinoma, grade 1, estrogen-receptor positive, progesterone-receptor positive, Her2-neu negative. The disease is >2 mm from all inked margins. There are two sentinel nodes with no abnormal pathology
- pT1cN0Mx, stage IA
- Adjuvant radiation therapy is recommended
- "Suitable" candidate for breast brachytherapy per ASTRO consensus guidelines [16]

Use of Image Guidance

- Patient undergoes placement of balloon applicator 1 week after lumpectomy under ultrasound guidance
- CT scan is obtained to confirm appropriate placement
- Target (lumpectomy cavity, clips, seroma) identified
- Organs at risk (heart, skin, and ribs) identified
- Large air cavity identified on CT scan (Fig. 7.7, left)
- The applicator was adjusted and air was suctioned through the vacuum port of the applicator
- Repeat CT scan confirmed placement and decreased size of the air cavity deep to the applicator (Fig. 7.7, right)

Dosage Used

- 3.4 Gy per fraction × 10 fractions

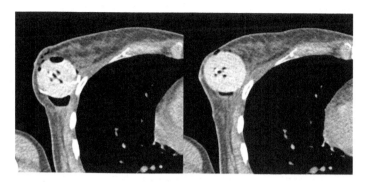

FIG. 7.7. Axial CT images of a large air cavity identified after balloon applicator placement (*left*) and a representative image after air suctioning through the vacuum port (*right*)

- Fractions delivered BID for 5 days
- Balloon catheter removed on the final day after the final fraction

Dose Distribution

- Axial CT image of a left breast cancer with balloon applicator and corresponding isodose lines demonstrating typical plan appearance (Fig. 7.8)

Breast Case Study 7.2: Breast Brachytherapy with SAVI

Sixty-one-year-old female with infiltrating ductal carcinoma of the left breast, Stage IA, T1cN0 ER+PR+HER2/neu-, status post-lumpectomy, and sentinel lymph node biopsy. She underwent a left breast lumpectomy, and final pathology confirmed a 1.6-cm infiltrating ductal carcinoma, SBR grade 2, with high-grade DCIS. One sentinel lymph node was sampled and was negative for evidence of metastatic disease

Discussion: She is a candidate for breast conservation therapy with lumpectomy followed by whole breast radiotherapy or accelerated partial breast irradiation. The patient chooses APBI with the SAVI device

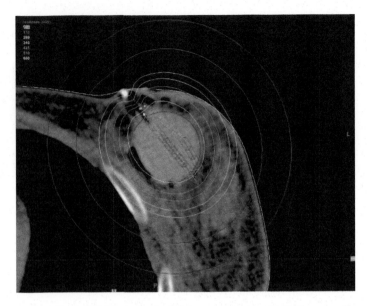

FIG. 7.8. Axial CT image of a left breast cancer with balloon applicator and corresponding isodose lines demonstrating typical plan appearance

Procedure with Image Guidance: We performed the SAVI brachytherapy with local sedation under ultrasound guidance in the department.

Treatment plan: We planned for a total dose of 3400 cGy in 340 cGy HDR per fraction using a 6-1 mini SAVI applicator given her pre-brachytherapy CT scan volume and measurements.

The SAVI catheter applicator size was verified. Using the SAVI treatment planning procedure and checklist (in the clinical appendix), the treatment plan was generated. The SAVI was drawn due to a reference of metal clips on catheters 2, 4, and 6.

The normal tissues are drawn, such as the lung, heart if the tumor is left-sided, ribs, and skin. The SAVI, PTV, and PTV evaluation structures are drawn after referencing the appropriate radiographic imaging as shown in Fig. 7.9. Using a geometric optimization, a treatment plan is generated and reviewed. The

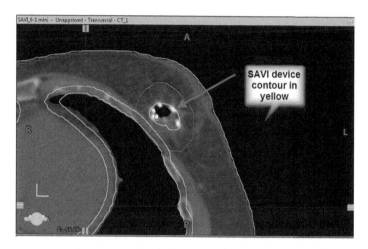

FIG. 7.9. SAVI device contour on the CT planning scan

normal tissue maximum doses are reviewed including the V200, V150, D90, and D95. A dose volume histogram is referenced for the PTV evaluation structure and normal critical structures. 340 cGy prescribed to the surface of the PTV evaluation volume for a total dose of 3400 cGy, as shown in Fig. 7.10. The plan was generated and approved by the attending physician. Then, the physicist performed a second check for quality assurance.

Breast Case Study 7.3: Breast Brachytherapy with Interstitial

Forty-seven-year-old female with a history of a left breast, low grade DCIS, status post-lumpectomy with final pathology showing low grade DCIS, cribriform pattern, measuring 0.15 cm, with 3 mm negative margins.

Discussion: We discussed the pathophysiology of DCIS, the natural history, and current recommendations. She is a candidate for breast conservation therapy with lumpectomy followed by whole breast radiotherapy, or accelerated partial breast irradiation.

Procedure with Image Guidance: At the pre-brachytherapy CT scan, she had a small cavity, less than 1 cm that had partially

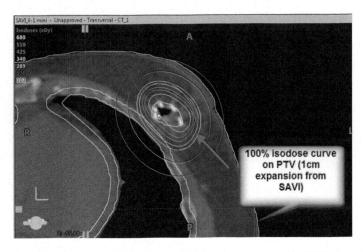

FIG. 7.10. Isodose distribution, 100 % isodose line on the PTV contour, which is 1 cm from the SAVI device

closed as shown in Fig. 7.11. Due to the small cavity and irregularity of the target volume, we treated her with freehand interstitial brachytherapy using an ultrasound technique. The patient was placed in the supine position. Bimanual palpation of the breast revealed a scar around the nipple areola complex. A sterile marking pen was used to mark the optimal needle locations in the breast. An ultrasound was used to verify the lumpectomy cavity posterior to the nipple.

Local anesthesia was used in the dermis, subcutaneous breast tissue, and deep breast tissue.

Using manual palpation and breast ultrasound guidance, the first interstitial needle was placed. Then, a plastic catheter was placed into the needle and the needle was removed. The catheter was advanced into the breast tissue. There were two planes used. There were five needles and catheters placed in the deep plane, and four in the anterior plane, for a total of eight catheters.

Once the catheters were placed, secure buttons and rubber stoppers were placed on the catheters to ensure stability of the catheters in the breast.

Treatment Plan: The preplan template for needle placement was referenced. The number of interstitial catheters and

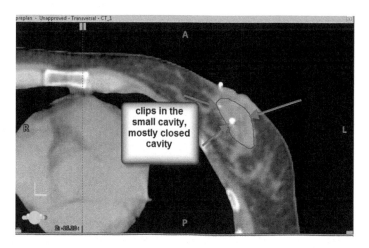

FIG. 7.11. Clips in the small lumpectomy cavity, with the majority of the cavity closed and unable to accommodate a multichannel single entry catheter

sequence was noted and referenced to the setup photographs and simulation template.

The CT images were imported into the treatment planning system. The catheter buttons and catheters were localized and drawn. The simulation and template worksheet was referenced again. The normal tissues were drawn, such as the lung, ribs, and skin. The lumpectomy cavity was drawn after referencing the clinical examination and the appropriate radiographic imaging, such as the pretreatment and pre-brachytherapy imaging. Using volumetric optimization and specified dwell weighting, a treatment plan was generated and reviewed as shown in Fig. 7.12. The normal tissue maximum doses were reviewed. An equivalent dose calculation table was used and a dose volume histogram was constructed. Dose optimization was carried out to ensure an appropriate dose to the gross tumor volume and high risk clinical target volume as well as keeping the appropriate dose constraints on the normal tissues. 340 cGy was prescribed to the PTV. The plan was generated and approved by the attending physician. The physicist then performed a second check for quality assurance.

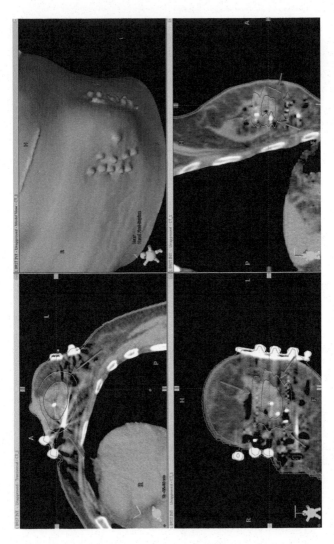

Fig. 7.12. The *arrows* pointing to the PTV which is a 1.5 cm expansion of the cavity. The skin render shows the two plane implant with four catheters in each plane

Appendix B: Breast Brachytherapy (example SAVI) Procedure Checklists

Jyoti Mayadev, Sonja Dieterich, Stanley Benedict, Robin Stern

Department of Radiation Oncology
SAVI General Workflow Procedure

I.   Introduction
  A. The SAVI (**S**trut **A**djustable **V**olume **I**mplant) device is used to delivery accelerated partial breast irradiation (APBI) via HDR brachytherapy. The device consists of a central catheter and 6-10 peripheral catheters surrounding the central catheter. The device is inserted into the lumpectomy cavity by a physician generally within 6 weeks of the lumpectomy procedure. Prescription is 3.4 Gy/fx to the outer surface of the PTV_Eval structure (see below) BID for 10 fractions delivered in 5 contiguous treatment days (excluding weekends).
II. Pre-insertion evaluation
  A. A CT of the lumpectomy cavity is obtained in the Radiation Oncology department no more than 72 hours before planned insertion of the SAVI device.
  B. The lumpectomy cavity is evaluated for volume, length, and size to determine the appropriate device size.
  C. The optimal insertion angle and point of entry on the skin is determined.
III. Insertion
  A. The SAVI device is inserted by the attending physician.
  B. The patient will be given the SAVI Expansion Tool with instructions to bring it with her to simulation.
IV. CT Simulation
  A. The Simulation Procedure is described in Clinical Practice>HDR Brachytherapy> SAVI >SAVI Simulation Procedure
V.   Treatment Planning
  A. The Treatment Planning Procedure is described Treatment Planning Procedure located at Clinical Practice >HDR Brachytherapy >SAVI >SAVI Treatment Planning Procedure
VI. Treatment
  A. Pre-treatment QA is performed at least every treatment day before the first fraction to insure no change in the SAVI device position.
    1. Visual marks on the patient/device and skin-to-handle distance are checked for consistency.
    2. Surviews are obtained and compared to Surviews taken at simulation for consistency.
  B. SAVI catheters are connected to the HDR afterloader, the length verified by measurement and treated per departmental procedures.
VII. Removal of device
  A. The SAVI device is removed by the physician after the last fractional treatment.

Department of Radiation Oncology
SAVI Pre-Implantation Procedure

I.   Perform CT evaluation of the lumpectomy cavity no more than 72 hours prior to insertion of the SAVI device.
II.   Patient does not have to be in treatment position. Arms may be up or down.
III. Scan parameters:
    A.   3mm contiguous slices (helical scan)
    B.   scan the entire cavity plus at least 2 cm margin superiorly and inferiorly
    C.   breath hold if possible
IV.   Send images to BrachyVision for evaluation.
V.   Radiation Oncologist contours the cavity.
VI.   Determine and record volume, length of long axis, and length of short axis of the contoured cavity. The radiation oncologist uses these parameters to determine the SAVI applicator size.
VII. The radiation oncologist evaluates the images set for best insertion angle and point of entry on the skin.

Department of Radiation Oncology
SAVI Breast Simulation Procedure

I. Required equipment:

    A. GammaMedplus source guide tubes with locking mechanism, 200 mm interstitial, one for each peripheral lumen of the applicator (7 for 6-1 applicators, 9 for 8-1 applicator, 11 for 10-1 applicator).

    B. 1 GammaMedplus source guide tube with locking mechanism, 250 mm interstitial

    C. GammaMedplus 1300mm length gauge

    D. GammaMedplus 250mm length cutting gauge

    E. GammaMedplus 200mm length cutting gauge

II. Position patient in treatment position with ipsilateral arm up.

III. Position the patient so the lasers intersect as close to the SAVI as possible. Mark the patient at the projection of the lasers.

IV. Acquire AP and lateral Surviews of the breast.

V. Insert a dummy marker cable into the central catheter. This step can be performed before the Surviews are acquired, at the discretion of the attending physician.

VI. Perform CT scan with the following parameters:

    A. Axial (not helical) scan

    B. 2 mm contiguous slices

    C. breath hold if possible

    D. scan at least the entire breast. Sup/inf borders to be specified by radiation oncologist.

VII. Radiation oncologist evaluates the images for placement and expansion of the SAVI. Radiation oncologist and/or surgeon adjusts the device if and as needed. Repeat Surviews and CT after adjustment.

    A. If additional expansion is needed, remove the catheter protector from the central catheter. Carefully insert the SAVI Expansion Tool over the central catheter until properly engaged into the fitting of the SAVI device. Turn the Expansion Tools as needed.

VIII. On the Simulation Worksheet, mark device size and relative positioning on the figures.

IX. Mark the SAVI white ring and the skin in a continuous line for rotational assessment at the position of one of the catheters. Record catheter number on Simulation Worksheet.

X. Push the white ring against the skin and measure ring-to-hub distance using the marks on the SAVI central catheter. Record on the Simulation Worksheet.

XI. Export CT data to BrachyVision for planning.

XII. Keep Surview images at the CT console for the length of the treatment for pre-treatment evaluation.

XIII. Check catheter lengths
   A. Arms can be lowered for patient comfort.
   B. Remove catheter protectors from all the SAVI device catheters.
   C. Connect the source guide tubes to the SAVI catheters.
      1. Connect the 250mm guide tube to the central catheter.
      2. Connect a 200mm guide tube to each of the peripheral catheter.
   D. Use the length gauge to check the length of each catheter+guide tube. Record results on Simulation Worksheet.
      1. If length too long (>1301 mm), trim the SAVI catheter.
         a. Use the appropriate length cutting gauge to mark the catheter at the proper length.
         b. Cut the catheter at the mark.
         c. Use the end of the cutting gauge to open the cut end of the catheter.
         d. Reconnect guide tube and recheck length.
      2. If length too short (< 1299 mm), that catheter can not be used for treatment. Tape the catheter protector in place within the catheter to "seal off" catheter.
      3. If one or more catheters are too short, the radiation oncologist may choose to replace entire SAVI device.

XIV. Disconnect source tubes. Remove the Expansion Tool if it was used, and replace the catheter protectors.

XV. Re-bandage or re-dress the SAVI-skin entrance site.

XVI. Store the Expansion Tool in a safe place in the HDR treatment or console room.

XVII. Dosiemtrist checks quality of images in Brachyvision before patient is released from the department.

SAVI™ Simulation Worksheet

Place label here

Sim Date: _____

Therapists: _____

Site: Left ☐   Right ☐   Breast

Device Configuration:

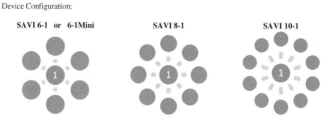

SAVI 6-1 or 6-1Mini   **SAVI 8-1**   **SAVI 10-1**

Skin mark placed along catheter #: _____

Do not use any catheter which fails the length check.
Tape catheter protector into catheter.

A=Ring-Hub index

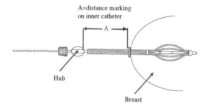

A=distance marking on inner catheter

Hub

Breast

Catheter #	Length Check	
	Pass	Fail
1		
2		
3		
4		
5		
6		
7		
8		
9		
10		
11		

Initial	Task
	Place dummy wire in central catheter before CT scan
	Dosimetrist checked image quality in BrachyVision before releasing the patient

Department of Radiation Oncology
SAVI Breast Treatment Planning Procedure

I. Import the simulation CT into Brachyvision.

II. Radiation oncologist contours the following structures using the structure template "SAVI" (Insert/New Structures from Template):

   A. Body = surface of the skin

   B. SAVI = extent of the SAVI device.

      1. Encloses invaginated tissue.

      2. Contour distally to the end of the metal band and proximally to where the peripheral struts rejoin the shaft.

      3. Contour around the device struts.

   C. Lung = lung/chest wall interface. Can be drawn using auto-contour (right click, "flood fill". "Post process" to remove uncontoured pockets.).

   D. Invag = tissue invaginating into the applicator.

   E. Air = air within the PTV (see step III.A) but outside the struts of the applicator. The oncologist may opt not to draw this structure if s/he judges the volume to be small enough to meet the conformity requirement (see step IV). Contour air using variable brush. "Avoid painting over" SAVI.

III. Create the following structures from the above:

   A. Chest wall = 0.5 cm positive 3D expansion of Lung ("Extract Wall" from LUNG; outer margin 0.5 cm, inner magin 0 cm). Alternately, the physician may draw the Chestwall contours.

   B. Skin = 0.2 cm rind **inside** of body touching the skin. ("Extract Wall" from BODY; Outer margin 0 cm, inner margin 0.2 cm). Create by 0.2 cm 3D expansion of Body then subtract Body. (Note: this is different from the vendor's recommendation of defining the rind outside the body, so that the max dose to the structure would represent max dose ot the skin surface.)

   C. PTV = 1.0 cm positive 3D expansion of SAVI structure excluding Chestwall and volume outside of Body. ("Margin fro Structure" from SAVI, 1 cm, check box for "avoid structure", enter CHESTWALL". In "Post Processing", clean-up by checking box "remove parts outside of" BODY, hit "Apply". Note: MD may further edit the PTV based on the patient's anatomy and surgical margins.

    D. PTV_Eval = PTV minus SAVI and plus Invag ("Boolean Operators": (PTV sub SAVI) or INVAG)

IV. Check conformity index

    A. If Air structure not drawn, note on the Pre-Plan Check Sheet and skip to step V.

    B. Determine volume of PTV_Eval and Air structures.

    C. Calculate (Air volume) / (PTV_Eval volume) and record on the Pre-Plan Check Sheet

        1. If ratio < 10%, meets conformity requirements.

        2. If ratio > 10%, physician decides whether to

            a. Redefine SAVI structure to include Air, re-expand to define new PTV and new PTV_Eval, **or**

            b. wait 1-2 days for air to escape and repeat CT-simulation.

 V. Insert new plan. Select technique = "Intracavitary" and prescribe 340 cGy/fraction for 1 fraction.

VI. Define the applicators in software.

    A. Rotate and shift the views such that the entire axis of the SAVI device is clearly visible on two of the orthogonal views. These are "full length" views, and the third view will be a "head-on" view of the device.

    B. Page through the head-on view and identify catheters #2, #4, and #6. See Figure 1 and Figure 2.

        1. The integrated marker on catheter #2 is the most distal marker

        2. The integrated marker on catheter #4 is the marker nearest the center.

        3. The integrated marker on catheter #6 is the most proximal marker.

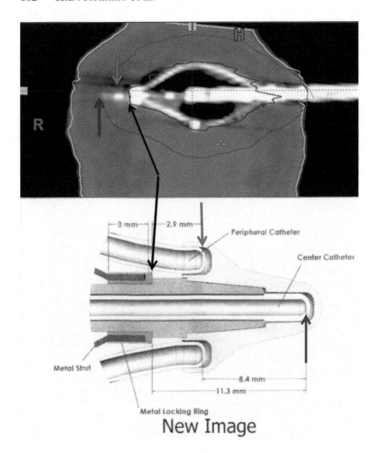

FIG. I. (revised per manufacturer 7/31/2014)

C. On one of the full length views, identify the bright metal band at the distal tip of the device. Use the measure tool to measure **11.3 mm** along the central axis beyond the distal edge of the metal band. Move the orthogonal plane selector/indicator so the line is at the **11.3 mm** position. (**bold** are revised values per manufacturer 7/31/2014)

D. Move the measure tool to measure **2.9 mm** along the central axis beyond the distal edge of the metal band. On both full-length views, insert a short reference line perpendicular to the central axis at this distance. Delete the measurement line.

E. Insert a new Applicator. Confirm ID is "Applicator1", channel number = 1, applicator length = 130 cm, step size = 0.5 cm, and first source posn = 0 cm. On one full length view, draw the applicator tip at the **11.3 mm** position marked with the view selector/indicator line and draw the applicator along the central catheter to beyond where the proximal ends of the peripheral catheter rejoin the central catheter.

F. Change the head-on view to show the marker on catheter #4. This view should be at approximately the center of the SAVI device.

G. Rotate the head-on view until catheter #2 is visualized fully along its entire length in one of the full-length views.

　　1. If the catheter has some out-of-plane curvature it might not be possible to visualize the entire catheter at once. In this case, it is necessary to rotate the views slightly tofully identify the catheter when defining the applicator.

H. In the full length view, insert a new applicator. Confirm ID is "Applicator2", channel number = 2, applicator length = 130 cm, step size = 0.5 cm, and first source posn = 0 cm. Put the tip at the **2.9 mm** reference line at the outer surface of the central axis. Draw the applicator along but just outside the nitinol strut visible in the images.

I. Repeat steps G-H for each additional catheter, confirming the appropriate applicator name and channel number.

　　1. Do not create an applicator for any catheter that did not pass the length test performed during simulation.

J. Verify proper definition of applicators by displaying 3D image in upper right window and turning off all structures. One by one and in sequence, highlight each applicator in the head-on view and verify the position of the selected applicator (in red) in the 3D display.

VII. Create dwell positions by selecting Planning/Applicator/Fit Soure Positions Inside Structure. Select "Fit all applicators" and PTV_Eval.

VIII. Run optimization.

    A. Select Planning/Modify Dose/Volume Optimization.

    B. Check "surface" box next to PTV.

    C. Change objectives to 340 cGy +/-17 cGy (this is equivalent to +/-5%).

    D. Click Optimize.

IX. If necessary, use the Dose Shaper tool to reduce dose to skin and chestwall.

    A. Select Dose Shaper tool, the right click and set slider bar all the way to the right towards "Local".

X. Evaluate the plan using DVH and dose display tools. Goals are:

    A. PTV_Eval: 95% of volume receives >95% of prescribed dose

    B. Volume of PTV_Eval receiving ≥200% of Rx dose must be < 20 cc

    C. Volume of PTV_Eval receiving ≥150% of Rx dose must be < 50 cc

XI. Modify plan with Dose Shaper tool as needed to obtain acceptable plan.

XII. Save plan, print to pdf, import into MOSAIQ. Dosimetrist and physician approve the plan.

XIII. Export plan to the treatment console.

XIV. Authorized Medical Physicist second-checks the plan, approves the plan pdf, and completes the "2nd Physics Check – Brachytherapy" QCL..

    A. Check includes verification of:

        1. Rx in MOSAIQ specifies 3.4 Gy/fx to the surface of PTV_Eval for 10 fractions BID and is approved by the Authorized User radiation oncologist

        2. PTV_Eval defined correctly

        3. conformity ratio < 10%

        4. definition of applicators, including name, channel, location of tip, position of applicator

        5. planned dose agrees with Rx

        6. plan achieves dosimetric goals

SAVI™ Pre-Treatment QA Checksheet

Patient: _____   MRN: _____

- Place patient in treatment position on immobilization device (i.e. Vac-Loc or Breast Board) for pre-fraction orthogonal images, *assuring replication of position prior to each treatment*.
- Remove all dressings prior to any images.
- Verify continuity of mark on skin/SAVI disk for rotational consistency. Tolerance ±10°.
- Confirm index from ring to SAVI hub and compare to reference from simulation. Tolerance ±2 mm.
- Obtain AP and Lateral Surviews. Compare to images taken during simulation. Tolerance ±10°. (Optional at physician's discretion for PM).

Enter initials

	Fraction	1	2	3	4	5	6	7	8	9	10
Therapist	Date										
	Time (AM or PM)										
	Mark on skin at catheter # ___										
	Ring-hub index: ___										
	Initials										
MD	Review AP Surview										
	Review Lat Surview										

Department of Radiation Oncology
SAVI Breast Pre-Treatment Quality Assurance and Treatment Delivery

I. Verification of the position of the SAVI device must be performed at least before the first treatment fraction each day. Verification consists of radiographic as well as visual checks as defined below.

II. Pre-treatment QA

    A. Position the patient on the CT-sim couch in treatment position. Align marks on patient to lasers.

    B. Confirm that the line drawn on SAVI white ring and skin during simulation is unbroken. Record and initial on Pre-Treatment QA Check Sheet.

    C. Measure distance from skin surface to catheter handle, record and initial on Pre-Treatment QA Check Sheet. Measured distance should be within +2 mm of simulation measurement.

    D. Acquire AP and lateral Surviews.

    E. The attending physician compares the Surviews to Surviews taken at time of simulation to evaluate for movement or rotation of the SAVI device relative to the patient anatomy. Rotation difference should be < 10 degrees. The attending physician initials the Pre-Treatment QA Check Sheet.

    F. If all pre-treatment QA test results are acceptable, the treatment may proceed.

    G. Treatment and treatment QA will be performed in accordance with departmental procedures for HDR treatment (see GammaMed HDR Brachytherapy Procedures and HDR Treatment Check Procedure).

    H. Position patient in the HDR treatment room in treatment position.

    I. Remove the catheter protectors from each catheter of the SAVI device.

    J. Carefully insert the SAVI Expansion Tool over the central catheter until properly engaged into the fitting of the SAVI device.

    K. Connect the source guide tubes to the SAVI device catheters

        1. Connect the 250mm guide tube to the central catheter.

        2. Connect a 200mm guide tube to each of the peripheral catheters.

    L. Perform a length check on each catheter + guide tube. All must pass for treatment to be delivered.

M. Connect guide tubes to the channel connectors on the HDR afterloader, making sure catheter #1 is connected to channel #1, etc. for all catheters.

N. The Authorized Medical Physicist checks the guide tube connection prior to initiation of treatment.

O. The therapist, Authorized Medical Physicist, and Authorized User physician perform pre-treatment checks in accordance with departmental procedures for HDR treatment (see HDR Treatment Check Procedure). These procedures include a documented procedural pause before initiation of treatment delivery.

P. Deliver treatment in accordance with departmental procedures for HDR treatment.

Q. Perform post-treatment checks in accordance with departmental procedures.

R. Disconnect the guide tubes from the SAVI device catheters, remove the Expansion Tool, and insert the catheter protectors into the catheters.

S. Store the Expansion Tool in a safe site in the HDR treatment or console room.

T. Re-bandage or re-dress the SAVI-skin entrance site.

III. Emergency

A. In case of the source fails to return to the safe during treatment, follow departmental emergency procedures (Emergency Procedures for GammaMed Plus HDR in Case the Source Fails to Return to the Safe). See SAVI Emergency Removal Procedure if emergent removal of the SAVI device is required.

Department of Radiation Oncology
SAVI Emergency Removal

I.   This procedure specifies how to emergently remove the SAVI device in the event that the active source can not be retracted during treatment delivery. Departmental emergency procedures (Emergency Procedures for GammaMed Plus HDR in Case the Source Fails to Return to the Safe) will be followed.

II. To remove the SAVI device, the Authorized User physician will:

A.   Grasp the white handle (marked with a "1") on the central catheter shaft between thumb and forefingers of one hand. If desired, use the other hand to move the transfer tubes away from the central catheter.

B.   Using the other hand, grasp the expansion tool, which is on the central catheter, between the transfer tube and the white handle.

C.   Confirm the expansion tools is properly seated and ready to be used to collapse the SAVI device.

D.   Quickly rotate the expansion tool **COUNTER-CLOCKWISE** four (4) full turns.

E.   Rotate the entire SAVI device a half turn in either direction.

F.   Continue rotation the expansion tool COUNTER-CLOCKWISE until the SAVI device is completely collapsed (between 4 and 8 more rotations depending on size of SAVI device). An audible and/or tactile "click" confirms the applicator is completely closed.

G.   Move one hand to breast at incision site and place it so the catheter exit site is between the thumb and pointer finger.

H.   Pull device from breast using the other hand, giving a slight rotation as it is withdrawn from the breast.

I.   Deposit the device, with transfer tubes still attached, into the emergency pig.

Radiation Oncology Breast Interstitial High Dose Rate Implantation

Physician:

Date of Planning Scan: _____   Laterality: _____

Number of catheters inserted: _____   Needle length: _____

Pt's Label Here

Friction caps

Cleaning caps

Record Reference Length

Catheter	1	2	3	4	5	6	7	8	9	10	11	12	13	14	15	16	17	18	R.T.T. Initials
Date • Fx																			
Reference (+/- 1mm) 1																			
2																			
3																			
4																			
5																			
6																			
7																			
8																			
9																			
10																			

References

1. Huang E, Buchholz TA, Meric F, Krishnamurthy S, Mirza NQ, Ames FC, et al. Classifying local disease recurrences after breast conservation therapy based on location and histology: new primary tumors have more favorable outcomes than true local disease recurrences. Cancer. 2002;95(10):2059–67.
2. Keisch M, Arthur D, Patel R, Rivard M, Vicini F. American Brachytherapy Society (ABS) Task Group for breast brachytherapy; February 2007. https://http://www.american-brachytherapy.org/guidelines/abs_breast_brachytherapy_task-group.pdf. [updated February 2007; cited 1 October 2015].
3. Trifiletti D, Showalter TN, Libby B, Brenin DR, Schroen AT, Reardon KA, et al. Intraoperative breast radiation therapy with image guidance: findings from CT images obtained in a prospective trial of intraoperative high-dose-rate brachytherapy with CT on rails. Brachytherapy. 2015;14(6):919–24.
4. NSABP. B-39, RTOG 0413: a randomized Phase III study of conventional whole breast irradiation versus partial breast irradiation for women with stage 0, I, or II breast cancer. Clin Adv Hematol Oncol. 2006;4(10):719–21.
5. Shah C, Vicini F, Wazer DE, Arthur D, Patel RR. The American Brachytherapy Society consensus statement for accelerated partial breast irradiation. Brachytherapy. 2013;12(4):267–77.
6. Chuba PJ, Hamre MR, Yap J, Severson RK, Lucas D, Shamsa F, et al. Bilateral risk for subsequent breast cancer after lobular carcinoma-in-situ: analysis of surveillance, epidemiology, and end results data. J Clin Oncol. 2005;23(24):5534–41.
7. Shah C, Wilkinson JB, Shaitelman S, Grills I, Wallace M, Mitchell C, et al. Clinical outcomes using accelerated partial breast irradiation in patients with invasive lobular carcinoma. Int J Radiat Oncol Biol Phys. 2011;81(4):e547–51.
8. Ott OJ, Hildebrandt G, Potter R, Hammer J, Hindemith M, Resch A, et al. Accelerated partial breast irradiation with interstitial implants: risk factors associated with increased local recurrence. Int J Radiat Oncol Biol Phys. 2011;80(5):1458–63.
9. Strnad V, Hildebrandt G, Potter R, Hammer J, Hindemith M, Resch A, et al. Accelerated partial breast irradiation: 5-year results of the German-Austrian multicenter phase II trial using interstitial multicatheter brachytherapy alone after

breast-conserving surgery. Int J Radiat Oncol Biol Phys. 2011;80(1):17–24.

10. Polgar C, Van Limbergen E, Potter R, Kovacs G, Polo A, Lyczek J, et al. Patient selection for accelerated partial-breast irradiation (APBI) after breast-conserving surgery: recommendations of the Groupe Europeen de Curietherapie-European Society for Therapeutic Radiology and Oncology (GEC-ESTRO) breast cancer working group based on clinical evidence (2009). Radiother Oncol. 2010;94(3):264–73.

11. Smith TE, Lee D, Turner BC, Carter D, Haffty BG. True recurrence vs. new primary ipsilateral breast tumor relapse: an analysis of clinical and pathologic differences and their implications in natural history, prognoses, and therapeutic management. Int J Radiat Oncol Biol Phys. 2000;48(5):1281–9.

12. Fowble B, Solin LJ, Schultz DJ, Rubenstein J, Goodman RL. Breast recurrence following conservative surgery and radiation: patterns of failure, prognosis, and pathologic findings from mastectomy specimens with implications for treatment. Int J Radiat Oncol Biol Phys. 1990;19(4):833–42.

13. Faverly DR, Burgers L, Bult P, Holland R. Three dimensional imaging of mammary ductal carcinoma in situ: clinical implications. Semin Diagn Pathol. 1994;11(3):193–8.

14. Schroen AT, Brenin DR, Kelly MD, Knaus WA, Slingluff Jr CL. Impact of patient distance to radiation therapy on mastectomy use in early-stage breast cancer patients. J Clin Oncol. 2005;23(28):7074–80.

15. Voti L, Richardson LC, Reis I, Fleming LE, Mackinnon J, Coebergh JW. The effect of race/ethnicity and insurance in the administration of standard therapy for local breast cancer in Florida. Breast Cancer Res Treat. 2006;95(1):89–95.

16. Hershman DL, Buono D, McBride RB, Tsai WY, Joseph KA, Grann VR, et al. Surgeon characteristics and receipt of adjuvant radiotherapy in women with breast cancer. J Natl Cancer Inst. 2008;100(3):199–206.

17. Showalter SL, Grover S, Sharma S, Lin L, Czerniecki BJ. Factors influencing surgical and adjuvant therapy in stage I breast cancer: a SEER 18 database analysis. Ann Surg Oncol. 2013;20(4):1287–94.

18. Correa C, Harris E, Leonardi MC, Smith B, Taghian AG, et al. Accelerated Partial Breast Irradiation: Executive summary for the update of an ASTRO Evidence-Based Consensus Statement. PRO 2016; in press.

19. The American Society of Breast Surgeons. Consensus statement for accelerated partial breast irradiation; 2008. https://http://www.breastsurgeons.org/statements/PDF_Statements/APBI_statement_revised_100708.pdf. [cited 10 April 2015].

20. Wilkinson JB, Beitsch PD, Shah C, Arthur D, Haffty BG, Wazer DE, et al. Evaluation of current consensus statement recommendations for accelerated partial breast irradiation: a pooled analysis of William Beaumont Hospital and American Society of Breast Surgeon MammoSite Registry Trial Data. Int J Radiat Oncol Biol Phys. 2013;85(5):1179–85.

21. Shaitelman SF, Vicini FA, Beitsch P, Haffty B, Keisch M, Lyden M. Five-year outcome of patients classified using the American Society for Radiation Oncology consensus statement guidelines for the application of accelerated partial breast irradiation: an analysis of patients treated on the American Society of Breast Surgeons MammoSite Registry Trial. Cancer. 2010;116(20):4677–85.

22. McHaffie DR, Patel RR, Adkison JB, Das RK, Geye HM, Cannon GM. Outcomes after accelerated partial breast irradiation in patients with ASTRO consensus statement cautionary features. Int J Radiat Oncol Biol Phys. 2011;81(1):46–51.

23. Beitsch P, Vicini F, Keisch M, Haffty B, Shaitelman S, Lyden M. Five-year outcome of patients classified in the "unsuitable" category using the American Society of Therapeutic Radiology and Oncology (ASTRO) Consensus Panel guidelines for the application of accelerated partial breast irradiation: an analysis of patients treated on the American Society of Breast Surgeons MammoSite(R) Registry trial. Ann Surg Oncol. 2010;17 Suppl 3:219–25.

24. Christoudias MK, Collett AE, Stull TS, Gracely EJ, Frazier TG, Barrio AV. Are the American Society for Radiation Oncology guidelines accurate predictors of recurrence in early stage breast cancer patients treated with balloon-based brachytherapy? Int J Surg Oncol. 2013;2013:829050.

25. Stull TS, Catherine Goodwin M, Gracely EJ, Chernick MR, Carella RJ, Frazier TG, et al. A single-institution review of accelerated partial breast irradiation in patients considered "cautionary" by the American Society for Radiation Oncology. Ann Surg Oncol. 2012;19(2):553–9.

26. Strnad V, Hannoun-Levi JM, Guinot JL, Lossi K, Kauer-Dorner D, Resch A, et al. Recommendations from GEC ESTRO Breast Cancer Working Group (I): target definition and target delineation for accelerated or boost Partial Breast Irradiation using

multicatheter interstitial brachytherapy after breast conserving closed cavity surgery. Radiother Oncol. 2015;115(3):342–8.

27. Major T, Gutierrez C, Guix B, van Limbergen E, Strnad V, Polgar C, et al. Recommendations from GEC ESTRO Breast Cancer Working Group (II): target definition and target delineation for accelerated or boost partial breast irradiation using multicatheter interstitial brachytherapy after breast conserving open cavity surgery. Radiother Oncol. 2016;118(1):199–204.

28. Shah C, Wobb J, Manyam B, Khan A, Vicini F. Accelerated partial breast irradiation utilizing brachytherapy: patient selection and workflow. J Contemp Brachyther. 2016;8(1):90–4.

29. Vicini FA, Keisch M, Shah C, Goyal S, Khan AJ, Beitsch PD, et al. Factors associated with optimal long-term cosmetic results in patients treated with accelerated partial breast irradiation using balloon-based brachytherapy. Int J Radiat Oncol Biol Phys. 2012;83(2):512–8.

30. Rabinovitch R, Winter K, Kuske R, Bolton J, Arthur D, Scroggins T, et al. RTOG 95-17, a Phase II trial to evaluate brachytherapy as the sole method of radiation therapy for Stage I and II breast carcinoma—year-5 toxicity and cosmesis. Brachytherapy. 2014;13(1):17–22.

31. Fisher B, Land S, Mamounas E, Dignam J, Fisher ER, Wolmark N. Prevention of invasive breast cancer in women with ductal carcinoma in situ: an update of the National Surgical Adjuvant Breast and Bowel Project experience. Semin Oncol. 2001;28(4):400–18.

32. Fisher B, Anderson S, Bryant J, Margolese RG, Deutsch M, Fisher ER, et al. Twenty-year follow-up of a randomized trial comparing total mastectomy, lumpectomy, and lumpectomy plus irradiation for the treatment of invasive breast cancer. N Engl J Med. 2002;347(16):1233–41.

33. Early Breast Cancer Trialists' Collaborative Group, Darby S, McGale P, Correa C, Taylor C, Arriagada R, et al. Effect of radiotherapy after breast-conserving surgery on 10-year recurrence and 15-year breast cancer death: meta-analysis of individual patient data for 10,801 women in 17 randomised trials. Lancet. 2011;378(9804):1707–16.

34. Polgar C, Fodor J, Major T, Nemeth G, Lovey K, Orosz Z, et al. Breast-conserving treatment with partial or whole breast irradiation for low-risk invasive breast carcinoma—5-year results of a randomized trial. Int J Radiat Oncol Biol Phys. 2007;69(3):694–702.

35. Polgar C, Major T, Fodor J, Sulyok Z, Somogyi A, Lovey K, et al. Accelerated partial-breast irradiation using high-dose-rate interstitial brachytherapy: 12-year update of a prospective clinical study. Radiother Oncol. 2010;94(3):274–9.

36. Shah C, Antonucci JV, Wilkinson JB, Wallace M, Ghilezan M, Chen P, et al. Twelve-year clinical outcomes and patterns of failure with accelerated partial breast irradiation versus whole-breast irradiation: results of a matched-pair analysis. Radiother Oncol. 2011;100(2):210–4.

37. Shah C, Wilkinson JB, Lyden M, Beitsch P, Vicini FA. Predictors of local recurrence following accelerated partial breast irradiation: a pooled analysis. Int J Radiat Oncol Biol Phys. 2012;82(5):e825–30.

38. Shah C, Badiyan S, Ben Wilkinson J, Vicini F, Beitsch P, Keisch M, et al. Treatment efficacy with accelerated partial breast irradiation (APBI): final analysis of the American Society of Breast Surgeons MammoSite breast brachytherapy registry trial. Ann Surg Oncol. 2013;20(10):3279–85.

39. Kamrava M, Kuske RR, Anderson B, Chen P, Hayes J, Quiet C, et al. Outcomes of breast cancer patients treated with accelerated partial breast irradiation via multicatheter interstitial brachytherapy: The Pooled Registry of Multicatheter Interstitial Sites (PROMIS) experience. Ann Surg Oncol. 2015;22 Suppl 3:404–11.

40. Strnad V, Ott OJ, Hildenbrandt G, Kauer-Dorner D, Knauerhase H, Major T, et al. 5-year results of accelerated partial breast irradiation using sole interstitial multicatheter brachytherapy versus whole-breast irradiation with boost after breast-conserving surgery for low-risk invasive and in-situ carcinoma of the female breast: a randomised, phase 3, non-inferiority trial. Lancet. 2016;387(10015):229–38.

41. Benitez PR, Keisch ME, Vicini F, Stolier A, Scroggins T, Walker A, et al. Five-year results: the initial clinical trial of MammoSite balloon brachytherapy for partial breast irradiation in early-stage breast cancer. Am J Surg. 2007;194(4):456–62.

42. Yashar CM, Scanderbeg D, Kuske R, Wallace A, Zannis V, Blair S, et al. Initial clinical experience with the Strut-Adjusted Volume Implant (SAVI) breast brachytherapy device for accelerated partial-breast irradiation (APBI): first 100 patients with more than 1 year of follow-up. Int J Radiat Oncol Biol Phys. 2011;80(3):765–70.

43. Vicini F, Beitsch P, Quiet C, Gittleman M, Zannis V, Fine R, et al. Five-year analysis of treatment efficacy and cosmesis by the American Society of Breast Surgeons MammoSite Breast Brachytherapy Registry Trial in patients treated with accelerated partial breast irradiation. Int J Radiat Oncol Biol Phys. 2011;79(3):808–17.
44. Cuttino LW, Arthur DW, Vicini F, Todor D, Julian T, Mukhopadhyay N. Long-term results from the Contura multilumen balloon breast brachytherapy catheter phase 4 registry trial. Int J Radiat Oncol Biol Phys. 2014;90(5):1025–9.

Chapter 8
Eye Plaque Brachytherapy

Tijana Skrepnik, John Gloss, Cameron Javid, and Baldassarre Stea

Introduction

- Uveal melanoma is the most common primary malignant intraocular neoplasm
- It arises from melanocytes of the uveal tracts
- Comprises approximately 1500 of the 2400 cases of all primary ocular and orbital malignant tumors in the US per year with an incidence of 5.1 per million [1]
- Majority of cases are diagnosed incidentally on routine ophthalmology exam or once visual symptoms arise

T. Skrepnik, MD • J. Gloss, PSM • B. Stea, MD, PhD (✉)
Department of Radiation Oncology, Banner University
Medical Center, University of Arizona, 1501 N. Campbell Ave,
Tucson, AZ 85724, USA
e-mail: skrepnik@email.arizona.edu johnegloss@email.arizona.edu;
bstea@email.arizona.edu

C. Javid, MD, FACS
Department of Ophthalmology, University of Arizona,
1501 N. Campbell Ave, Tucson, AZ 85724, USA

Retina Associates, 6561 E Carondelet Dr, Tucson, AZ 85710, USA
e-mail: cgjavid@gmail.com

© Springer International Publishing AG 2017   197
J. Mayadev et al. (eds.), *Handbook of Image-Guided
Brachytherapy*, DOI 10.1007/978-3-319-44827-5_8

- Presenting symptoms consist of flashes of light, floaters, decreased visual acuity, visual field deficits
- Rarely patients present with eye pain and redness (due to necrotic or large tumors causing retinal detachment and inflammation)

Rationale for Brachytherapy

- Treatment options for ocular melanoma include enucleation, laser photocoagulation, transpupillary thermotherapy, proton beam radiotherapy, and episcleral plaque brachytherapy
- Until the 1980s, enucleation was the standard of care for all choroidal melanoma patients
- The COMS trial, a randomized, prospective study that evaluated the effectiveness of globe-conserving episcleral plaque brachytherapy versus enucleation [2], had a major impact on the treatment of this disease. This trial results showed equivalent survival for the two treatment approaches but the plaque therapy offered the potential for vision preservation
- Plaque brachytherapy for appropriately selected patients (medium-sized tumors with an apical height of 2.5–10 mm and maximum basal diameter of ≤16 mm) remains the recommended treatment of ocular melanoma today

Goals of Brachytherapy

- Goals of plaque brachytherapy are preservation of function (vision), control of disease, and cosmesis (retention of the eye)
- Radioactive plaque brachytherapy is primarily indicated for small uveal tumors (<10 mm in diameter) that demonstrate growth over time and for all medium-sized tumors, based on COMS size criteria (10–16 mm in basal diameter)

- The most commonly used isotope in North America is I-125 (gamma emitter) because of the higher penetration in thicker lesions as well as its ready availability, relative safety, and adoption in many treatment centers [3]
- Other isotopes used for the same purpose are ruthenium-106, iridium-192, strontium-90, and palladium-103
- Local control: the COMS medium-sized tumor study [2] demonstrated that ~90 % of tumors are controlled at 5 years after plaque treatment
- COMS also reported only 10.3 % treatment failures, defined as tumor growth, recurrence, extra-scleral extension, or enucleation due to pain and other factors
- Maintenance of visual acuity: the COMS medium-sized study demonstrated that 83 % and 57 % of patients retained vision better than 20/200 at 1- and 3-years follow-up

Pertinent Anatomy for Brachytherapy

- Figure 8.1 depicts a schematic diagram of the human eye [4]
- The globe is a round structure approximately 25–30 mm in diameter
- The uveal tract (the middle layer of the eyeball) located between the sclera externally and the retinal neuroepithelial tissue internally is the site of origin of choroidal melanomas
- The uvea is divided into three contiguous parts: the pigmented iris, the muscular ciliary body, and the vascular choroid. The intervening stroma is comprised of melanocytes from the neural crest
- Ocular melanomas arise most commonly from the choroid layer, less commonly from the ciliary body and rarely from the iris
- Choroidal melanomas are typically larger and more likely to metastasize as compared with ciliary body or iris melanoma

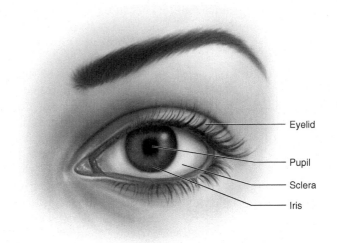

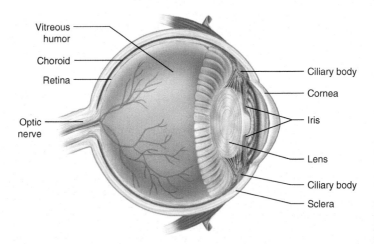

Fig. 8.1. Anatomy of the eye

Pathology

- Table 8.1 presents some quick facts for choroidal melanoma [5, 6]

Rationale for Brachytherapy

- Table 8.2 presents the rationale for using I-125 plaque brachytherapy based on COMS data for medium-sized lesions [2, 7]

Selection Criteria

Selection for Implantation

- Selection for implantation of radioactive plaque in the treatment of ocular tumors is based on tumor size, location, and extent of disease
- Standard plaque size varies from 10 to 22 mm in diameter
- An experienced ocular oncologist's clinical exam combined with ultrasonography and fundus photography enables accurate measurements down to less than 1 mm accuracy
- Important to select the plaque that covers the tumor with a 2–3 mm safety margin extending around the tumor; thus the largest tumor that could be implanted should not exceed 18 mm in the basal diameter
- For example, for a 12 mm (basal diameter) choroidal melanoma, a 16 mm plaque in diameter should be used to adequately treat this tumor
- Prior to implantation, ocular oncologist performs a multitude of tests in the office looking for documented growth, high-risk characteristics of the tumor, or occasionally biopsy-positive confirmation

TABLE 8.1 Quick facts for choroidal melanoma

Quick facts for choroidal melanoma	
Cell of origin	Uveal melanocytes from the neuroectoderm, located in intervening stroma of the choroidal layer
Pathologic subtypes	**Spindle Cell (Grade 1)**: Fusiform shape, less pronounced atypia, resemble migrating neural crest cells
	• Spindle A: long, grooved nuclei; inconspicuous nucleoli, *very low* potential for metastasis, some consider them nevoid cells
	• Spindle B: plump, prominent nucleoli
	• **Best survival**
	Mixed (Grade 2): Both spindle and epithelioid characteristics
	Epithelioid (Grade 3): Ovoid shaped, anaplasia common, larger tumors, prominent nucleoli, resemble primitive neural crest cells
	• **Worst survival**

Macroscopic appearance	Oval, dome-shaped
	Most commonly present as mushroom or collar-button/stud shaped. Collar button shapes tend to be thicker and have poor visual outcomes
Poor prognostic factors	**Location**: Near fovea/macula, extrascleral extension, optic nerve invasion, tumor margin anterior to equator
	Size: Larger tumors (thickness >5 mm), rapidly growing
	Pathology: Epithelioid subtype, necrosis, prominent nucleoli, high Ki67
	Genetics: Chromosome 3 monosomy (high metastatic potential), Chromosome 5 trisomy
	Necrosis 7–10 % of patients have significant necrosis and these tumors do poorly (swift growth)
Patterns of spread	Intraocular: Vitreous seeding (Bruch's membrane rupture, rare). Spread through retina is rare
	Extrascleral extension (15 %)
	Hematogenous Metastases (91–95 % to liver), lung (24–28 %), bone (16 %), and brain (4 %)

Table 8.2 Rationale for brachytherapy

Rationale for using I-125 plaque brachytherapy	COMS data for medium-sized lesions
Equivalent survival to enucleation compared with I-125 plaque at 12 year follow up (FUP)	1. 5 Years overall survival (unadjusted): 81 % vs. 82 % ($p = 0.48$)
	2. 5 Years rate of all-cause mortality: 19 % vs. 18 %
	3. 12 Years rate of all-cause mortality: 41 % and 43 %
	4. Risk of death ratio plaque/enucleation: 0.99
No increase in rate of death from metastasis with plaque versus enucleation at 12 year FUP	1. 5 Years melanoma-specific mortality: 11 % and 10 %
	2. 5 Years estimated risk ratio death plaque/enucleation: 0.91
	3. 10 Years melanoma-specific mortality: 17 % and 18 %
	4. 12 Years melanoma-specific mortality 17 % and 21 %
Low risk of treatment failure (Local failure, LF)	1. 5 Years risk of treatment failure: 10.3 %
	2. Tumor regression rate 89.7 %
High retention rate of globe at 5 years [2]	1. 5 Years globe retention rate ~88 %

When to Implant

- Radioactive plaque implantation for ocular tumors, in general, is performed when documented growth is observed, or
- When a patient has one or more high-risk characteristics in the setting of choroidal melanoma, or in the presence of positive biopsy findings
- High risks features include loss of vision or changes in vision as a sign a tumor may require treatment
- Conditions such as choroidal melanoma or choroidal hemangioma, etc., may be treated with primary brachytherapy, reserving external beam radiation treatment for conditions such as choroidal metastatic disease or ocular lymphoma

Clinical Guidelines to Judge Readiness for Implantation

- Documented growth and/or high-risk features are used to judge readiness for implantation combined with the patient's motivation to proceed (preserve the eye) and a thorough understanding that the purpose of radioactive plaque implantation is to prevent metastatic spread of tumors or to reduce visually debilitating symptoms and visual loss including metamorphopsia (distortion of the visual fields)

Medical Operability, Anesthesia Consent, Guidelines for Anticoagulation

- Radioactive plaque implantation is usually performed under general anesthesia and it is removed under local anesthesia involving retro-bulbar block
- Preoperative guidelines require anesthetic clearance by the patient's primary care physician to undergo general and local anesthesia

- Patients on anticoagulation need to be transitioned to a low molecular weight heparin or instructed to hold anticoagulation for a period of time preprocedure
- In patients with cardiac procedures such as cardiac stents within the last year, this may be difficult as anticoagulation cannot be discontinued temporarily in most patients and patients must assume an increased risk of intraoperative bleeding during the informed consent process

Image Guidance Utilization

Use of Image Guidance Preprocedure

- The ocular oncologist utilizes many ancillary tests in the diagnosis of ocular tumors; however, the most important would be the visual appearance and the experience of the ocular oncologist visualizing the tumor
- Ancillary tests to confirm the diagnosis may include fundus photography, fundus fluorescein angiography, IC-Green angiography, ultrasonography, enhanced depth imaging, OCT (optical coherent tomography), UBM (ultrasound biomicroscopy) for anterior tumors, and occasionally fine-needle aspiration biopsy (FNAB)
- Fortunately, ocular oncology is unique as most diagnoses of tumors can be made without FNAB by an experienced ocular oncologist
- The exact size of the tumor down to a fraction of a millimeter cannot be overstated to aid in the proper selection and sizing of the radioactive plaque implantation

Commonly Used Image Guidance

- The BIO (binocular indirect ophthalmoscopy) is a procedure performed by the ocular oncologist in the office, utilizing a headlight and special optics, examining the patient in the supine position through a dilated eye with a 20 diopter handheld condensing lens
- This procedure allows complete access in visualization of the entire posterior segment of the eye, examining the retina, choroid, optic nerve vessels, macula, extending all the way to the ora serrata (origin of the retina) with techniques such as scleral depression
- This technique, combined with an experienced ocular oncologist, is the single most important modality for correct diagnosis
- Fundus photography (Fig. 8.2a) is also quite useful for documentation and measurement, if the lesions are in the posterior pole rather than the far periphery of the eye. It can also be very helpful monitoring the patient every few months or years to document subtle growth
- The cons of this technique are that it involves a well-trained ocular photographer or certified retinal angiographer
- Fundus auto-fluorescence can be helpful, although not pathognomonic in certain ocular tumors, as it may show intrinsic circulation to highly vascular tumors and aid in defining the tumor borders
- Retinal ICG (Indo-cyanine Green) angiography penetrates deeper into the choroid and can be useful in evaluating the vascularity of tumors or choroidal flow in conditions such as choroidal hemangioma. The cons are the cost of the fundus camera and a well-trained ultrasonographer for proper usage
- B, A-scan ultrasonography is an office-based procedure using ultrasound that is extremely helpful in ocular oncology. It is very useful in calculating the height of the tumor down to a fraction of a millimeter

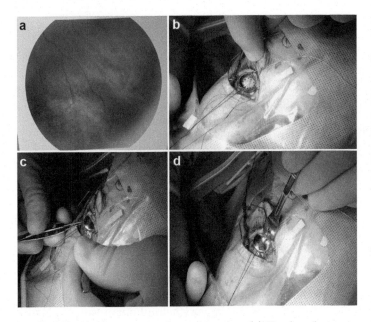

Fɪɢ. 8.2. Brachytherapy eye plaque insertion. (**a**) Fundus photography showing the choroidal melanoma. (**b**) Dummy plaque in place with the tumor outlined on the sclera by the *dots*. (**c**) Insertion of the radioactive gold plated plaque. (**d**) Radioactive plaque firmly sutured in place

as well as the intrinsic makeup of the tumor based on reflectivity curves suggesting a homogeneous or heterogeneous cellular architecture. This technique also helps with diagnosing fluid or shallow exudative retinal detachment which may be associated with ocular tumors as well as extra-scleral extension

Use of Image Guidance During Procedure

- The main use of image guidance during the operative procedure is the binocular indirect ophthalmoscope combined with the 20 diopter lens, visualizing the tumor and providing intraoperative localization

- Although not required, intraoperative ultrasonography has been shown to be helpful to confirm the exact placement and adequate coverage of radioactive plaques intraoperatively
- In addition to intraoperative ultrasonography, future areas of development include intraoperative OCT

Guidelines for Implantation

Preprocedure Advice, Procedural Positioning, Exam Assessment

- Once the proper diagnosis has been made, the procedure is carried out in the operating room. The patient is supine under general anesthesia, with the eye well dilated, and after the timeout and informed consent has been verified, exam again is performed in the operating room to verify correct eye location and extent of tumor

Procedure Tips

- Precise localization of the tumor is the key to allow accurate placement of the radioactive plaque and thus to ensure complete coverage of all borders of the tumor. Failure to do so may result in tumor recurrence
- A widely dilated pupil is paramount for adequate visualization of the posterior segment of the globe
- After the conjunctiva is open at 360° and the rectus muscles are isolated with a 2-0 silk suture allowing rotation of the globe during the visualization done with BIO, a surgical pen is used to mark the borders of the tumor on the sclera utilizing transpupillary illumination
- Prior to placement of the plaque, it is common practice to perform a fine needle aspiration biopsy (transvitreous or transscleral) with a 27-gauge needle attached to

a small syringe. This specimen is commonly used to provide prognostic information such as whether the patient is in a low-, medium-, or high-risk group for metastatic spread

- Recent GEP (gene expression profiling) methodology has been extremely useful in providing postoperative counseling. This information not only changes the frequency of systemic tumor surveillance, monitoring liver and lung in the setting of choroidal melanoma, but also gives highly accurate prognostic information regarding 5-year metastatic-free data
- Some centers also use chromosome 3 and 8 analysis, which can stratify melanomas into low or high risk for future systemic spread
- Rarely, FNAB may be used to confirm the primary diagnosis
- In the case of very posterior plaques, the indirect ophthalmoscope and use of a scleral marker may be required to mark edges of the tumor for proper localization.

Verification of Brachytherapy

- Verification of brachytherapy adequacy is performed by first suturing a "dummy" plaque (hollow plaque of same dimensions as the radioactive plaque) to the sclera with 2.0 silk sutures, utilizing the scleral markers as a guidance (Fig. 8.2b)
- Once this is performed, additional transillumination can be used to confirm precise localization as well as good tumor coverage by the plaque
- Sometimes due to posterior location, all borders cannot be confirmed. In these cases, making sure the anterior and lateral borders have adequate coverage with a properly sized plaque will suffice
- Once verification is completed, the "dummy" plaque is removed and the gold-plated radioactive plaque is

firmly sutured to the globe utilizing the same sutures used for the "dummy" plaque (Fig. 8.2c, d)

- It is important that the radioactive plaque be firmly attached to the globe, making sure extraocular tissue is not in between the sclera and the plaque which will cause tilting of the plaque and alter the radiation dose
- Sometimes extraocular muscles need to be temporarily removed in order to provide adequate plaque placement. Then, at the time of plaque removal, muscles may be placed back into their original position. Failure to place the muscle in its exact position may result in postoperative double vision (see section on "Toxicity")
- In cases of anteriorly placed plaques, conjunctiva or sterilized pericardium may be used to cover the plaque to aid in patient comfort
- For iris melanomas, temporary tarsorrhaphy (suturing the eyelid closed) may be required to aid in patient comfort during the several days the plaque is left in place
- Verification is done by the ocular oncologist and the radiation oncologist
- Laser indirect ophthalmoscope or intraoperative ultrasound can also be used if available

Evaluation of Implantation

- Plaques that are initially well localized can become displaced away from the sclera during the time the plaque is in place (up to 7 days); this displacement will invariably reduce radiation dose to the tumor, thus potentially causing a local recurrence. It is therefore important to firmly secure the plaque placement with at least three sutures. The availability of intraoperative ultrasound for postimplant evaluation may reduce the risk of local failure

212   T. Skrepnik et al.

Treatment Planning

Optimal Brachytherapy Dose

- COMS guidelines recommend prescribing *85 Gy to 5 mm from the inner sclera for tumors <5 mm in apical height and to the tumor apex for tumors ≥5 mm in apical height*
- The ABS 2013 guidelines report typical dose prescriptions of *70–100 Gy to the tumor apex* (Fig. 8.3a–d)

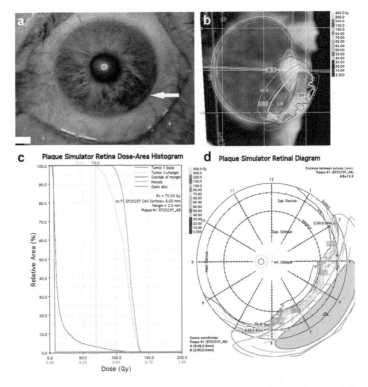

FIG. 8.3. Treatment plan for an iris melanoma eye plaque. (**a**) Melanoma of the iris shown by the *arrow*. (**b**) Isodose lines superimposed on a CT scan of the globe. (**c**) Dose volume histogram corresponding to the implant. (**d**) Isodose lines superimposed on a retinal diagram

- A recent publication from our group has shown that dosing to the tumor apex even for tumors <5 mm in apical height results in similar tumor control probability but with improved toxicity profile (better preservation of vision) [8]
- Dose rates of 0.60 Gy/h–1.05 Gy/h are recommended which results in 3–7 consecutive days of treatment [9]
- Mainly I-125 and Pd-103 (both gamma emitters) plaques are used in North America, but Ru-106 (beta emitter) is also common in Europe
- Isotope selection does affect the dose distribution and delivery time. For example, the use of Pd-103 may deliver a lesser dose to normal structures due to the lower energy photon spectrum [10]

Use of Image Guidance for Target Volume Delineation

- The fundus diagram created from ultrasound and photographic images provides the tumor orientation within the eye, tumor dimensions, and basal diameter of the tumor
- In addition, the location (coordinates) of the sclera, macula, fovea, optic nerve, lens, and opposite eye wall locations should be included
- These coordinates are then entered into the treatment planning system
- Additional imaging including CT and MRI can be performed, but the 2013 ABS consensus guidelines suggest that additional imaging does not provide superior tumor measurements [11]

Optimization of Target Volume

- The tumor apex is used as the prescription point, but adjustments may be made to ensure the prescription isodose line encompasses the maximum dimensions of the tumor

- Plaque size (ranging from 10 to 22 mm) is selected to provide adequate margin to the peripheral dimensions of the tumor (usually 2 mm)
- Doses to normal ocular structures (see section on "Use of Image Guidance for Target Volume Delineation") should be reported

Seed Loading and Optimal Dose Distribution

- The number of radioactive seeds loaded in the plaque is a function of the plaque size, ranging from 5 seeds for a 10 mm plaque to 24 seeds for a 20 mm plaque (Fig. 8.4)
- The seed coordinates for COMS standard eye plaques are predetermined based on the plaque size [12]
- Traditional treatment planning software can be used with seed characterization in water phantoms, but custom plaque software does exist (Fig. 8.4)
- Extra care must be taken when using heterogeneity corrections as the dose distribution can vary up to 20 % compared to traditional dose prescriptions [10]

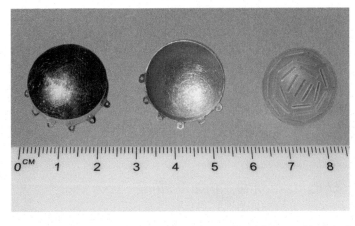

FIG. 8.4. Picture of a 20 mm plaque. Top view of the gold plated plaque (*left*); plaque inverted showing the side in contact with the sclera (*center*); Silastic seed carrier insert (*right*)

Toxicity

- Toxicity associated with I-125 plaque brachytherapy is related to the total dose, dose rate, and dose volume as well as tumor factors such as size and location of the tumor
- Side effects are usually delayed and increase with follow-up time, therefore shorter follow-up biases the reported outcomes
- Side effects can be grouped by anterior vs. posterior segment complications
- Range for each toxicity and general time of onset was summarized by Wen et al. and are listed as follows [13]

Anterior Segment Complications

- Iris neovascularization: 4–23 % at a mean 26.7 months after treatment
- Neovascular glaucoma: 2–45 % from 2 to 58 months after treatment
- Any type of glaucoma: 60 % at 5 years
- Radiation-induced cataract: 68 % vision limiting cataract underwent cataract surgery (COMS). Cumulative dose ≥24 Gy had 5 years cataract incidence of 92 % compared with 65 % for <12Gy

Posterior Segment or Intraocular Complications

- Hemorrhage (vitreous, retinal, choroidal): 2–21 %
- Secondary retinal detachment: rare
- Radiation retinopathy: 10–63 %
- Radiation maculopathy: 13–52 % at 25.6 months after treatment; the risk increases to 63 % when dose to macula >90Gy [14]
- Optic neuropathy: 8–16 %; larger tumors carry greater risk: 39 % at 3 years and 46 % at 5 years; risk is 50 % if tumor <4 mm from disc margin

- Scleral atrophy: 0–33 % in posterior plaques
- Diplopia: 1.7–10 %, mostly occurring in first year after treatment

Decreased Visual Acuity

- Risk depends on initial visual acuity and the dose to macula/fovea, optic disc, and nerve
- COMS incidence of 20/200 or worse acuity at 1- and 3-years 17 % and 43 %, respectively
- COMS loss of ≥6 Snellen lines at 1-, 2-, and 3-years posttreatment: 18 % and 34 %, 49 %. Worse with age >50 years, tumor thickness >5 mm, and proximity to the foveal avascular zone

Enucleation Secondary to Complications (Blind, Painful Eye) or Recurrence

- COMS reported a 12.5 % rate of enucleation for complications related to apical tumor height >5 mm, vitreous opacification and distance to foveola

Damage to Fellow Eye

- The COMS study [15] revealed minimal damage to the fellow eye with a mean change in visual acuity from baseline: 1 letter (0.2 lines) or less. The 5- and 10-year incidence of significant cataract or cataract surgery in fellow eye: 8 % and 15–18 %

References

1. Singh AD, Turell ME, Topham AK. Uveal melanoma: trends in incidence, treatment, and survival. Ophthalmology. 2011;118(9): 1881–5.
2. Jampol LM, et al. The COMS randomized trial of iodine 125 brachytherapy for choroidal melanoma. IV. Local treatment

failure and enucleation in the first 5 years after brachytherapy. COMS report no.19. Ophthalmology. 2002;109(12):2197–206.

3. Finger PT. Radiation therapy for choroidal melanoma. Surv Ophthalmol. 1997;42:215–32.

4. Diagram courtesy of Cancer.gov. http://www.cancer.gov/types/ retinoblastoma/patient/retinoblastoma-treatment-pdq. Accessed 23 Nov 2015.

5. Greven KM, Greven CM. Chapter 29: Orbital, ocular and optic nerve tumors. In: Gunderson LL, Tepper JE, editors. Clinical radiation oncology. Philadelphia: WB Saunders; 2012. p. 529–42.

6. McCartney A. Pathology of ocular melanomas. Br Med Bull. 1995;51(3):678–93.

7. The Collaborative Ocular Melanoma study Group. The COMS randomized trial of iodine 125 brachytherapy for choroidal melanomas: V. Twelve-year mortality rates and prognostic factors: COMS report no.28. Arch Ophthalmol. 2006;124(12):1684–93.

8. Vonk DT, Kim Y, Javid C, Gordon JD, Stea B. Prescribing to tumor apex in episcleral plaque iodine-125 brachytherapy for medium-sized choroidal melanoma: a single-institutional retrospective review. Brachytherapy. 2015;14:726–33.

9. Nag S, Quivey JM, Earle JD, et al. American Brachytherapy Society. The American Brachytherapy Society recommendations for brachytherapy of uveal melanomas. Int J Radiat Oncol Biol Phys. 2003; 56:544–55.

10. Rivard MJ, Chiu-Tsao S-T, Finger PT, et al. Comparison of dose calculation methods for brachytherapy of intraocular tumors. Med Phys. 2011;38:306–16.

11. American Brachytherapy Society level 1 consensus statement regarding the use of plaque brachytherapy for choroidal melanoma. Brachytherapy. 2013;13(1):1–14.

12. Chiu-Tsao S-T, Astrahan MA, Finger PT, et al. Dosimetry of 125I and 103Pd COMS eye plaques for intraocular tumors: report of Task Group 129 by the AAPM and ABS. Med Phys. 2012;39: 6161–84.

13. Wen JC, Oliver SC, McCannel TA. Ocular complications following I-125 brachytherapy for choroidal melanoma. Eye. 2009; 23(6):1254–68.

14. Stack R, Elder M, Abdelaal A, Hidajat R, Clemett R, et al. New Zealand experience of I125 brachytherapy for choroidal melanoma. Clin Experiment Ophthalmol. 2005;33(5):490–4.

15. Collaborative Ocular Melanoma Study Group. Ten-year follow up of fellow eyes of patients enrolled in COMS randomized trials: COMS report no. 22. Ophthalmology. 2004;111(5):966–76.

Chapter 9
Head and Neck Brachytherapy

D. Jeffrey Demanes

Introduction

Rationale for Brachytherapy (BT)

- Higher tumor doses are delivered to more specific targets with brachytherapy than with EBRT
- Brachytherapy, however, requires anesthesia and has some procedural risks
- Outcomes with brachytherapy depend on implant quality and good clinical management
- The reader should consult the ABS [1] and GEC-ESTRO [2], and other listed references [3–6]
- Image guidance may refer to the use of imaging during the implant procedure or its use during treatment planning and dosimetry

D.J. Demanes, MD, FACRO, FACR, FASTRO (✉)
Division of Brachytherapy, Department of Radiation Oncology,
UCLA David Geffen School of Medicine, Los Angeles, CA, USA
e-mail: jeffreydemanes@gmail.com

© Springer International Publishing AG 2017   219
J. Mayadev et al. (eds.), *Handbook of Image-Guided Brachytherapy*, DOI 10.1007/978-3-319-44827-5_9

Goal of Brachytherapy: Definitive, Postoperative, Salvage

- Brachytherapy may be used in any primary or recurrent (H&N) cancer, wherever carriers and radiation sources can be safely inserted
- Treatment must be offered in the context of the patients' overall health, smoking and alcohol history, HPV/P16 status, and psychosocial circumstances
- Brachytherapy optimizes the dosimetry to enhance local tumor control and to maximize preservation of organ function
- The relative risks and benefits of surgery, external radiation with or without chemotherapy, and brachytherapy should always be considered
- Brachytherapy may be an alternative or adjuvant to surgery.
    - As an alternative, it avoids the morbidity associated with tissue removal and reconstruction
    - As adjuvant, it enhances surgery by eradicating persistent disease at the surgical margins
- The decision to use BT in combination with EBRT or by itself depends primarily upon the likelihood of regional spread of disease. When used with EBRT, brachytherapy offers the precision high dose boost needed to control gross disease
- Disease control, functional outcome, and the occurrence complications depend upon nature and extent of disease, dosimetry, comorbidity, and the use of surgery or chemotherapy
- Cosmetic results with brachytherapy are typically good
- Brachytherapy is often used to salvage local tumor recurrences after prior radiation because sufficient dose can still be delivered to a localized target without exceeding normal tissue tolerance

- Head and neck BT is mostly performed as an interstitial (IS) implant with afterloading. Virtually any soft tissue can be implanted with the tube and button afterloading technique
- The implant design, catheter distribution, and dosimetry are always customized to accommodate the individual clinical circumstances
- The complexity and risk of the procedure are related to the lesion size, anatomic location, and the relationship of the implant to bone and vascular structures. In general, the salivary glands can be ignored, but the mandible and blood vessels must be managed as organs at risk

Timing Brachytherapy

- Brachytherapy may be done before or after EBRT
- The advantage of doing BT first is the extent of the lesion is most readily apparent, the surrounding tissue has not been affected by radiation, and the logistics for scheduling procedures in the operating room are easier
- The benefit to doing it after EBRT is induction of regression and control of microscopic disease
- When BT is performed with surgery, catheters can be inserted during operative exposure or they can be placed at a later date for close or positive margins

Brachytherapy Source Loading Methods

- Afterloading BT: Source loading may be done with manual afterloading low dose rate (LDR) or robotic afterloading either as high dose rate (HDR) or pulsed dose rate (PDR). Although there is a rich history of LDR BT, most modern H&N BT is now done with robotic afterloading due to radiation safety considerations and improved ability to provide nursing care [7]

- Permanent seeds [8–10]: Permanent seeds may be used in the H&N region when the lesion volume accommodates the sources or there is a surface onto which a seed embedded mesh can be applied. Permanent seed implants are most commonly used to treat recurrent disease presenting in a definable soft tissue volume and in locations where afterloading may be more difficult to accomplish. The advantage of seeds is their simplicity and efficiency of source delivery
- Intraoperative Brachytherapy [11–13]: The implant can be done with surgery as an open procedure where sources are placed with visual guidance directly on or in the tumor and where normal tissue can be displaced away from the sources. Treatment can be delivered as intraoperative radiation therapy (IORT) with (1) HDR in a shielded operating room or (2) electronically generated low-energy radiation sources (ELS) in an operating room without special shielding

Pertinent Anatomy for Brachytherapy

- Head and neck anatomy is complex, highly functional, and of major cosmetic importance
- As with all invasive procedures BT is constrained by bones, nerves, and vascular anatomy. To safely do BT, the anatomy and relationship of the disease to the carotid arteries must be understood (Fig. 9.1a–e)
- The common carotid bifurcates at about the level of the hyoid bone. The internal carotid then takes a more posterior course, so it is posterior to the vertebrate in the coronal plane at the base of skull. The carotid artery is thus more exposed in the lower neck and more protected in the upper neck
- The vessels are more vulnerable if the patient has had a radical neck dissection

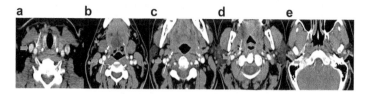

FIG. 9.1. Serial axial angiographic CT images showing normal course of common carotid artery (CCA), internal carotid artery (ICA), external carotid artery (ECA), and internal jugular vein (IJV). (**a**) Level A (Larynx): CCA (*long-white arrow*) just medial to the IJV (*fat blue arrow*). Sometimes a more medial CCA produces an abnormal hypopharynx contour. (**b**) Level B (Hyoid at carotid bifurcation): ICA (*long-white arrow*) ECA (*short white arrow*) Dilated proximal ICA = carotid bulb. ICA typically posterior-lateral to ECA just beyond bifurcation (sometimes it is initially more medial). (**c**) Level C (Tongue): ICA (*long-white arrow*) medial to IJV. ECA (*short-white arrow*) is anterior and medial to ICA. (**d**) Level D (Uvula at Ramus Mandible): ICA (*white arrow*) moved slightly more medial (which is common in older patients and occasionally there is even a tortuous redundant loop). (**e**) Level E (Base skull): ICA entering the carotid canal (*white arrow*) posterior to anterior line of the vertebral body

- The mandible affects access to soft tissues, and it must be protected from excessive radiation doses. The courses of the cranial nerves are less apparent, but the injury to hypoglossal nerve or the sympathetic chain from BT can become clinically apparent
- The relationship of the lesion to airway and alimentary tract adds another level of complexity to BT procedures

Pathology

- Squamous cell carcinoma is the typical histology of cancers treated with BT
- Lesions of the lip and oral cavity are mostly well differentiated and those of the pharynx are moderate or poorly differentiated

- Poorly differentiated lesions have a greater chance of lymphatic spread and respond better to chemoradiation therapy
- The connection of human papilloma virus (HPV) to squamous cell carcinoma of the oropharynx has altered our concept of the squamous cancer of the oropharynx, and it is changing the way these H&N cancers are managed [14–16]
- It appears that lower doses of radiation (dose de-escalation) are sufficient for HPV positive cases. There may be implications for the use of BT in oropharynx cancer
- Although surgery is the mainstay of treatment, other histology such as adenocarcinoma, melanoma, and sarcoma are sometimes treated with BT [17–20].

Rationale for Image Guidance in Brachytherapy

- Image guidance may describe guidance of needle or catheter placement or simulation and dosimetry
- Some H&N lesions, such as lip and small oral cavity cancers, are directly visible during the implant procedure. Even so, it is helpful to have 3D images of the final catheter positions prior to leaving the operating suite
- The challenge to the application of image guidance in H&N BT is the absence of 3D imaging tools in the operating room where most H&N implant procedures are performed
- This situation may be changing as portable 3D scan imaging devices become available
- For larger lesions of the tongue and less accessible sites such as oropharynx or deep in the neck, it is helpful to image the implant at the time of the procedure
- Discovery of poor catheter distributions during postoperative CT simulation is disappointing and detrimental. It is far better to know and adjust the implant catheter in the operating room before discontinuation of anesthesia

Selection Criteria for Brachytherapy (Table 9.1)

■ Brachytherapy is indicated for the delivery of a localized dose of radiation to improve local disease control and to decrease side effects

■ Brachytherapy alone may be used for lip, oral, and other anterior cancers of the H&N with limited likelihood of lymphatic spread

■ It is used with EBRT for larger oral lesions and for most lesions of the pharynx where lymphatic spread is more common

Brachytherapy Alone (Monotherapy)

Early Cancers of Lip, Buccal Mucosa, Nasal Vestibule, and Oral Cavity [5, 21–31]

■ Monotherapy BT is performed as a single interstitial implant followed by source loading over several days

■ It is the equivalent of a wide local excision without lymph node dissection, so its success is predicated upon the disease being localized

■ The indications are small lesion size, accessible location, and favorable histology. Stage T1 or small T2, anterior (lip, nasal vestibule, and oral cavity) and well-differentiated lesions without perineural invasion or lymphovascular involvement are good candidates for brachytherapy alone. Some studies suggest lymph nodes should be treated in T2 cancers [32]

■ The implant should encompass the primary disease with a 1–1.5 cm margin in all dimensions

■ Image guidance during catheter placement may be omitted for readily accessible lesions, but 3D imaging dosimetry should be applied whenever possible (Fig. 9.2a, b)

■ Postoperative monotherapy can also be used in cases with close or positive margins [30]. Wound healing

TABLE 9.1 Indications for brachytherapy and the GEC-ESTRO recommendations (references include LDR and HDR*)

Primary site	BT alone	BT + EBRT	Dose (EQD2 α/β 10)	Local control	STN or BI*
Lip [21–28]	<5 cm	<5 cm	BT 60–70 EBRT + BT 75	90% T1–2 BT alone	2–10% STN
Buccal [30, 111]	T1–2N0	T3	BT 65–70 EBRT 45–50 + BT 25–30	85% BT alone	<10% STN
Oral tongue [24–26, 29, 33, 35, 82, 83, 114, 116–120, 122–123]	T1–2N0	T3–4	BT 65–70 EBRT 45–50 + BT 25–30 (postop EBRT 50–60 + BT 10–25)	90% T1–2 BT alone	10–20% STN 5–10% BI
Floor of mouth [21, 23, 124]	T1–2N0 <3 cm	T2>3 cm T3–4N0	BT only 65 EBRT 45–50 + BT 15–25 (Postop EBRT 50–60 + BT 10–25)	90% T1–2 BT alone	10–30% STN 5–10% BI
Oropharynx [36–40, 75–77, 82, 126–129]	T1N0 Selected	T1–4N+ <5 cm	EBRT 45–50 Tonsil + BT 25–30 BOT + BT 30–35	T1–2 80–90% T3–4 65–80%	20–25% STN <5% BI

Nasopharynx [41–45, 88, 130]	NA	T1–2	EBRT T1 60, T2 70 +HDR 3Gy×6 fx (EQD2 16.3)	90% EBRT+BT	NA
Nasal and paranasal [91, 93, 94, 127, 131–135]	T1	T2–4	EBRT 40–50+BT (dose?)	Highly variable circumstances	NA
	Small T2?		BT alone for positive margins		
Salvage [9, 34, 46–64]	Common	Variable	BT alone 50–60	50–70% BT alone	10–30%

EBRT external beam radiation therapy, *BT* brachytherapy, *STN* soft tissue necrosis, *BI* bone injury

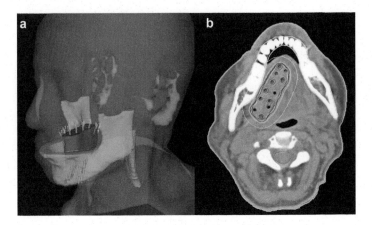

FIG. 9.2. Virtual 3D image of oral tongue implant (**a**) and 3D-CT treatment planning showing axial isodose distribution (**b**)

should be sufficiently complete to avoid tissue breakdown, especially where there are grafts or free-flaps. Under usual circumstances 4–6 weeks after surgery is a reasonable interval to wait to do BT

Brachytherapy with External Beam

Locally Advanced Oral Cavity Not Suitable for BT Alone [24, 33–35]

- These lesions are larger, more deeply invasive, and often have an endophytic component; the risk of regional lymph node spread or perineural invasion is substantial
- BT with EBRT allows localized dose escalation for enhanced tumor control and less dose to the mandible, salivary glands, and taste buds
- Surgical resection of the lesion followed by BT and EBRT is another common strategy for locally advanced disease, but it is associated with more functional impairment of the tongue than single modality therapy of smaller lesions [30, 34]

- The indications for postoperative BT are lympho-vascular invasion, perineural invasion, and positive or close surgical margins

Oropharynx Cancer (OPC): Base Tongue, Tonsil, Soft Palate, and Pharynx [36–40]

- OPC usually presents as adenopathy or as a locally advanced primary
- The main role of BT in oropharynx is as a boost to EBRT
- The use of BT with EBRT for tonsil and base of tongue cancer results in excellent functional outcomes and good preservation of quality of life [37]
- Combined EBRT and BT for soft palate has the advantage of preserving the soft palate, and it usually obviates the need for a prosthetic device
- The use of BT in OPC cancer minimizes damage of the pharyngeal constrictors
- Tracheostomy is often, but not always, performed to protect the airway during BT in the OPC

Nasopharynx (NPC)

- Brachytherapy boost of early (T1 or T2) disease with little or no bone erosion and no intracranial extension is performed by outpatient placement of an intraluminal applicator under local anesthesia [41–43]
- In more advanced disease, the use of BT is less likely to impact the outcome because base of skull or intracranial extension precludes disease encompassing anatomic access [44, 45]

Hypopharynx, Larynx, and Trachea

- Lesions of the hypopharynx and larynx are technically challenging for BT due to the less accessible location, laryngeal cartilage, and vascular anatomy

- For the most part these cancers are treated with either surgery or EBRT or a combination of the two
- Brachytherapy is used in selected cases as salvage or for palliation
- With image guidance these lesions may become more amenable to BT
- Outpatient intraluminal BT is another approach applicable to trachea cancer and stomal recurrences (usually palliative circumstances)

Salvage of Previously Irradiated Patients

- Local recurrence and new primaries in previously irradiated patients are common in H&N cancer
- Normal tissue tolerance places limits on additional radiation therapy, so BT has been used when the disease is amenable and the patient's general condition allows a procedure to be performed. The surgical option should always be considered and the condition of the previously irradiated tissues assessed before proceeding with salvage radiation therapy
- It can be applied to recurrent disease at the primary site, lymph nodes, or other soft tissue locations
- Doses to the normal tissues, especially the spinal cord, need to be reviewed so that treatment can be delivered with due consideration for normal tissue tolerance
- Salvage interstitial implants can be complicated and challenging [9, 34, 46–65]

When to Implant (Post EBRT, During EBRT)

- Interstitial BT may be performed before or after EBRT, whereas intraluminal applications can be done at any point in relation to EBRT
- Bulky, friable, or exophytic lesions may be reduced in size and made more amenable to BT by pretreatment with EBRT

- Lesions with extensive nodal involvement or a propensity for microscopic nodal spread such as lesions of the oropharynx are also probably best treated with EBRT before BT
- On the other hand, lesions of the lip and oral cavity treated with combined therapy may be implanted before EBRT when the lesion is well defined and better targeted. Additionally adjacent tissues, not having been previously irradiated, are in better condition
- BT is not typically given as preoperative therapy, but there may be some indications
- Intraoperative placement of BT catheters is another useful strategy as described before

Clinical Guidelines to Judge Readiness for Implantation

- Chemotherapy should be discontinued before BT to avoid metabolic perturbations and blood count depression that will complicate the procedure
- Patients treated with EBRT without chemotherapy prior to BT will need about 2 weeks for recovery of acute radiation effects
- Patients who have both radiation and chemotherapy will need about 3 weeks

Perioperative Considerations: Medical Clearance, Anesthesia Evaluation, Consent, Preoperative Testing

- Head and neck BT is technically challenging because it involves the airway, affects access to nutrition, and it can damage vital neurovascular structures
- Prerequisite are history and physical examination, medication review, and evaluation of co-morbid conditions such as cardiovascular disease, chronic lung disease, hypertension, and diabetes that directly affect the risks and safety of the procedure

- Preoperative blood counts and basic chemistry panels are the minimum standard; guidelines for preoperative CXR and EKG should follow institutional anesthesia policies
- Medical clearances for the procedure should be obtained and the risks of anesthesia evaluated with special attention to securing and managing the airway
- Consent should always include possible tracheostomy in the event of unexpected airway impairment
- The initial nature and extent of the lesion and its status at the time of BT should be reevaluated before the procedure
- Also vascular anatomy should be reviewed and considered as part of planning the procedure
- Prior radiation or surgery may affect the anatomy and vulnerability of the major vessels
- *Pretreatment* dental evaluation and management should include preparation of fluoride trays, treatment of gingival disease, and performance of necessary tooth repairs and extractions
- Custom prosthetic devices to displace or shield normal tissue can be fabricated to improve dosimetry and protect the mandible [5, 66–69]
- Unless there are strong indications, extractions *after* radiation therapy are to be avoided
- Standardized preoperative and postoperative order templates are recommended for quality assurance
- Intraoperative antibiotics are recommended. The author prefers to continue antibiotics the entire duration that the implant is in the patient
- Postoperative orders must address:
  - Activity
  - Pain control—(usually PCA with hydromorphone)
  - Airway management and oral care (suctioning, cleaning, rinses, etc.)
  - Feeding (NG, PEG, NPO, etc.)—wait 24 h postop to start feeding
  - Antibiotics

- Preventative measures: fall precautions, decubitus ulcers, deep vein thrombosis
- IV fluids and I&O monitoring
- Management of underlying medical conditions (diabetes, hypertension, etc.)
- Steroids and antacids to prevent stress ulcer or reflux
- Applicator, oral, and tracheostomy care should be meticulous
- Emergency tracheostomy tray in room at all times

Image Guidance Utilization

Use of Image Guidance Preprocedure

- Images of the H&N typically include CT or MRI or PET-CT or all three
- These images define the extent of the primary lesion and the presence of regional perineural or lymphatic spread. Staging studies directly affect the treatment strategy and help define the radiation therapy targets

Brachytherapy Clinical Target Volume (CTV)

- To achieve a successful outcome with BT alone, the implant must encompass the gross tumor and any adjacent microscopic subclinical disease
- When combining BT with EBRT the implant may be less concerned with the microscopic margins
- GEC-ESTRO [70] definitions of gross tumor volumes (GTV) and clinical tumor volumes (CTV):
  - iGTV = initial gross tumor volume (pretreatment clinical and imaging staging)
  - Brachytherapy volumes (at time of BT after initial EBRT—restaging)
    - rGTV = residual GTV

- HR-CTV = high-risk CTV includes some margin around the rGTV
- IR-CTV = intermediate risk CTV = iGTV
- LR-CTV = low-risk CTV = regions at risk for initially harboring microscopic disease

- H&N BT is usually done in the operating room without 3D image guidance because such imaging is typically not available
- As a result, the author prefers to implant a larger volume approximating the original disease (iGTV), i.e., the IR-CTV or at least generously encompass residual disease (rGTV) with a margin, i.e., the HR-CTV. It is better to insert more catheters and to be able to later decide what is the optimal treatment volume during 3D image-based treatment planning

Implant Quality and the Need to Fully Encompass the Lesion

- For most H&N BT, the goal is to create a homogenous dose distribution with a margin around the periphery of the lesion
- It is best achieved when the target volume is fully encompassed by catheters
- Failure to implant the entire lesion results in markedly higher doses within the target volume (i.e., poor dose homogeneity) and higher doses to adjacent normal tissues
- Poorly spaced peripheral catheters can also lead to scalloping of the dose margin, which may result in inadequate target coverage
- Uniform peripheral catheter spacing is most important for smaller implants. Catheter spacing for larger implants is less important because of the smoothing effect on dosimetry of the additional source positions. Intercatheter spacing may also be increased from 1 cm to 1.5 cm for the same reason. Correct catheter spacing in H&N cancer reduces complication rates [71–73]

- When inserting catheters, there is a tendency (especially in the oral tongue) to have the planes converge at depth, even though they appear to be properly spaced at the entrance and exit sites
- It is therefore important to place the medial plane needles sufficiently medial (separated from the lateral plane) in the tissue to achieve proper spacing between the planes along their entire length
- Placement of additional (third) medial row of catheters is preferable to having an implant of insufficient thickness or volume
- Dose uniformity can be achieved by HDR dwell time modulation in cases where there are too many catheters too close together, but it cannot compensate as well for too few or widely spaced catheters
- Additional needle and catheter insertions are much less harmful to the patient in the long run than inadequate dosimetry (poor target coverage or excessive hot spots)

The Four Types and Utility of Image Guidance during Procedure

Fluoroscopy

- Limited role for H&N BT guidance because it is a 2D modality

Ultrasound

- Useful around the major blood vessels in the neck
- Impediments are the presence of the mandible and the difficulty in placing a probe in the proper orientation (right angle) to the catheter trajectory
- Ultrasound is most useful during implantation of adenopathy of the lower neck where the major vessels can be seen and avoided (Fig. 9.3)

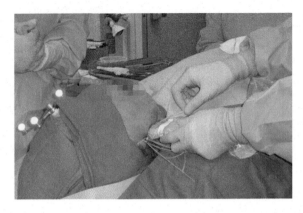

FIG. 9.3 Ultrasound guidance of a neck and pharynx implant (also with CT-surface anatomy fusion image guidance—note reflectors affixed to forehead)

CT Scan

■ Potentially valuable tool for guiding and checking catheter placement during the implant. CT is not yet readily available in operating rooms where most H&N BT procedures are performed, and it does not allow actual real-time guidance

■ The lack of its availability in the OR is a matter of resource allocation and technology development. A new generation of portable CT scans is now available (Fig. 9.4)

MRI Scan

■ Less available than CT scan for intraoperative guidance but it provides the best information soft tissue anatomy. MRI is now being used for targeted biopsies and ablations, but for the most part they are not available to BT specialists

■ The ability to do real-time imaging for catheter placement is an advantage of MRI

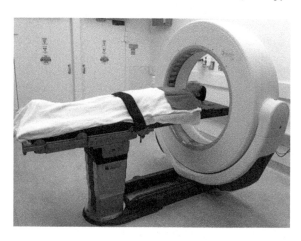

FIG. 9.4 Example of a portable CT that can be used in the operating room for image guidance and simulation radiography during head and neck brachytherapy

■ A lack of clarity and distortion of brachytherapy needles is a disadvantage

Guidelines for Implantation for Complex Interstitial Brachytherapy [1, 2]

Preprocedure Advice

Tracheostomy and Airway Management

■ Interstitial BT catheters can impair access to the airway
■ There must be a plan on how to secure the airway at the beginning of the procedure (direct, fiberoptic, transoral, or transnasal intubation)
■ The patient should not be paralyzed until there is certainty that the airway can be secured
■ Standard direct intubation or video assisted transoral intubation are performed for easier airways. Oral intubation is done when it is followed by tracheostomy

- However, oral intubation without tracheostomy impedes the BT procedure, so nasal intubation using a right angle endotracheal (RAE) tube is preferred if tracheostomy is not going to be performed
- If intubation is not feasible, an "awake" tracheostomy can be done under local anesthesia with the patient sedated
- The decision to do a tracheostomy to protect the airway during BT depends upon the risk of subsequent airway obstruction from the applicator, secretions, edema, or postoperative bleeding. A prophylactic tracheostomy is recommended for posterior (pharynx) implants, large or friable lesions, extensive implants or any circumstance that might make urgent intubation difficult (trismus, dental status, distorted airway, or the affect on tissue of prior therapy)
- A cuffed fenestrated (size 6 or 8) tracheostomy tube is recommended (facilitates implant removal and decannulation)
- In patients with prior tracheostomy or a tracheal stoma, a cuffed "Armor" tube can be used

Positioning and Patient Setup

- Patient position is supine, arms tucked, with a role behind the shoulders to elevate the head into the sniffing position
- If patient has tracheostomy, turn OR table 180° to bring the airway tubing out of operative field

Procedure Tips

Needles and Catheters

- Open-ended 17-gauge, 15 cm long, 30° beveled needles are recommended for implantation
- Once inserted into the skin, the needles can be carefully advanced (not stabbed) through the tissue, so they can be moved past rather than through the vessels

- Sharper needles are more likely to enter vessels and they are more dangerous for the physician
- It is safest to insert needles and replace them with catheters one needle at a time
- Once the needle is in position and the bevel tip is visible, the leader of the catheter can be "directly" inserted until it comes out through the skin
- The needle is removed and the catheter pulled, so the button (with a size 1 silk tie attached to the side hole) is snug on the mucosal surface. Color-coded fixing buttons are threaded over the catheters for external fixation
- Silk ties (to facilitate removal) are attached to the internal button exit the mouth; they are gathered and covered with a ¼ in. Penrose drain and attached externally, so they cannot be swallowed
- Edema that may occur during the implant can affect the process of catheter insertion and impact both dosimetry and clinical management

Leader-In-Wire

- When the bevel end of the trocar is not visible, the leader-in-wire technique can be used to load the catheter [74]. It involves inserting a 27-gauge wire into the external portion end of the needle until it exits internally from the bevel. After directing the wire out the oral cavity, a catheter leader can be threaded to replace the needle. Please see the reference for a detailed description

Palatal Arch (Double Leader)

- Implantation of midline structures requires a pair of implant needles inserted symmetrically on either side of the neck or face whose beveled ends meet near the midline. A catheter with leaders on both ends (double leader catheters) can be inserted to create an arch. Please see references [48, 75–77]

Bone, Tissue Displacement, and Mandible Shielding

- The mandible is an obstacle to catheter placement, and it is at risk for radiation injury
- Catheter kinking (prevents source insertion) must be avoided by limiting catheter curvature. *Internal end-to-end button fixation* is one such solution [78, 79]
- The mandible should be protected during oral cavity implants with some form of tissue displacement or shielding

Catheter Entry Site Design, Spacing, and Stabilization

- Needle entry sites design in H&N can be challenging because of variability of the target, bony anatomy, and the need to avoid vascular structures
- Tentative catheter entry sites should be marked on the skin
- A method has been developed using *round* perforated 10 French Jackson–Pratt drains to help space (1–1.5 cm) and stabilize BT catheters [80]

Implant Removal

- Catheter removal is relatively painless, but preparation must be made to manage patient's anxiety, secretions, and especially hemorrhage. *Always have an assistant available!*
- Anterior lesions can be done at the bedside, but deeper lesions are best removed under anesthesia in the operating room with paralysis
- The most accessible (anterior) and least likely to bleed catheters are removed first and deeper catheters last. Catheters should be removed one at a time
- Tugging on silk ties helps identify internal to external connections and is used to pull the catheter out through the mouth

- The skin is depressed slightly so the catheter can be cut below the relaxed level to avoid pulling the contaminated end of the catheter through the tissue
- Bleeding is best controlled by tapenade with a fingertip placed precisely on the bleeding site rather than by packing
- Direct laryngoscopy after removal confirms hemostasis and is used to assess the tissue condition and airway status
- Antibiotic ointment is applied to catheter exit sites and the freshly cleaned tracheostomy
- The nasogastric feeding tube can be removed immediately or later, depending upon circumstances

Individual Site Tips and Suggestions

Lip and Buccal Mucosa

- Implantation (catheter placement) can be done without image guidance
- Do not under dose the surface (vermillion lip, or mucosa)
- Custom surface applications or interstitial device or a combination can be used [81]
- Posterior buccal lesions are encompassed with either posterior looping or crossing catheters
- Implant displacement from gingiva and bone with generic or custom prosthetic devices reduces mandible dose [5, 66–69]

Oral Tongue

- The plastic tube with button and the hairpin guide gutter techniques are well described [24, 74, 82–85]
- The implant should begin with the lateral plane starting with the most anterior position, especially if the lesion is near the tip
- A finger in the floor of mouth is used to guide the needle along the undersurface of the tongue, so it exits

at the junction with the dorsum (where the mucosa changes from smooth to rough)

- In order not to stick the guiding finger, needle advancement and palpation are not done simultaneously
- Internal catheter spacing is approximately 1 cm or button to button
- Entry spacing will vary according to the anatomical access
- It is best to have some space (0.5 cm) between the catheters and the mandible
- In order to avoid catheter convergence deep in the tongue, the second plane of catheters should enter the skin and be directed more medially than might be thought, before heading superiorly out the dorsum

Floor of Mouth (FOM)

- FOM is challenging because of the thinness of the mucosa and closeness to the mandible
- Lesions involving the gingiva should be managed surgically, but when surgery is not an option, BT catheters can be placed on the lesion ≈ 5 mm from the gingival surface. Sloping anatomy means the needles must not enter the skin too close to the edge of the mandible or they will exit the mucosa too close to the attachment of the tongue
- Gingival extension can be encompassed by wrapping catheters (kinking can be a problem) or by using stacked internal buttons, so the source projects well above the floor of mouth mucosa [78, 86]

Base Tongue

- BT poses a greater airway risk for OP than OC and thus prophylactic tracheostomy is advisable
- BOT implant design must account for anatomy by spacing catheters 1.5–2 cm apart on the skin in the transverse plane and allowing them to converge to 1 cm spacing at the mucosa

- The deepest catheters are inserted first because reaching these locations with the palpating finger become increasingly difficult as catheters are added. See section in this chapter on Wire in Leader Technique [74]

Tonsil

- The ramus of the mandible impedes access to the tonsil. This barrier can be circumvented by the use of looping or a dual catheter technique as mentioned previously
- The anterior loop is limited superiorly by the maxilla and zygoma and inferiorly by the body of the mandible
- Extension to the BOT or lateral pharyngeal wall can be implanted with the single leader catheters
- The risk of bleeding is greater for tonsil than BOT because of proximity to major blood vessels

Hard and Soft Palate (HP and SP)

- The SP is implanted with 3–4 double leader palatal arch catheters with the first entry 1 cm below and slightly posterior to the angle of the mandible [75–77]
- The examining finger must be inserted into the nasopharynx behind the soft palate to appreciate the correct trajectory through the lateral pharyngeal fold (posterior pillar) then up and along the free border of the SP
- It exits near the midline to meet its counterpart before loading the double leader catheter
- The second catheter runs about 1 cm anterior through the anterior tonsillar pillar into the SP
- If there is room, a third catheter can be inserted behind the mandible
- The most anterior catheter is inserted in front of the angle of the mandible at the junction of the ramus and the body where it passes posterior to the maxillary tubercle at the HP–SP junction

- HP lesions are usual surgical, but they can be implanted with a modified palatal arch technique by threading the internal portion of the catheters through Jackson–Pratt drains, which can be sutured to the soft palate. Alternatively, a removable prosthodontics applicator can be used for daily outpatient treatment delivery [87]

Nasopharynx (NP) and Posterior Pharynx Wall (PPW)

- Early NPC may be managed with IC-BT boost; more extensive disease (primary or recurrent) often requires complex IS-BT. Deep invasion into the skull base or through the foramen is beyond the dosimetry range of curative transcutaneous BT
- *Lateral transcutaneous approach*: 15 cm implant needles are either inserted on either side of the face to meet in the midline (arch technique), or alternatively, a single 20 cm needle can be passed entirely across the pharynx to exit the contralateral face (like the pencil in Grant's Atlas of Anatomy) [88]. The first catheter skin entry site is below the zygoma through the mandibular notch traverses the superior naso-pharynx above the torus tuberous. (The wire-in-leader technique for paired arch needles is technically challenging at this level of the NP). A second needle is inserted just behind the head of the mandible 1 cm posterior and inferior to the first needle. It crosses at the junction of the roof and posterior wall. Forward thrust of the jaw facilitates needle insertion. More inferiorly the large vessels may be within the needle trajectory. Thicker tissue inferiorly may require supplemental unilateral tube and button catheters
- The *endoscopic approach* consists of direct visualization of the lesion with a rigid scope and the guided placement of specially formatted curved catheters based upon CT or MRI image guidance [89, 90]

Nasal Vestibule

- Lesions of the nasal vestibule (columella, nasal alae, and distal nasal cavity) may be implanted with free-hand tubes and buttons or with a template (or Jackson–Pratt drain technique) using closed ended catheters with obturators [31, 91, 92]
- The principles of catheter spacing are the same as for other sites, but the presence of cartilage and bone affect the implant execution of this region

Paranasal Sinuses

- Surgery is the treatment of choice in most cases
- BT may be intraoperative or postoperative
- Intraoperative treatment can be given in a shielded operating room or with an electronically generated device with low shielding requirements [93]
- Alternatively afterloading catheters can be inserted at the time of the procedure and fractionated treatment delivered later as usual [94]

Peristomal Recurrence

- Recurrent cancer involving a tracheal stoma can be treated with intraluminal or IS BT catheters [95, 96]
- The airway must be protected

Cervical Adenopathy [36, 38, 46, 47, 50–52, 56–59, 61–64, 97]

- Implantation may be intraoperative with immediate or delayed source delivery or transcutaneous with treatment delivered over a period of time after the insertion procedure
- A variety of techniques have been employed including tube and button and permanent seeds

Lower and Mid Neck

- Lower neck adenopathy can be implanted with tangential (to the vertical axis of the spine) skin-to-skin catheter placement (Fig. 9.5a, b)

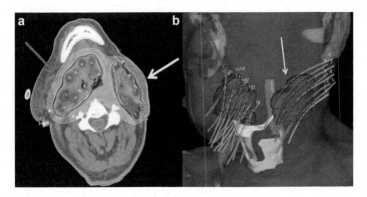

Fig. 9.5 (**a**, **b**) Extensive tongue cancer with implantation of primary and contralateral mid cervical adenopathy

- In the low neck, the great vessels are anteriorly situated, and they may traverse the intended implant target volume
- In the nonoperated neck, it is possible to place multiple planes catheters sometimes both deep and superficial to the vessels to encompass adenopathy
- Intraoperative ultrasound and CT image guidance and proper needle insertion technique are measures to avoid penetrating the vessels
- Prior neck dissection, ulcerated lesions, and prior irradiation significantly increase the risk of vascular injury

Upper Neck

- Upper cervical adenopathy is not amenable to implantation by a tangential approach. The lower border of the mandible generally demarcates where the tangential technique is no longer applicable
- The upper neck is best implanted with a "transpharyngeal" approach (Case Study 9.1). A prophylactic tracheostomy is advisable. The carotid artery curves posterior in the upper neck: at the base of skull, it is posterior to the vertebral body and behind the plane of implantation
- CT image guidance may be helpful, but the mandible usually interferes with ultrasound guidance

- Needles are inserted perpendicular to the skin and directed into pharynx (mucosal surface)
- Two or more planes of single leader tube and button catheters with silk ties are either loaded directly or with the wire-in-leader technique. Upper neck implants should be removed in the operating room

Verification of Brachytherapy with Visual and Imaging

- Visual verification in H&N BT is an intrinsic part of the implant process
- Image verification of catheter positions generally happens after the patient leaves the operating room when modifications of the implant can no longer be made
- As noted earlier, inserting extra catheters or planes of catheters offers some measure of protection for avoiding implanting an insufficient target volume
- The preferred methodology would be to verify with a 3D image (CT or MRI) while the patient is still under anesthesia and the situation is amenable to making improvements
- Such equipment will hopefully soon become available for image guidance during H&N BT and for facilitating simulation radiography and dosimetry prerequisites to starting therapy

Evaluation of Implantation

- Head and neck implants are evaluated with 3D CT or MRI simulation
- The implanted volume can be viewed in relationship to the original extent of disease (iGTV) by fusion technology
- Changes in real time can be done using ultrasound or fluoroscopy but these modalities provide only limited data about tumor coverage, catheter relationships, and proximity of the implant to organs at risk

Distribution of Implant

- The physician draws the CTV, with or without fusion, using the available clinical and radiographic information
- The catheter distribution and coverage of the CTV will determine the quality of the dosimetry. CTVs that are entirely encompassed by the catheter array will have good dosimetry when using HDR technology, even if catheter spacing is somewhat uneven so long as there are no large areas vacant of catheters
- Precise documentation of the relationship of the implant to normal structures such as the mandible, eyes, and the spinal cord will be important for applying proper dose constraints to these structures
- When using HDR fraction size as well as total dose needs to be taken into consideration when calculating normal tissue tolerance

Ultrasound and CT Guidance

- See Figs. 9.3 and 9.4

Treatment Planning Considerations

- Treatment planning in H&N is complicated because variable clinical circumstances; primary versus recurrent disease, variable histology, diverse lesion size and location, and intricate relationships to normal structures

Head and Neck Brachytherapy Doses (Table 9.2)

- The practitioner must choose the best treatment schedule based upon the site, size, location, and character of the lesion and the relationship to nor-

TABLE 9.2 Dose and fractionation by treatment site

Site	Stage	EBRT EQD2	LDR Gy	HDR Dose×Fx	HDR Gy	BT α/β 10≈EQD2	EBRT+BT EQD2	Comments
Lip	T1N0		60–65	4 Gy×12	48	56 Gy		9 fractions<5 days
				(5 Gy×9)	(45)			12 fractions>5 days
	T2N0		65–70	4.25 Gy×12	51	60 Gy		
				(5.25×9)	(47.25)			
	T3-4 or N+	50 Gy	25–30	4 Gy×6	24	28 Gy	75–80 Gy	
Buccal	T1N0		65–70	4.25 Gy×12	51	60 Gy		Poorer prognosis than lip
				(5.25×9)	(47.25)			
	T2N0		65–75	4.5 Gy×12 65	54	65 Gy		Higher doses
				(5.5 Gy×9)	(49.5)			
	T3-4 or N+	50 Gy	25–30	4 Gy×6	24	28 Gy	75–80 Gy	

(continued)

TABLE 9.2 (continued)

Site	Stage	EBRT EQD2	LDR Gy	HDR Dose×Fx	HDR Gy	BT α/β 10≈EQD2	EBRT+BT EQD2	Comments
FOM	T1N0		60–65	4 Gy×12	48	56 Gy		Higher morbidity than OT
				(5 Gy×9)	(45)			Surgery if close to mandible
	T2N0		65–70	4.25 Gy×12	51	60 Gy	65–70 Gy	
				(5.25×9)	(47.25)			
	T3-4 or N+	50 Gy	20–25	4 Gy×5	20	23 Gy	70–75 Gy	
OT	T1N0		65–70	4.25 Gy×12	51	60 Gy		Higher doses than FOM
				(5.25×9)	(47.25)			
	T2N0		65–70	4.5 Gy×12	54	65 Gy		
				(5.5 Gy×9)	(49.5)			
	T3-4 or N+	50 Gy	25–30	4 Gy×6	24	28 Gy	75–85 Gy	

PostOp	LN (−)		50–60	4.5 Gy × 9	40.5	49 Gy		Evaluate primary margins, LNs, and surgery findings
				(5.25 Gy × 7)	36.75	47 Gy		
Lip/OC	LN (+)	50–55 Gy	15–25	4 Gy × 4	16	19 Gy	60–75 Gy	
				(3.75 Gy × 5)	18.75	21 Gy		
OP	Tonsil & SP	50–55 Gy	20–25	4 Gy × 4	16	19 Gy	75–80 Gy	Lower doses for HPV positive
				(3.75 Gy × 5)	18.75	21 Gy		
	Base tongue	50–55 Gy	25–30	4 Gy × 5	20	23 Gy	75–85 Gy	
				3.75 Gy × 6	22.5	26 Gy		
*NP	T1	60 Gy	n/a	3 Gy × 6	18	20 Gy	80 Gy	With chemotherapy
	T2	70 Gy	n/a	4 Gy × 3	12	14 Gy	84 Gy	
Nasal	T1-2N0		60–65	4 Gy × 12	48	56 Gy		Limited data
				(5 Gy × 9)	(45)			
	T3 or N+	50 Gy	15–20				65–80 Gy	Risk cartilage injury

(continued)

TABLE 9.2 (continued)

Site	Stage	EBRT EQD2	LDR Gy	HDR Dose × Fx	HDR Gy	BT α/β 10≈EQD2	EBRT+BT EQD2	Comments
Sinus	T1-2N0 close/+ margins		50-60	4.5 Gy×9	40.5	49 Gy		Limited data
				(5.25 Gy×7)	36.75	47 Gy		
	T3-4 or N+	50–60 Gy						
Salvage	rTXN0		50-60	4 Gy×12	56	56 Gy		Extremely variable circumstances
				4.75 Gy×9	53	49 Gy		
				(5.75 Gy×7)	53	47 Gy		
	rTXN+	50 Gy	20-25	4 Gy×5	20	23 Gy	70-80 Gy	

*Nasopharynx = intracavitary

Disclaimer—None of the protocols presented in this chapter are intended as recommendations for specific patients. They are rough guides based upon the available literature and the author's experience. Clinicians must use their own experience and judgment

mal structures such as the mandible, spinal cord, eye, etc

■ Dose selection may be affected by the size of the GTV and CTV

■ The patient's general condition, comorbidity status, and dental health factor into treatment planning

Monotherapy

■ LDR doses recommended in the literature are in the range of 60–70 Gy

■ HDR dose are EQD2 equivalent or slightly less. HDR is typically given in 3–4 Gy per fraction in US and Europe or 5–6 Gy per fraction in Asia

■ Two dose fractionation examples (from many possible alternatives) are presented in Table 9.2

Boost

■ LDR doses are usually in the range of 15–30 Gy

■ HDR is given to about the same EQD2 typically in 4–6 fractions at 3–5 Gy per fraction depending upon the EBRT dose

■ HDR is commonly given in twice daily fractions for H&N

Use of Image Guidance for Target Volume Delineation

■ Simulation radiography for H&N cancer is mostly performed on CT scanners but MRI is also suitable (where the GTV may be more apparent)

■ The author currently tends to err on the side of larger implants because the consequences of local recurrence are worse than those of soft tissue necrosis

Optimization of Target Volume: Point Based, Volume Based [98, 99]

- In some forms of image-guided BT relatively few catheters are inserted in the center of a lesion and a large dose gradient from the middle to the periphery of the tumor is acceptable. In H&N BT, however, this approach would likely result in unacceptably high rates of soft tissue necrosis
- The concept in H&N, as stated before, is to fully encompass the lesion with a uniform array of catheters, so a relatively homogeneous dose distribution can be achieved. The CTV should thus be volume based
- Interstitial H&N BT is best planned using 3D images and volume based calculations with V100, V150, D90, D100, and OAR dose constraints using $D_{0.1cm^3}$, D_{1cm^3}, and D_{2cm^3} parameters

Optimal Dose Distribution with Isodose Curves

- Curative therapy will include CTV goals of dose to 90 % of the CTV (D90) > than 100 % of the prescription dose and volume of the 100 % isodose (V100) should encompass >90 % of the CTV
- The primary OARs are the spinal cord, brain stem, eyes, and mandible
- Consideration should also be given to major blood vessels and cranial nerves, but the latter are hard to delineate with CT images alone
- The commonly used dose homogeneity factor of volume of the target that receives 150 % of the prescription dose (V150) ranges from 20 to 35 % in most cases where a generous array of catheters encompasses the target
- Higher V150 can be expected when the implant fails to encompass the lesion or there are large portions of the CTV without catheters

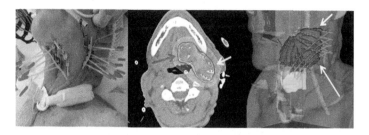

Fig. 9.6. Base of tongue cancer with simultaneous implantation of primary and upper cervical adenopathy

Dose Distributions

■ See Case Study 9.1 in Fig. 9.6

Toxicity

Toxicity Side Effect Review

■ BT results in comparatively few of the side effects commonly associated with EBRT such as xerostomia, loss of taste acuity, proclivity to dental caries, and injury to pharyngeal musculature

■ The BT procedure itself may present challenges with regard to airway management and patient comfort, but because there is no incision, recovery is usually rapid. The incidence of procedural complications is low, if proper quality and safety measures are followed [73, 100]

■ Acute radiation injury is localized, and it advances and recedes over about 2–3 weeks after treatment delivery

■ Clinically significant late complications include soft tissue necrosis (STN), bone injury (BI), and cranial neuropathy (CN)

- STN may be superficial ulceration or deep necrosis leading to fistula with the need for major medical and surgical intervention. The onset may be delayed 6–12 months or longer after completion of therapy and take many months to resolve
- BI may similarly be limited to transient bone exposure of relatively health alveolar bone or it may progress to osteoradionecrosis (ORN). Various definitions of ORN have been proposed, most of which include persistent bone exposure over a period of months, bone sequestration, and radiographic evidence of bone devascularization. Good BT dosimetry and the use of spacers to separate and shields to protect the mandible are effective prophylactic measures. The incidence of ORN has been decreasing in recent years due to improved technology; it is estimated to be about 3 % [101, 102]
- Cranial neuropathy (most apparent in XII and sympathetic chain) is another potential morbidity associated with IS-BT
- Accelerated carotid artery atherosclerosis is dose-dependent effect of radiation therapy to the neck if CT is done around the major vessels [103, 104]

Toxicity Rates of STN and BI

- Toxicity rates are extremely variable depending upon the clinical circumstances and definitions of toxicity (see Table 9.1 and accompanying references)
- STN ranges from 5 to 30 %
- BI occurs mostly when lesions are close to bone (particularly the mandible)

Toxicity Management

- Acute radiation mucositis managed with oral and dental hygiene, frequent oral rinses, good nutrition, local and systemic pain medication, and if needed, good tracheostomy wound care

- It is best to avoid using dentures (especially mandibular) for an extended period after BT and to have soft well-fitted dentures once they are resumed
- Early detection of STN allows institution of enhanced oral hygiene and the use of medications (such as a trial of antibiotics, and the use of pentoxifylline 400 mg and vitamin E 400 mg three times daily) [105, 106]
- Progression would lead the author to obtain consultation for hyperbaric oxygen (HBO) treatment [107, 108]

Conclusions and Future Developments

- Brachytherapy is a safe and effective treatment for many H&N cancers
- HDR, LDR, and PDR source loading appear to be equally effective, but there are few direct outcome comparisons. The advantage of HDR and PDR is the radiation safety
- HDR involves once or usually twice-daily treatment, so it is the most convenient in terms of nursing and patient management
- Image guidance and brachytherapy navigation are important future developments currently under investigation for H&N cancer

Acknowledgement Dr. Demanes wishes to thank Ming Zhang BS for his extensive and valuable contributions this work. He organized the references, edited and proofread the manuscript, and assisted in preparation of the figures and tables.

Appendix

Head and Neck Case Study 9.1: Interstitial Implant Base of Tongue and Adenopathy (3D-CT Simulation)

A 72-year-old male nonsmoker with a 2.5 cm HPV positive LEFT base of tongue with an associated 3 cm necrotic level II lymph node. It was a T2N2a (MRI and PET-CT) poorly differentiated squamous cell carcinoma that extended to the pharyngeal wall. His disease was diagnosed 1-year prior to starting radiation therapy, as he initially pursued alternative treatments. He received 50 Gy EBRT to the primary site and both necks without chemotherapy. The primary and neck node implant was performed without image guidance 2 weeks after EBRT. The dosimetry is shown in Fig. 9.6. The HDR dose was $3.75 \times 5 = 18.75$ Gy.

Head and Neck Case Study 9.2: Implant Navigation for Recurrent Neck Cancer

Seventy-one-year-old male with history of T1N0 poorly differentiated SCC RIGHT oral tongue with perineural invasion treated with hemiglossectomy and 63 Gy postoperative EBRT to primary and ipsilateral neck. One year later, he developed ipsilateral recurrent matted adenopathy, which was treated with neck dissection. One more year passed until he developed symptomatic unresectable RIGHT parapharyngeal mass and perivascular adenopathy. PET-CT was suspicious limited for contralateral adenopathy. He was treated with chemoradiation of 50 Gy EBRT to both necks and the tongue followed by image-guided BT using electromagnetic navigation (ENM) for catheter insertion to avoid vascular injury and target guidance. A preplan dosimetry profile was created from clinical examination and PET-CT findings (Fig. 9.7). The implant was done under ultrasound guidance

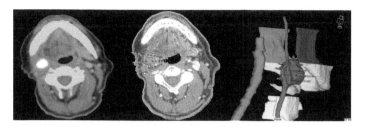

FIG. 9.7. Unresectable recurrent tongue cancer with prior radiation therapy involving deep perivascular soft tissue. Preplanning PET-CT, catheter trajectories, and virtual image of proposed catheter distribution in relation to CTV and carotid artery

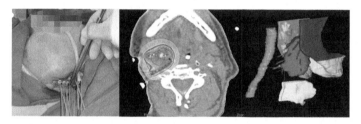

FIG. 9.8. Actual implant of same patient completed implant, postimplant dosimetry, and virtual image

and ENM. The carotid artery was successfully avoided and the catheter distribution achieved satisfactory coverage of the clinical target volume (Fig. 9.8).

References

1. Nag S, Cano ER, Demanes DJ, Puthawala AA, Vikram B, Society AB. The American Brachytherapy Society recommendations for high-dose-rate brachytherapy for head-and-neck carcinoma. Int J Radiat Oncol Biol Phys. 2001;50(5):1190–8.
2. Mazeron JJ, Ardiet JM, Haie-Meder C, Kovacs G, Levendag P, Peiffert D, et al. GEC-ESTRO recommendations for brachytherapy for head and neck squamous cell carcinomas. Radiother Oncol. 2009;91(2):150–6.

3. Demanes DJ. Head and neck brachytherapy: a description of methods and a summary of results. In: Brachytherapy: an international perspective; 2016. p. 71–143.

4. Demanes DJ, DiGiaimo R, Menchaca-Garcia C, Syverson T. Chapter 15: Foundations of brachytherapy practice. In: Brachytherapy: application and techniques. 2nd ed. New York: Demos Medical Publishing; 2015.

5. Gerbaulet A, Potter R, Mazeron JJ, Meertens H, Limbergen EV, Ash D, et al. GEC ESTRO handbook of brachytherapy. Leuven: ACCO; 2002.

6. Harrison LB, Sessions RB, Kies MS. Head and neck cancer: a multidisciplinary approach. 4th ed. Philadelphia: Lippincott Williams & Wilkins; 2013.

7. Aronowitz JN. Afterloading: the technique that rescued brachytherapy. Int J Radiat Oncol Biol Phys. 2015;92(3):479–87.

8. Vikram B, Hilaris BS, Anderson L, Strong EW. Permanent Iodine-125 implants in head and neck cancer. Cancer. 1983;51:1310–4.

9. Ashamalla H, Rafla S, Zaki B, Ikoro NC, Ross P. Radioactive gold grain implants in recurrent and locally advanced head-and-neck cancers. Brachytherapy. 2002;1:161–6.

10. Zhu L, Jiang Y, Wang J, Ran W, Yuan H, Liu C, et al. An investigation of 125I seed permanent implantation for recurrent carcinoma in the head and neck after surgery and external beam radiotherapy. World J Clin Oncol. 2013;11(1):60.

11. Nag S, Schuller D, Pak V, Grecula J, Bauer C, Young D. IORT using electron beam of HDR brachytherapy for previously unirradiated head and neck cancers. Front Radiat Ther Oncol. 1997;31:112–6.

12. Morikawa LK, Zelefsky MJ, Cohen GN, Zaider M, Chiu J, Mathur N, et al. Intraoperative high-dose-rate brachytherapy using dose painting technique: evaluation of safety and preliminary clinical outcomes. Brachytherapy. 2013;12(1):1–7.

13. Teckie S, Scala LM, Ho F, Wolden S, Chiu J, Cohen GN, et al. High-dose-rate intraoperative brachytherapy and radical surgical resection in the management of recurrent head-and-neck cancer. Brachytherapy. 2013;12(3):228–34.

14. Fakhry C, Westra WH, Li S, Cmelak A, Ridge JA, Pinto H, et al. Improved survival of patients with human papillomavirus-positive head and neck squamous cell carcinoma in a prospective clinical trial. J Natl Cancer Inst. 2008;100(4):261–9.

15. Ang KK, Harris J, Wheeler R, Weber R, Rosenthal DI, Nguyen-Tan PF, et al. Human papillomavirus and survival of patients with oropharyngeal cancer. N Engl J Med. 2010;363:24–35.
16. Tornesello ML, Perri F, Buonaguro L, Ionna F, Buonaguro FM, Caponigro F. HPV-related oropharyngeal cancers: from pathogenesis to new therapeutic approaches. Cancer Lett. 2014;351(2):198–205.
17. Shibuya H, Takeda M, Matsumoto S, Hoshina M, Suzuki S, Takagi M. The efficacy of radiation therapy for a malignant melanoma in the mucosa of the upper jaw: an analytic study. Int J Radiat Oncol Biol Phys. 1993;25:35–9.
18. Zhang J, Zhang JG, Song TL, Zhen L, Zhang Y, Zhang KH, et al. 125I seed implant brachytherapy-assisted surgery with preservation of the facial nerve for treatment of malignant parotid gland tumors. Int J Oral Maxillofac Surg. 2008;37(6):515–20.
19. Stannard CE, Hering E, Hough J, Knowles R, Munro R, Hille J. Post-operative treatment of malignant salivary gland tumours of the palate with iodine-125 brachytherapy. Radiother Oncol. 2004;73(3):307–11.
20. Meng N, Zhang X, Liao A, Tian S, Ran W, Gao Y, et al. Management of recurrent alveolar soft-part sarcoma of the tongue after external beam radiotherapy with iodine-125 seed brachytherapy. Head Neck. 2014;36(12):E125–8.
21. Beauvois S, Hoffstetter S, Peiffert D, Luporsi E, Carolus JM, Dartois D, et al. Brachytherapy for lower lip epidermoid cancer: tumoral and treatment factors influencing recurrences and complications. Radiother Oncol. 1994;33(3):195–203.
22. Guibert M, David I, Vergez S, Rives M, Filleron T, Bonnet J, et al. Brachytherapy in lip carcinoma: long-term results. Int J Radiat Oncol Biol Phys. 2011;81(5):e839–43.
23. Lapeyre M, Peiffert D, Malissard L, Hoffstetter S, Pernot M. An original technique of brachytherapy in the treatment of epidermoid carcinomas of the buccal mucosa. Int J Radiat Oncol Biol Phys. 1995;33(2):447–54.
24. Pernot M, Hoffstetter S, Peiffert D, Aletti P, Lapeyre M, Marchal C, et al. Role of interstitial brachytherapy in oral and oropharyngeal carcinoma: reflection of a series of 1344 patients treated at the time of initial presentation. Otolaryngol Head Neck Surg. 1996;115:519–26.
25. Yamazaki H, Inoue T, Koizumi M, Yoshida K, Kagawa K, Shiomi H, et al. Comparison of the long-term results of

brachytherapy for T1-2N0 oral tongue cancer treated with Ir-192 and Ra-226. Anticancer Res. 1997;17(4A):2819–22.

26. Khalilur R, Hayashi K, Shibuya H. Brachytherapy for tongue cancer in the very elderly is an alternative to external beam radiation. Br J Radiol. 2011;84(1004):747–9.

27. Kakimoto N, Inoue T, Inoue T, Murakami S, Furukawa S, Yoshida K, et al. High-dose-rate interstitial brachytherapy for mobile tongue cancer: influence of the non-irradiated period. Anticancer Res. 2006;26:3933–8.

28. Akiyama H, Yoshida K, Shimizutani K, Yamazaki H, Koizumi M, Yoshioka Y, et al. Dose reduction trial from 60 Gy in 10 fractions to 54 Gy in 9 fractions schedule in high-dose-rate interstitial brachytherapy for early oral tongue cancer. J Radiat Res. 2012;53(5):722–6.

29. Matsumoto K, Sasaki T, Shioyama Y, Nakamura K, Atsumi K, Nonoshita T, et al. Treatment outcome of high-dose-rate interstitial radiation therapy for patients with stage I and II mobile tongue cancer. Jpn J Clin Oncol. 2013;43(10):1012–7.

30. Lapeyre M, Bollet MA, Racadot S, Geoffrois L, Kaminsky MC, Hoffstetter S, et al. Postoperative brachytherapy alone and combined postoperative radiotherapy and brachytherapy boost for squamous cell carcinoma of the oral cavity, with positive or close margins. Head Neck. 2004;26(3):216–23.

31. Levendag PC, Nijdam WM, van Moolenburgh SE, Tan L, Noever I, van Rooy P, et al. Interstitial radiation therapy for early-stage nasal vestibule cancer: a continuing quest for optimal tumor control and cosmesis. Int J Radiat Oncol Biol Phys. 2006;66(1):160–9.

32. Bansal A, Ghoshal S, Oinam AS, Sharma SC, Dhanireddy B, Kapoor R. High-dose-rate interstitial brachytherapy in early stage oral tongue cancer—15 year experience from a tertiary care institute. J Contemp Brachytherapy. 2016;8(1):56–65.

33. Bourgier C, Coche-Dequeant B, Fournier C, Castelain B, Prevost B, Lefebvre JL, et al. Exclusive low-dose-rate brachytherapy in 279 patients with T2N0 mobile tongue carcinoma. Int J Radiat Oncol Biol Phys. 2005;63(2):434–40.

34. Grabenbauer GG, Rodel C, Brunner T, Schulze-Mosgau S, Strnad V, Muller RG, et al. Interstitial brachytherapy with Ir-192 low-dose-rate in the treatment of primary and recurrent cancer of the oral cavity and oropharynx. Review of 318 patients treated between 1985 and 1997. Strahlenther Onkol. 2001;177(7):338–44.

35. Kakimoto N, Inoue T, Inoue T, Murakami S, Furukawa S, Yoshida K, et al. Results of low- and high-dose-rate interstitial brachytherapy for T3 mobile tongue cancer. Radiother Oncol. 2003;68(2):123–8.

36. Puthawala AA, Syed AM, Eads DL, Gillin L, Gates TC. Limited external beam and interstitial 192 Iridium irradiation in the treatment of carcinoma of the base of the tongue: a ten year experience. Int J Radiat Oncol Biol Phys. 1988;14(5):839–48.

37. Harrison LB, Zelefsky MJ, Armstrong JG, Carper E, Gaynor JJ, Sessions RB. Performance status after treatment for squamous cell cancer of the base of tongue—a comparison of primary radiation therapy versus primary surgery. Int J Radiat Oncol Biol Phys. 1994;30(4):953–7.

38. Demanes D, Ruwanthi P, Cmelak A, Cruz R, Rodriguez R. Brachytherapy and external radiation for carcinoma of the base of tongue: implantation of the primary tumor and cervical adenopathy. Int J Brachytherapy. 2000;16:211–23.

39. Barrett WL, Gleich L, Wilson K, Gluckman J. Organ preservation with interstitial radiation for base of tongue cancer. Am J Clin Oncol. 2002;25(5):485–8.

40. Gibbs IC, Le Q-T, Shah RD, Terris DJ, Fee WE, Goffinet DR. Long-term outcomes after external beam irradiation and brachytherapy boost for base-of-tongue cancers. Int J Radiat Oncol Biol Phys. 2003;57(2):489–94.

41. Levendag P, Peters R, Meeuwis CA, Visch LL, Spikema D, de Pan C, et al. A new applicator design for endocavitary brachytherapy of cancer in the nasopharynx. Radiat Oncol. 1997;45(1):95–8.

42. Leung TW, Wong VY, Sze WK, Lui CM, Tung SY. High-dose-rate intracavitary brachytherapy boost for early T stage nasopharyngeal carcinoma{private}. Int J Radiat Oncol Biol Phys. 2008;70(2):361–7.

43. Wu J, Guo Q, Lu JJ, Zhang C, Zhang X, Pan J, et al. Addition of intracavitary brachytherapy to external beam radiation therapy for T1-T2 nasopharyngeal carcinoma. Brachytherapy. 2013;12(5):479–86.

44. Levendag PC, Keskin-Cambay F, de Pan C, Idzes M, Wildeman MA, Noever I, et al. Local control in advanced cancer of the nasopharynx: is a boost dose by endocavitary brachytherapy of prognostic significance? Brachytherapy. 2013;12(1):84–9.

45. Rosenblatt E, Abdel-Wahab M, El-Gantiry M, Elattar I, Bourque JM, Afiane M, et al. Brachytherapy boost

in loco-regionally advanced nasopharyngeal carcinoma: a prospective randomized trial of the International Atomic Energy Agency. Radiat Oncol. 2014;9:67.

46. Vikram B, Strong EW, Shah JP, Spiro RH, Gerold F, Sessions RB, et al. Intraoperative radiotherapy in patients with recurrent head and neck cancer. Am J Surg. 1985;150(4):485–7.

47. Park RI, Liberman FZ, Lee DJ, Goldsmith MM, Price JC. Iodine-125 seed implantation as an adjunct to surgery in advanced recurrent squamous cell cancer of the head and neck. Laryngoscope. 1991;101:405–9.

48. Peiffert D, Pernot M, Malissard L, Aletti P, Hoffstetter S, Kozminski P, et al. Salvage irradiation by brachytherapy of velotonsillar squamous cell carcinoma in a previously irradiated field: results in 73 cases. Int J Radiat Oncol Biol Phys. 1994;29(4):681–6.

49. Nag S, Schuller DE, RodríguezVillalba S, MartínezMonge R, Grecula J. Intraoperative high dose rate brachytherapy can be used to salvage patients with previously irradiated head and neck recurrences. Rev Med Univ Navarra. 1999;43(2):56–61.

50. Zelefsky M, Zimberg S, Raben A, et al. Brachytherapy for locally advanced and recurrent lymph node metastases. J Brachytherapy Int. 1998;14:123.

51. Puthawala A, Syed AM, Gamie S, Chen YJ, Londrc A, Nixon V. Interstitial low-dose-rate brachytherapy as a salvage treatment for recurrent head-and-neck cancers: long-term results. Int J Radiat Oncol Biol Phys. 2001;51(2):354–62.

52. Nutting C, Horlock N, A'Hern R, Searle A, Henk JM, Rhys-Evans P, et al. Manually after-loaded 192Ir low-dose rate brachytherapy after subtotal excision and flap reconstruction of recurrent cervical lymphadenopathy from head and neck cancer. Radiother Oncol. 2006;80(1):39–42.

53. Klein M, Menneking H, Langford A, Koch K, Stahl H. Treatment of squamous cell carcinomas of the floor of the mouth and tongue by interstitial high dose rate irradiation using iridium192. Int J Oral Maxillofac Surg. 1998;27(1):45–8.

54. Glatzel M, Buntzel J, Schroder D, Kuttner K, Frohlich D. High-dose-rate brachytherapy in the treatment of recurrent and residual head and neck cancer. Laryngoscope. 2002;112(8):1366–71.

55. Hepel JT, Syed AM, Puthawala A, Sharma A, Frankel P. Salvage high-dose-rate (HDR) brachytherapy for recurrent head-and-neck cancer. Int J Radiat Oncol Biol Phys. 2005;62(5):1444–50.

56. Pellizzon AC, dos Santos Novaes PE, Conte Maia MA, Ferrigno R, Fogarolli R, Salvajoli JV, et al. Interstitial high-dose-rate brachytherapy combined with cervical dissection on head and neck cancer. Head Neck. 2005;27(12):1035–41.

57. Narayana A, Cohen GN, Zaider M, Chan K, Lee N, Wong RJ, et al. High-dose-rate interstitial brachytherapy in recurrent and previously irradiated head and neck cancers—preliminary results. Brachytherapy. 2007;6(2):157–63.

58. Kupferman ME, Morrison WH, Santillan AA, Roberts D, Diaz Jr EM, Garden AS, et al. The role of interstitial brachytherapy with salvage surgery for the management of recurrent head and neck cancers. Cancer. 2007;109(10):2052–7.

59. Perry DJ, Chan K, Wolden S, Zelefsky MJ, Chiu J, Cohen G, et al. High-dose-rate intraoperative radiation therapy for recurrent head-and-neck cancer. Int J Radiat Oncol Biol Phys. 2010;76(4):1140–6.

60. Martinez-Monge R, Pagola Divasson M, Cambeiro M, Gaztanaga M, Moreno M, Arbea L, et al. Determinants of complications and outcome in high-risk squamous cell head-and-neck cancer treated with perioperative high-dose rate brachytherapy (PHDRB). Int J Radiat Oncol Biol Phys. 2011;81(4):e245–54.

61. Bartochowska A, Wierzbicka M, Skowronek J, Leszczynska M, Szyfter W. High-dose-rate and pulsed-dose-rate brachytherapy in palliative treatment of head and neck cancers. Brachytherapy. 2012;11(2):137–43.

62. Rudzianskas V, Inciura A, Juozaityte E, Rudzianskiene M, Kubilius R, Vaitkus S, et al. Reirradiation of recurrent head and neck cancer using high-dose-rate brachytherapy. Acta Otorhinolaryngol Ital. 2012;32(5):297–303.

63. Scala LM, Hu K, Urken ML, Jacobson AS, Persky MS, Tran TN, et al. Intraoperative high-dose-rate radiotherapy in the management of locoregionally recurrent head and neck cancer. Head Neck. 2013;35(4):485–92.

64. Strnad V, Lotter M, Kreppner S, Fietkau R. Re-irradiation with interstitial pulsed-dose-rate brachytherapy for unresectable recurrent head and neck carcinoma. Brachytherapy. 2014;13(2):187–95.

65. Rudzianskas V, Inciura A, Vaitkus S, Padervinskis E, Rudzianskiene M, Kupcinskaite-Noreikiene R, et al. Reirradiation for patients with recurrence head and neck squamous cell carcinoma: a single-institution comparative study. Medicina (Kaunas). 2014;50(2):92–9.

66. Tamamoto M, Fujita M, Yamamoto T, Hamada T. Techniques for making spacers in interstitial brachytherapy for tongue cancer. Int J Prosthodont. 1996;9(1):95–8.
67. Miura M, Takeda M, Sasaki T, Inoue T, Nakayama Y, Fukuda H, et al. Factors affecting mandibular complications in low dose rate brachytherapy for oral tongue carcinoma with special reference to spacer. Int J Radiat Oncol Biol Phys. 1998;41(4):763–70.
68. Fujita M, Yutaka H, Kashiwado K, Akagi Y, Kashimoto K, Hiriu H, et al. Interstitial brachytherapy for stage I and II squamous cell carcinoma of the oral tongue: factors influencing local control and soft tissue complications. Int J Radiat Oncol Biol Phys. 1999;44(4):767–75.
69. Libby B, Sheng K, McLawhorn R, McIntosh A, Van Ausdal RG, Martof A, et al. Use of megavoltage computed tomography with image registration for high-dose rate treatment planning of an oral tongue cancer using a custom oral mold applicator with embedded lead shielding. Brachytherapy. 2011;10(4):340–4.
70. Haie-Meder C, Potter R, Van Limbergen E, Briot E, De Brabandere M, Dimopoulos J, et al. Recommendations from Gynaecological (GYN) GEC-ESTRO Working Group (I): concepts and terms in 3D image based 3D treatment planning in cervix cancer brachytherapy with emphasis on MRI assessment of GTV and CTV. Radiother Oncol. 2005;74(3):235–45.
71. Simon JM, Mazeron JJ, Pohar S, Le Péchoux C, Crook JM, Grimard L, et al. Effect of intersource spacing on local control and complications in brachytherapy of mobile tongue and floor of mouth. Radiother Oncol. 1993;26:19–25.
72. Pernot M, Aletti P, Carolus JM, Marquis I, Hoffstetter S, Maaloul F, et al. Indications, techniques and results of postoperative brachytherapy in cancer of the oral cavity. Radiat Oncol. 1995;35:186–92.
73. Pernot M, Luporsi E, Hoffstetter S, Peiffert D, Aletti P, Marchal C, et al. Complications following definitive irradiation for cancers of the oral cavity and the oropharynx (in a series of 1134 patients). Int J Radiat Oncol Biol Phys. 1997;37(3):577–85.
74. Demanes DJ, Rodriguez RR, Syed N, Puthawala A. Wire in leader technique: a method for loading implant catheters in inaccessible sites. J Brachytherapy Int. 1997;13(4).
75. Mazeron JJ, Belkacemi Y, Simon JM, Le Pechoux C, Martin M, Haddad E, et al. Place of Iridium 192 implantation in definitive

irradiation of faucial arch squamous cell carcinomas. Int J Radiat Oncol Biol Phys. 1993;27:251–7.

76. Nose T, Koizumi M, Nishiyama K. High-dose-rate interstitial brachytherapy for oropharyngeal carcinoma: results of 83 lesions in 82 patients. Int J Radiat Oncol Biol Phys. 2004;59(4):983–91.

77. Patra NB, Goswami J, Basu S, Chatterjee K, Sarkar SK. Outcomes of high dose rate interstitial boost brachytherapy after external beam radiation therapy in head and neck cancer—an Indian (single institutional) learning experience. Brachytherapy. 2009;8(2):248–54.

78. Sethi T, Ash DV, Flynn A, Workman G. Replacement of hairpin and loop implants by optimised straight line sources. Radiat Oncol. 1996;39:117–21.

79. Nag S, Martinez-Monge R, Zhang H, Gupta N. Simplified non-looping functional loop technique for HDR brachytherapy. Radiat Oncol. 1998;48:339–41.

80. Demanes DJ, Friedman JM, Park SJ, Steinberg ML, Hayes Jr JK, Kamrava MR. Brachytherapy catheter spacing and stabilization technique. Brachytherapy. 2012;11(5):392–7.

81. Feldman J, Appelbaum L, Sela M, Voskoboinik N, Kadouri S, Weinberger J, et al. Novel high dose rate lip brachytherapy technique to improve dose homogeneity and reduce toxicity by customized mold. Radiat Oncol. 2014;9:271.

82. Mazeron JJ, Crook JM, Benck V, Marinello G, Martin M, Raynal M, et al. Iridium 192 implantation of T1 and T2 carcinomas of the mobile tongue. Int J Radiat Oncol Biol Phys. 1990;19:1369–76.

83. Ash D, Gerbaulet A. Chapter 9: Oral tongue cancer. In: GEC ESTRO handbook of brachytherapy; 2002. p. 237–51.

84. Marsiglia H, Haie-Meder C, Sasso G, Mamelle G, Gerbaulet A. Brachytherapy for T1-T2 floor-of-the-mouth cancers; the Gustave-Roussy Institute experience. Int J Radiat Oncol Biol Phys. 2002;52(5):1257–63.

85. Ngan RKC, Wong RKY, Tang F. Interstitial brachytherapy for early oral tongue cancer using iridium hairpin or wire. J HK Coll Radiol. 2004;7(2):88–94.

86. Lapeyre M, Hoffstetter S, Peiffert D, Guerif S, Maire F, Dolivet G, et al. Postoperative brachytherapy alone for T1-2 N0 squamous cell carcinomas of the oral tongue and floor of mouth with close or positive margins. Int J Radiat Oncol Biol Phys. 2000;45(1):37–42.

268   D.J. Demanes

87. Kudoh T, Ikushima H, Kudoh K, Tokuyama R, Osaki K, Furutani S, et al. High-dose-rate brachytherapy for patients with maxillary gingival carcinoma using a novel customized intraoral mold technique. Oral Surg Oral Med Oral Pathol Oral Radiol Endod. 2010;109(2):e102–8.
88. Syed AM, Puthawala AA, Damore SJ, Cherlow JM, Austin PA, Sposto R, et al. Brachytherapy for primary and recurrent nasopharyngeal carcinoma: 20 years' experience at Long Beach Memorial. Int J Radiat Oncol Biol Phys. 2000;47(5):1311–21.
89. Kremer B, Kilmek L, Andreopoulos D, Mosges R. A new method for the placement of brachytherapy probes in paranasal sinus and nasopharynx neoplasm. Int J Radiat Oncol Biol Phys. 1999;43(5):995–1000.
90. Wan XB, Jiang R, Xie FY, Qi ZY, Li AJ, Ye WJ, et al. Endoscope-guided interstitial intensity-modulated brachytherapy and intracavitary brachytherapy as boost radiation for primary early T stage nasopharyngeal carcinoma. PLoS One. 2014;9(3):e90048.
91. Langendijk JA, Poorter R, Leemans CR, de Bree R, Doornaert P, Slotman BJ. Radiotherapy of squamous cell carcinoma of the nasal vestibule. Int J Radiat Oncol Biol Phys. 2004;59(5): 1319–25.
92. Allen MW, Schwartz DL, Rana V, Adapala P, Morrison WH, Hanna EY, et al. Long-term radiotherapy outcomes for nasal cavity and septal cancers. Int J Radiat Oncol Biol Phys. 2008;71(2):401–6.
93. Nag S, Tippin D, Grecula J, Schuller D. Intraoperative high-dose-rate brachytherapy for paranasal sinus tumors. Int J Radiat Oncol Biol Phys. 2004;58(1):155–60.
94. Teudt IU, Meyer JE, Ritter M, Wollenberg B, Kolb T, Maune S, et al. Perioperative image-adapted brachytherapy for the treatment of paranasal sinus and nasal cavity malignancies. Brachytherapy. 2014;13(2):178–86.
95. Bartochowska A, Skowronek J, Wierzbicka M, Leszczynska M, Szyfter W. The role of high-dose-rate and pulsed-dose-rate brachytherapy in the management of recurrent or residual stomal tumor after total laryngectomy. Laryngoscope. 2013;123(3):657–61.
96. Doyle LA, Harrison AS, Cognetti D, Xiao Y, Yu Y, Liu H, et al. Reirradiation of head and neck cancer with high-dose-rate brachytherapy: a customizable intraluminal solution for postoperative treatment of tracheal mucosa recurrence. Brachytherapy. 2011;10(2):154–8.

97. Tselis N, Ratka M, Vogt HG, Kolotas C, Baghi M, Baltas D, et al. Hypofractionated accelerated CT-guided interstitial 192Ir-HDR-brachytherapy as re-irradiation in inoperable recurrent cervical lymphadenopathy from head and neck cancer. Radiother Oncol. 2011;98(1):57–62.

98. Lessard E, Pouliot J. Inverse planning anatomy-based dose optimization for HDR-brachytherapy of the prostate using fast simulated annealing algorithm and dedicated objective function. Med Phys. 2001;28(5):773–9.

99. Lessard E, Hsu IC, Pouliot J. Inverse planning for interstitial gynecologic template brachytherapy: truly anatomy-based planning. Int J Radiat Oncol Biol Phys. 2002;54(4):1243–51.

100. Bhandare N, Mendenhall WM. A literature review of late complications of radiation therapy for head and neck cancers: incidence and dose response. J Nucl Med Radiat Ther. 2012;S2:9.

101. Wahl MJ. Osteoradionecrosis prevention myths. Int J Radiat Oncol Biol Phys. 2006;64(3):661–9.

102. Suryawanshi A, Pawar V, Singh M, Dolas RS, Khindria R, Kumar SNS. Maxillofacial osteoradionecrosis. J Dent Res Rev. 2014;1(1):42.

103. Scott AS, Parr LA, Johnstone PA. Risk of cerebrovascular events after neck and supraclavicular radiotherapy: a systematic review. Radiother Oncol. 2009;90(2):163–5.

104. Xu J, Cao Y. Radiation-induced carotid artery stenosis: a comprehensive review of the literature. Interv Neurol. 2014;2(4):183–92.

105. Delanian S, Chatel C, Porcher R, Depondt J, Lefaix JL. Complete restoration of refractory mandibular osteoradionecrosis by prolonged treatment with a pentoxifylline-tocopherol-clodronate combination (PENTOCLO): a phase II trial. Int J Radiat Oncol Biol Phys. 2011;80(3):832–9.

106. Delanian S, Lefaix JL. Current management for late normal tissue injury: radiation-induced fibrosis and necrosis. Semin Radiat Oncol. 2007;17(2):99–107.

107. Shaw RJ, Dhanda J. Hyperbaric oxygen in the management of late radiation injury to the head and neck. Part I: treatment. Br J Oral Maxillofac Surg. 2011;49(1):2–8.

108. Shaw RJ, Butterworth C. Hyperbaric oxygen in the management of late radiation injury to the head and neck. Part II: prevention. Br J Oral Maxillofac Surg. 2011;49(1):9–13.

109. Mazeron JJ, Richaud P. Lip cancer, report of the 18th annual meeting of the European Curietherapy Group. J Eur Radiother. 1984;5:50–6.

110. Van Limbergen E, Ding W, Haustermans K, et al. Lip cancer: local control results of low dose rate brachytherapy. The GEC-ESTRO 1993 survey on 2800 cases. Annual GEC ESTRO meeting Venice 1993; 1993.

111. Gerbaulet A, Limbergen EV. Chapter 8: Lip cancer. In: GEC ESTRO handbook of brachytherapy; 2002. p. 227–36.

112. Ayerra AQ, Mena EP, Fabregas JP, Miguelez CG, Guedea F. HDR and LDR brachytherapy in the treatment of lip cancer: the experience of the Catalan Institute of Oncology. J Contemp Brachytherapy. 2010;2(1):9–13.

113. Ghadjar P, Bojaxhiu B, Simcock M, Terribilini D, Isaak B, Gut P, et al. High dose-rate versus low dose-rate brachytherapy for lip cancer. Int J Radiat Oncol Biol Phys. 2012;83(4):1205–12.

114. Guinot JL, Arribas L, Vendrell JB, Santos M, Tortajada MI, Mut A, et al. Prognostic factors in squamous cell lip carcinoma treated with high-dose-rate brachytherapy. Head Neck. 2014;36(12):1737–42.

115. Gerbaulet A. Chapter 11: Buccal mucosa cancer. In: GEC ESTRO handbook of brachytherapy; 2002. p. 265–73.

116. Shibuya H, Hoshina M, Takedo M, Matsumoto S, Suzuki S, Okada N. Brachytherapy for stage I & II oral tongue cancer: an analysis of past cases focusing on control and complications. Int J Radiat Oncol Biol Phys. 1993;26:51–8.

117. Matsuura K, Hirokawa Y, Fujita M, Akagi Y, Ito K. Treatment results of stage I and II oral tongue cancer with interstitial brachytherapy: maximum tumor thickness is prognostic of nodal metastasis. Int J Radiat Oncol Biol Phys. 1998;40(3):535–9.

118. Yoshimura R, Shibuya H, Hayashi K, Toda K, Watanabe H, Miura M. Disease control using low-dose-rate brachytherapy is unaffected by comorbid severity in oral cancer patients. Br J Radiol. 2011;84(1006):930–8.

119. Stannard C, Maree G, Tovey S, Hunter A, Wetter J. Iodine-125 brachytherapy in the management of squamous cell carcinoma of the oral cavity and oropharynx. Brachytherapy. 2014;13(4):405–12.

120. Strnad V, Lotter M, Kreppner S, Fietkau R. Interstitial pulsed-dose-rate brachytherapy for head and neck cancer—single-institution long-term results of 385 patients. Brachytherapy. 2013;12(6):521–7.

121. Guinot JL, Santos M, Tortajada MI, Carrascosa M, Estelles E, Vendrell JB, et al. Efficacy of high-dose-rate interstitial brachytherapy in patients with oral tongue carcinoma. Brachytherapy. 2010;9(3):227–34.

122. Umeda M, Komatsubara H, Ojima Y, Minamikawa T, Shibuya Y, Yokoo S, et al. A comparison of brachytherapy and surgery for the treatment of stage I-II squamous cell carcinoma of the tongue. Int J Oral Maxillofac Surg. 2005;34(7):739–44.

123. Yamazaki H, Inoue T, Yoshida K, Yoshioka Y, Furukawa S, Kakimoto N, et al. Comparison of three major radioactive sources for brachytherapy used in treatment of node negative T1-T3 oral tongue cancer: influence of age on outcome. Anticancer Res. 2007;27:491–8.

124. Gerbaulet A, Mazeron JJ, Ash D. Chapter 10: Flow of mouth cancer. In: GEC ESTRO handbook of brachytherapy; 2002. p. 253–64.

125. Mazeron JJ, Limbergen EV. Chapter 12: Oropharynx. In: GEC ESTRO handbook of brachytherapy; 2002. p. 275–87.

126. Rudoltz MS, Perkins RS, Luthmann RW, Fracke TD, Green TM, Moye L, et al. High-dose-rate brachytherapy for primary carcinomas of the oral cavity and oropharynx. Laryngoscope. 1999;109:1967–73.

127. Levendag P, Nijdam W, Noever I, Schmitz P, van de Pol M, Sipkema D, et al. Brachytherapy versus surgery in carcinoma of tonsillar fossa and/or soft palate: late adverse sequelae and performance status: can we be more selective and obtain better tissue sparing? Int J Radiat Oncol Biol Phys. 2004;59(3):713–24.

128. Cano ER, Lai SY, Caylakli F, Johnson JT, Ferris RL, Carrau RL, et al. Management of squamous cell carcinoma of the base of tongue with chemoradiation and brachytherapy. Head Neck. 2009;31(11):1431–8.

129. Takacsi-Nagy Z, Oberna F, Koltai P, Hitre E, Major T, Fodor J, et al. Long-term outcomes with high-dose-rate brachytherapy for the management of base of tongue cancer. Brachytherapy. 2013;12(6):535–41.

130. Chang JT, See L, Tang SG, Lee SP, Wang C, Hong JH. The role of brachytherapy in early-stage nasopharyngeal carcinoma. Int J Radiat Oncol Biol Phys. 1996;36(5):1019–24.

131. Karim AB, Kralendonk JH, Njo KH, Tabak JM, Elsenaar WH, van Balen AT. Ethmoid and upper nasal cavity carcinoma: treatment, results and complications. Radiother Oncol. 1990;19(2):109–20.

132. McCollough WM, Mendenhall NP, Parsons JT, Mendenhall WM, Stringer SP, Cassisi NJ, et al. Radiotherapy alone for squamous cell carcinoma of the nasal vestibule: management of the

primary site and regional lymphatics. Int J Radiat Oncol Biol Phys. 1993;26(1):73–9.

133. Tiwari R, Hardillo JA, Tobi H, Mehta D, Karim ABMF, Snow G. Carcinoma of the ethmoid: results of treatment with conventional surgery and post-operative radiotherapy. Eur J Surg Oncol. 1999;45:401–5.

134. Evensen JF, Jacobsen AB, Tausjo JE. Brachytherapy of squamous cell carcinoma of the nasal vestibule. Acta Oncol. 1996;35(S8):87–92.

135. Strege RJ, Kovacs G, Lamcke P, Maune S, Holland D, Eichmann T, et al. Role of perioperative brachytherapy in the treatment of malignancies involving the skull base and orbit. Neurosurg Q. 2007;17(3):193–207.

Chapter 10
Gastrointestinal Brachytherapy: Esophageal Cancer

Supriya K. Jain and Karyn A. Goodman

Introduction

Rationale for Brachytherapy in Esophageal Cancer

- According to the American Cancer Society, approximately 16,910 cases of esophageal cancer will be diagnosed in 2016 [1]
- Standard management of locally advanced esophageal cancer is concurrent chemoradiation both as definitive nonsurgical therapy [2–4] and as neoadjuvant treatment prior to surgery [5, 6]
  - However, local failure rates remain high, and esophageal cancer continues to have a poor prognosis despite years of effort in improving chemotherapy, surgery, and radiation therapy
  - Many patients present with advanced disease, and the location of the esophageal lesions and proximity

S.K. Jain, MD, MHS • K.A. Goodman, MD, MS (✉)
Department of Radiation Oncology, University of Colorado
School of Medicine, Aurora, CO, USA
e-mail: supriya.jain@ucdenver.edu; karyn.goodman@ucdenver.edu

© Springer International Publishing AG 2017   273
J. Mayadev et al. (eds.), *Handbook of Image-Guided Brachytherapy*, DOI 10.1007/978-3-319-44827-5_10

to nearby critical structures limit the ability to deliver therapeutic dose

- Elderly patients and patients with multiple comorbidities may not be good candidates for esophagectomy
- For patients who are treated nonsurgically with external beam radiation with or without chemotherapy, rates of disease persistence remain higher than 50 % [2–4]
- Patients who have received prior radiation have additional limitations on the delivery of additional radiation due to dose tolerance and surgically altered anatomy

- HDR endoluminal brachytherapy is an effective and well-tolerated treatment
- High-dose rate (HDR) endoluminal brachytherapy permits delivery of tumoricidal doses to superficial lesions of the esophagus while delivering much lower doses to surrounding tissue
- Brachytherapy techniques provide a superior means of delivering high doses of radiation to localized targets than external beam radiation
    - Dose delivery from radiation is dependent upon the inverse square law, which states that the radiation delivered to a point is proportional to the inverse square of the distance between the point and the source of radiation
    - By taking advantage of this law, when brachytherapy sources are placed within the esophagus in close proximity to the target lesion, very high doses of radiation are absorbed by malignant tissue physically near the source while doses to normal tissues outside the target receive doses of radiation much lower relative to that within the target
    - The radiation dose to nearby critical structures is therefore significantly less, and minimizing treatment uncertainty permits precise dose localization

and delivery of a more radiobiologically effective treatment in several large fractions
- Coupled with computer optimized inverse treatment planning algorithms, brachytherapy is well suited to deliver high doses of radiation to the esophageal lesion while limiting doses to nearby sensitive normal structures such as the spinal cord, lungs, heart, and other nearby tissues

HDR Endoluminal Brachytherapy in Esophageal Cancer

- Endoluminal high-dose rate (HDR) brachytherapy has been implemented in salvage treatment for locally recurrent esophageal cancer, in the primary management of patients who are not surgical candidates (as a boost for persistent disease after definitive chemoradiation) and as palliative treatment in stage IV disease
- It is particularly useful in the setting of re-irradiation as standard fields generally deliver significant dose to normal tissues including the lungs and the spinal cord
- The American Brachytherapy Society (ABS) has designed guidelines to assist in the use of HDR in the definitive and palliative treatment of esophageal cancers [7], including selection criteria to determine which patients could potentially benefit from endoluminal esophageal brachytherapy and the optimal applicator sizes:
  - Specified the use of an applicator with an external diameter of 6–10 mm and dosing regimens between 5 and 10 Gy per fraction in 1–4 fractions based on clinical scenario
  - With a prescription depth specified as 1 cm from the mid-source or mid-dwell without optimization and typical dose fall-off, the mucosal surfaces can receive doses in excess of 15 Gy per fraction using

the 6 mm applicator and assuming a 5-Gy fraction size

■ Dose-limiting toxicity of endoluminal HDR brachytherapy is late esophageal perforation or fistula

■ High rates of ulceration, stricture, and fistula have been observed at mucosal doses in excess of 15 Gy [8–10] using brachytherapy, which has curbed much of the interest in pursuing endoluminal brachytherapy as a treatment modality for esophageal cancer

■ At the same time, these and other studies with lower mucosal doses [11–13] suggest that there may be a benefit in terms of local control and symptomatic palliation

■ As such, there may be a point where the therapeutic ratio is of benefit to patients, and efforts to determine the optimal means of delivering sufficient prescription dose while maintaining a safe mucosal dose are justified

■ From the high-dose single fraction external beam radiosurgery experience for spine metastases, it has recently been shown that doses in excess of 15 Gy in a single fraction result in a significantly greater risk of ≥Grade 3 toxicity [14]

■ This suggests that optimal HDR techniques have large diameter applicators that allow delivery of adequate dose at prescription depth while limiting the mucosal dose to tolerable levels

■ These techniques would be used in conjunction with concurrent chemotherapy in inoperable patients, as a boost following definitive chemoradiation therapy or as a salvage treatment

■ There is an ongoing phase I clinical trial at Memorial Sloan Kettering Cancer Center (MSKCC) with several escalating dose levels to determine maximum deliverable tolerated dose with acceptable acute and late toxicity

Timing and Goal for Endoluminal Brachytherapy of Esophagus

- Definitive treatment (boost) for superficial primary esophageal tumor for nonsurgical candidates after combined chemoradiation therapy
- Salvage for locally recurrent esophageal cancer following chemoradiation therapy +/− surgical resection
- Palliative treatment for patients with stage IV disease
- Endoluminal brachytherapy may be delivered safely concurrent with capecitabine (preferred) or infusional 5-F luorouracil

Selection Criteria for Implantation (According to ABS Guidelines) [7]

- Good candidates for endoluminal HDR brachytherapy are patients with a primary tumor
  - ≤10 cm in length
  - Confined to the esophageal wall
  - Within the thoracic esophagus
  - Without regional lymph node or systemic metastases
- Contraindications for HDR Brachytherapy are patients with
  - Esophageal fistula
  - Cervical esophageal involvement (concern for the development of tracheoesophageal fistula)
  - Non-traversable esophageal stenosis

Medical Operability

- Comprehensive evaluation including
  - History and Physical examination
  - Performance status

- Weight
- Review of current medications
- Assessment of baseline comorbidities, including baseline pain assessment
- Laboratory assessment
- Evaluation by anesthesiologist

Applicator

- Size of applicator diameter is very important to decrease mucosal dose and yield low rates of toxicity
- Results of endoluminal brachytherapy for esophageal cancer at MSKCC demonstrate minimal toxicity with a 3-fraction approach using applicators with diameters >12 mm and limiting the mucosal dose to <12 Gy
- Applicators under 8 mm in diameter should not be used in the treatment of esophageal cancer (Table 10.1) [15]
- Typically, a bougie catheter (Fig. 10.1), similar to a Savary dilator catheter, with an internal lumen for insertion of a brachytherapy catheter has been used at MSKCC to center the brachytherapy catheter in the lumen
- A single-use applicator (the Esophageal Applicator) has been specifically designed for upper GI cancers (Ancer Medical, Hialeah, FL, USA) (Fig. 10.2a, b).
  - Flexible five-balloon self-centering applicator with one treatment catheter, 60 cm in length
  - Temporarily inserted into the esophageal tract to provide a pathway for the radioactive source guide-wire to deliver radiation to the clinician-specified target site
  - One catheter containing a central lumen for the passage of the radiation source guidewire. The central lumen (source lumen) of the device is configured to accept the radiation source from an HDR afterloader

TABLE 10.1 Calculated mucosal doses (assuming 5 cm treatment length, 5Gy/fx)

Applicator outer diameter (mm)	Prescribed to 10 mm from source		Prescribed to 5 mm from applicator surface	
	Max dose Gy (% prescription)	Central dose Gy (% prescription)	Max dose Gy (% prescription)	Central dose Gy (% prescription)
4	78 (1550 %)	32 (636 %)	43 (856 %)	23 (450 %)
5	53 (1054 %)	23 (458 %)	31 (628 %)	19 (372 %)
6	38 (768 %)	19 (372 %)	26 (524 %)	15 (308 %)
8	23 (454 %)	13 (266 %)	23 (460 %)	14 (272 %)
10	16 (314 %)	11 (216 %)	16 (314 %)	11 (216 %)
12	12 (232 %)	9 (176 %)	13 (266 %)	10 (200 %)
14	9 (178 %)	7 (148 %)	12 (232 %)	9 (188 %)
15	8 (158 %)	7 (138 %)	11 (226 %)	9 (185 %)
16	7 (144 %)	6 (128 %)	11 (218 %)	9 (183 %)
20	5 (104 %)	5 (100 %)	10 (192 %)	8 (162 %)

Used with permission from Folkert M, Cohen G, Wu A, et al. Endoluminal High-Dose-Rate Brachytherapy for Early Stage and Recurrent Esophageal Cancer in Medically Inoperable Patients, Brachytherapy 2013; 12:463–470

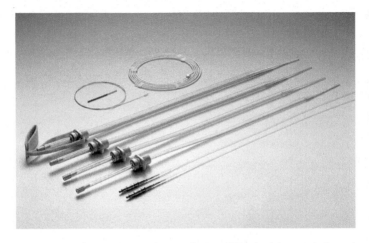

Fig. 10.1. Esophageal Bougie Applicator. (Used with permission of Varian Medical Systems, Palo Alto, CA, USA)

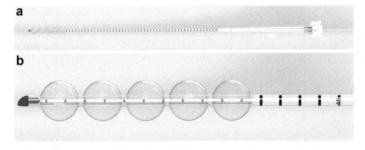

Fig. 10.2. The Esophageal Applicator (Ancer Medical, Nashua, NH) consists of a single treatment channel (**a**) and five distal balloons (**b**). (Used with permission of Ancer Medical, Hialeah, FL, USA)

- A series of five anatomically compliant balloons (baffles), 2 cm in diameter when maximally inflated, are sequentially placed 3 cm apart at the distal end of the applicator
- These balloons are covered by an outer compliant balloon liner (not shown in Fig. 10.2a, b). The balloons are inflated at the physician's discretion to

distend the esophagus at the treatment site to secure the applicator in the esophagus, and to center the source guidewire. This function aims to decrease the dose to the superficial mucosal layer. The balloons are inflated at the proximal end with individual (5) inflation tubes connected to stopcocks to accept syringes

- A second channel located along the side of the central source catheter provides the ability to utilize an esophageal guidewire to correctly locate the applicator in the esophagus via fluoroscopy guidance

- The applicator also incorporates X-ray markers to aid with positioning (Fig. 10.3) and is CT and MRI compatible

- CT-based planning can be performed (Fig. 10.4)

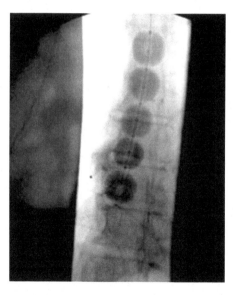

FIG. 10.3. The Esophageal Applicator also incorporates X-ray markers to aid with positioning using fluoroscopic imaging. (Courtesy of Gil'ad Cohen, PhD, Memorial Sloan Kettering Cancer Center, NY, NY)

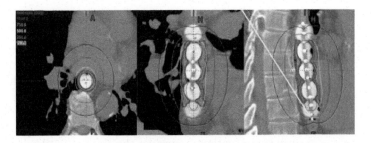

FIG. 10.4. CT-based planning is performed for high-dose rate brachytherapy using the Esophageal Applicator. Because of the nonuniform spacing between the source axis and tissue surface, optimization results in nonuniform dwell times. (Courtesy of Gil'ad Cohen, PhD, Memorial Sloan Kettering Cancer Center, NY, NY)

Guidelines for Implantation

- Outpatient procedure
- In operating room under general anesthesia with endotracheal intubation
- Three consecutive weekly sessions
- Concurrent chemotherapy with capecitabine

Procedure Advice

- Induction of general anesthesia with endotracheal intubation
- Verify the tumor extent endoscopically
- Identify the proximal and distal extent of the tumor fluoroscopically
- Place radiopaque fiducial markers on the skin surface (Fig. 10.5)
- Insert a guidewire through the scope into the stomach, and then remove the endoscope
- Insert the applicator into the esophagus over the guidewire into the treatment position (Fig. 10.6)
- If using the Ancer Esophageal Applicator, center the applicator by inflating the five balloons

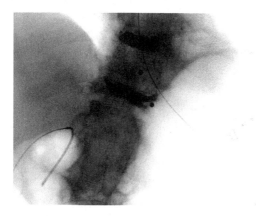

Fig. 10.5. Guidewire in the esophagus with externally placed BBs on the chest wall marking the extent of the tumor

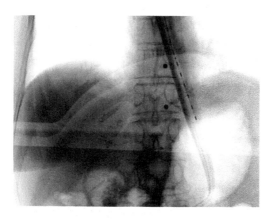

Fig. 10.6. Bougie catheter with dummy wire showing markers at 1 cm intervals in the esophagus. The externally placed BBs demarcate the extent of the tumor

- Remove the guidewire
- Visualize the applicator using the integrated X-ray markers and 10 % CT contrast in the balloons

Treatment Planning

- Using bougie catheter, plan is based on linear distance to cover the tumor region delineated by the external markers with additional margin (Fig. 10.7)
- If using the Ancer Esophageal Applicator, can perform a CT scan for treatment planning (Fig. 10.4)
- MRI-based simulation, if available, helps to improve soft tissue contrast for tumor delineation and allows for delivery of more conformal dose to target lesions
- Contour the target and surrounding healthy esophagus
- Dose is prescribed to a depth from the surface of the catheter, with prescription depth determined on the basis of clinical assessment of tumor thickness

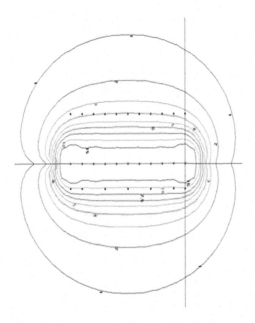

FIG. 10.7. 2D isodose contours for a single HDR treatment using the bougie applicator; dose was prescribed to 7 mm, with mucosal surface limited to 900 cGy

- Maximum tolerated dose is currently being determined in the setting of an ongoing phase I clinical trial (MSKCC)
  - Dose prescription and fractionation: 3 fractions at 5–6.5 Gy/fraction
- Treatment plan is generated to provide the specified dose
- Recommend dose constraint of mucosal surface dose to 8–10 Gy with an upper limit of 12 Gy (Table 10.1).

Treatment Delivery

- After review and approval of the plan, verify applicator positioning and connect patient to a remote afterloader in shielded room
- Clear room
- Deliver treatment
- Survey patient for residual activity
- Remove applicator
- Reverse anesthesia
- For the subsequent two weekly treatments, use the original CT or fluoroscopic-based plan
  - Insert the applicator under fluoroscopic guidance
  - Positioning of the applicator can be verified by matching the treatment length to fluoroscopically placed surface markers, and by measuring the insertion distance from the incisors using integrated insertion markers
  - For some patients, applicator positioning may also be verified with respect to a pre-implanted fiducial marker
  - After confirmation of applicator positioning, deliver treatment

Follow-Up and Assessment of Response

- Frequent follow-up is recommended to survey for potential recurrence
- Clinical Assessment of Response (Fig. 10.8a–c)
  - Follow-up by Radiation Oncology and Surgery departments every 2–3 months for the first 6 months, then every 6 months until 2 years after completion of brachytherapy
  - Evaluation by upper GI endoscopy with ultrasound at 3 and 9 months to assess response
  - During follow-up, any nodularity, mass, ulcer, or radiographic abnormality should prompt consideration of a biopsy
- Radiographic Assessment of Tumor Response After Brachytherapy
  - CT chest/abdomen imaging at 1, 3, 6, 9, and 12 months

Toxicity

- Acute Toxicity
  - Dysphagia
  - Cough

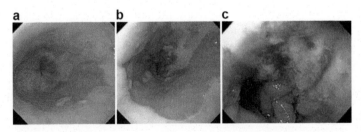

FIG. 10.8. Endoscopic view of (**a**) pretreatment residual tumor, (**b**) 1-week post first fraction (5 Gy), and (**c**) 3 months posttreatment (15Gy): mild asymptomatic stenosis at irradiated esophagojejunostomy site, consistent with radiation effect

- ■ Esophageal perforation
- ■ Esophageal ulceration
- ■ Fatigue
- ■ Sore throat from endotracheal intubation
- ■ Late Toxicity
  - ■ Chronic Dysphagia
  - ■ Esophageal stricture
  - ■ Esophageal perforation
  - ■ Esophageal ulceration
  - ■ Tracheoesophageal fistula

References

1. American Cancer Society. Cancer facts & figures 2016. Atlanta: American Cancer Society; 2016.
2. Herskovic A, Martz K, al-Sarraf M, et al. Combined chemotherapy and radiotherapy compared with radiotherapy alone in patients with cancer of the esophagus. N Engl J Med. 1992;326:1593–8.
3. al-Sarraf M, Martz K, Herskovic A, et al. Progress report of combined chemoradiotherapy versus radiotherapy alone in patients with esophageal cancer: an intergroup study. J Clin Oncol. 1997;15:277–84.
4. Cooper JS, Guo MD, Herskovic A, et al. Chemoradiotherapy of locally advanced esophageal cancer: long-term follow-up of a prospective randomized trial (RTOG 85-01). Radiation Therapy Oncology Group. JAMA. 1999;281:1623–7.
5. Tepper J, Krasna MJ, Niedzwiecki D, et al. Phase III trial of trimodality therapy with cisplatin, fluorouracil, radiotherapy, and surgery compared with surgery alone for esophageal cancer: CALGB 9781. J Clin Oncol. 2008;26:1086–92.
6. Stahl M, Walz MK, Stuschke M, et al. Phase III comparison of preoperative chemotherapy compared with chemoradiotherapy in patients with locally advanced adenocarcinoma of the esophagogastric junction. J Clin Oncol. 2009;27:851–6.
7. Gaspar LE, Nag S, Herskovic A, et al. American Brachytherapy Society (ABS) consensus guidelines for brachytherapy for esophageal cancer. Int J Radiat Oncol Biol Phys. 1997;38:127–32.

8. Hishikawa Y, Kurisu K, Taniguchi M, et al. High-dose-rate intra-luminal brachytherapy for esophageal cancer: 10 years experience in Hyogo College of Medicine. Radiother Oncol. 1991;21:107–14.

9. Gaspar LE, Winter K, Kocha WI, et al. A phase I/II study of external beam radiation, brachytherapy, and concurrent chemotherapy for patients with localized carcinoma of the esophagus (Radiation Therapy Oncology Group Study 9207). Cancer. 2000;88:988–95.

10. Sharma V, Mahantshetty U, Dinshaw KA, et al. Palliation of advanced/recurrent esophageal carcinoma with high-dose-rate brachytherapy. Int J Radiat Oncol Biol Phys. 2002;52:310–5.

11. Akagi Y, Hirokawa Y, Kagemoto M, et al. Optimum fractionation for high-dose-rate endoesophageal brachytherapy following external irradiation of early stage esophageal cancer. Int J Radiat Oncol Biol Phys. 1999;43:525–30.

12. Vuong T, Szego P, David M, et al. The safety and usefulness of high-dose-rate endoluminal brachytherapy as a boost in the treatment of patients with esophageal cancer with external beam radiation with or without chemotherapy. Int J Radiat Oncol Biol Phys. 2005;63:758–64.

13. Nonoshita T, Sasaki T, Hirata H, et al. High-dose-rate brachytherapy for previously irradiated patients with recurrent esophageal cancer. Radiat Med. 2007;25:373–7.

14. Cox BW, Jackson A, Hunt M, et al. Esophageal toxicity from high-dose, single-fraction paraspinal stereotactic radiosurgery. Int J Radiat Oncol Biol Phys. 2012;83:e661–7.

15. Folkert M, Cohen G, Wu A, et al. Endoluminal high-dose-rate brachytherapy for early stage and recurrent esophageal cancer in medically inoperable patients. Brachytherapy. 2013;12:463–70.

Chapter 11
Gastrointestinal Brachytherapy: Anal and Rectal Cancer

Supriya K. Jain and Karyn A. Goodman

Introduction

Rationale for Brachytherapy in Rectal Cancer

- According to the American Cancer Society, approximately 39,220 cases of rectal cancer are diagnosed annually in the United States [1]
- Standard management of rectal cancer
  - Stage I: Total mesorectal excision (TME) alone
  - Stage II–III: Neoadjuvant chemoradiation therapy (CRT) → TME → adjuvant chemotherapy
- Local recurrence rates after standard management are <10 % [2]
- TME provides excellent disease control in the management of primary rectal cancer; however, it may have an unfavorable impact on patients' functioning
  - Associated with potentially serious sequelae, with significant consequence on function and quality of life [2–5]

S.K. Jain, MD, MHS • K.A. Goodman, MD, MS (✉)
Department of Radiation Oncology, University of Colorado School of Medicine, Aurora, CO, USA
e-mail: Supriya.jain@ucdenver.edu; Karyn.goodman@ucdenver.edu

© Springer International Publishing AG 2017 289
J. Mayadev et al. (eds.), *Handbook of Image-Guided Brachytherapy*, DOI 10.1007/978-3-319-44827-5_11

- ▫ Surgery for low-lying rectal cancer can result in a permanent or temporary colostomy
- ▫ Can result in the development of permanent urinary incontinence, fecal incontinence, or sexual dysfunction [6–8]

- Approximately 20 % of patients have a pathologic complete response to preoperative chemoradiation, thus more recently, there has been interest in nonoperative management for patients who have a clinical complete response to CRT
- However, 80 % of patients may still harbor residual tumor cells and will benefit from surgical resection of the tumor
- While patients who have had a complete tumor response to CRT may experience excellent outcomes in the absence of TME, patients with biopsy-proven residual or recurrent disease after external beam radiation therapy ± chemotherapy are at high risk of local progression if surgery is omitted from their management
- Nonetheless, TME may not be performed either due to prohibitive surgical risk or patient refusal
  - Elderly patients and patients with multiple comorbidities may not be good candidates for radical rectal surgery
  - Some patients refuse any treatment that will leave them with a stoma, including standard-of-care TME
- Endorectal brachytherapy can be delivered to address local persistence or recurrence of disease in the rectal wall to improve local control for patients who are unable to undergo a radical rectal surgery or have refused a stoma. The goal is to deliver a high focal dose to the tumor cells and achieve a pathologic complete response

Rationale for Brachytherapy in Anal Cancer

- It is estimated that approximately 8080 people in the United States will be diagnosed with anal cancer in 2016 [1]
- Unlike rectal cancer, primary anal cancer is managed non operatively with chemoradiation alone
- The standard treatment, introduced by Nigro, involves concurrent external beam radiation therapy (EBRT), 5-Fluorouracil (5-FU), and mitomycin-C (MMC)
- Local failure after completion of this regimen ranges from approximately 10–25 %, with higher rates in patients unable to receive any component of the Nigro regimen. Some patients also have persistent disease after definitive chemoradiation
- Salvage of local recurrence or persistent disease is typically performed with an abdominoperineal resection (APR)
- If patients with persistent or locally recurrent anal cancer decline or are unfit for APR, endorectal/endoanal brachytherapy may represent an alternative option to provide local disease control

HDR Brachytherapy in Rectal and Anal Cancer

HDR Brachytherapy in the Management of Rectal Cancer

- The use of brachytherapy in the treatment of rectal cancer dates back to the early 1900s
  - One of the initial approaches involved application of a radium source internally, within the rectum [9, 10]

- Contact X-ray therapy, using a low-energy X-ray endorectal tube to deliver a high dose of radiation to the tumor, has demonstrated efficacy in controlling small, early-stage rectal tumors without external beam radiation. For many decades, contact X-ray therapy (CXRT) alone was used to effectively treat T1N0 rectal cancer [11, 12]. While this type of superficial radiotherapy does not utilize a radioactive source, the technique of applying high-dose radiotherapy directly to the tumor works in a way very similar to brachytherapy. CXRT is performed with a 50 kVp endorectal tube that delivers high doses of radiation to the tumor, while rapid dose falloff ensures low doses to deeper tissues. Because this approach provides only superficial dose, it is insufficient to control $\geq$T2 or node-positive disease. In this setting, a combination of CXRT and/or ^{192}Ir high-dose rate (HDR) brachytherapy with EBRT may be used to deliver adequate dose
- Many groups, especially in Europe, have reported on combination external beam radiotherapy followed by a "boost" to the tumor using brachytherapy in patients with locally advanced rectal cancer
  - French physician Jean Papillon (University of Lyon) was one of the first clinicians to combine endocavitary irradiation and EBRT. He treated 71 elderly patients with T2–T3 adenocarcinoma with cobalt arc therapy (30 Gy in 10 fractions over 13 days) followed 2 months later by CXRT (25 Gy) and an ^{192}Ir implant (20–30 Gy). The tumors were staged without imaging. Papillon reported that "the tolerance of this treatment was generally good. Benign and superficial radionecrosis, which healed spontaneously, was observed in five cases." At a minimum follow-up of 3 years, 46 patients (64.7 %) were alive and well, and 44 of these patients reported normal bowel function. The rate of cancer-specific death was 16 % at 5 years [13]

■ Maingon et al. reported on 151 rectal cancer patients
   who received radiotherapy alone with curative
   intent. By clinical examination, 76 (50 %) had T1
   lesions, 62 (41 %) T2, and 13 (9 %) T3. Of the 26
   patients evaluated by endorectal ultrasound
   (ERUS), 6 (23 %) had pelvic lymphadenopathy.
   CXRT was given to 129 patients (69 %), brachytherapy to 45 (30 %), and EBRT to 34 (22.5 %). No
   acute grade ≥3 toxicity was observed. Ten patients
   (7 %) experienced late grade ≥3 toxicity, 3 of whom
   required a colostomy (1 for rectal stenosis, 1 for
   rectal bleeding, and 1 for fecal incontinence). A
   clinical complete response was achieved in 93 % of
   patients at 3 months after treatment. Ultimately,
   local failure was observed in 50 cases (28 %). The
   risk of local recurrence increased with tumor size
   and tethering and with omission of EBRT. After
   salvage surgery, the local control rate for the entire
   cohort was 82 %. The 5-year disease-specific survival was 66 %. Of the 124 patients available for
   long-term follow-up, sphincter preservation was
   obtained in 104 (84 %), 102 (98 %) of whom had
   normal sphincter function [14]

■ Gerard et al. published a pilot study of 63 patients
   with T2-3N0-1M0, mid-to distal rectal cancer who
   were treated with radiotherapy alone. In this cohort,
   41 patients (65 %) had T2 disease, 22 (35 %) T3, 45
   (71 %) N0, and 18 (29 %) N1. Most patients
   (53/63 = 84 %) were staged by ERUS. All patients
   received CXRT (median 80 Gy in 3 fractions over
   21 days), followed by EBRT (39 Gy in 13 fractions
   over 17 days) with a concomitant boost (4 Gy in 4
   fractions). After a 4–6-week interval, all but 7
   patients received a low-dose rate ^{192}Ir implant
   (20 Gy over 22 h). There was no instance of grade
   ≥3 toxicity. Although most patients experienced
   acute proctitis, no treatment was interrupted
   because of intolerance or severe toxicity.
   Intermittent late rectal bleeding occurred in 24

patients (38 %), one of whom required occasional blood transfusions. Among the 39 living patients at the time of analysis, bowel function was scored as excellent in 19, good in 17, and fair in 3, based on the Memorial Sloan Kettering Cancer Center (MSKCC) scale. At a median follow-up time of 54 months, the rate of local tumor control was 63 %. Five patients required an abdominoperineal resection (APR), because they had residual disease at 2 months after treatment. Local recurrence was observed in 18 patients (28.5 %) who initially had a clinical complete response; 5 were salvaged by APR and 1 by a second course of CXRT. After primary or salvage treatment, the ultimate rate of pelvic control was 73 %. The 5-year overall survival rate was 64.4 % for the entire cohort and 78 % for the subset of 42 patients aged <80 years (84 % for T2 and 53 % for T3 lesions) [15]

■ Aumock et al. reported the experience at Washington University treating 199 patients with endocavitary RT±EBRT. The majority of tumors were freely mobile to palpation ($n=128$), ≤3 cm in greatest dimension ($n=136$), without clinical evidence of nodal metastases ($n=177$), and well to moderately differentiated ($n=190$). ERUS was used to evaluate 77 patients (39 %). Early during the study period, some patients received CXRT alone; however, an interim analysis revealed that tumor control improved with EBRT. Therefore, all patients treated after 1987 received EBRT (mean 45 Gy in 25 fractions) followed 6 weeks later by CXRT (mean 60 Gy divided in 2 fractions over 2 weeks). The primary toxicity was proctitis ($n=19$) that typically resolved within 10 months. Two patients required transfusions for rectal bleeding and 2 required dilation of a rectal stricture. Local recurrence was observed in 58 patients (29 %), 20 of whom were effectively salvaged surgically. Thus, after primary or salvage treatment, the ultimate pelvic control rate was 81 % [16]

■ Hoskin et al. reported on 50 patients who received endorectal HDR brachytherapy at a single institution. The majority of patients were elderly and frail (median age 82 years) and were therefore poor surgical candidates. Patients who had received prior CRT were treated to 12 Gy in 2 fractions ($n=18$); those who had not received prior EBRT were treated with a single 10 Gy fraction for palliation ($n=22$) or with 6 Gy fractions up to 36 Gy ($n=8$). Among the 25 patients with follow-up information, 14 achieved complete clinical regression, 7 partial (>50 %) regression, and 4 minimal (<50 %) regression. The authors reported significant palliation of mucous discharge, bleeding, pain, and diarrhea. In 2 patients who were treated palliatively with a single fraction of 10 Gy, the treatment was repeated 10 months later for recurrent symptoms and again provided good relief with no additional toxicity [17]

■ Taken together, these groups have shown that a combination of endorectal brachytherapy and EBRT is feasible and safe in the nonoperative management of rectal cancer

■ The most common side effect is acute and late proctitis Patients typically maintain good bowel function

■ Furthermore, these studies have demonstrated good rates of tumor control [13–17]

■ The feasibility and efficacy of endorectal brachytherapy have been evaluated in the preoperative setting.

  ■ Vuong et al. reported on 100 patients with T2 to early T4, operable rectal cancer treated with high-dose endorectal brachytherapy using 3-dimensional treatment planning (26 Gy in 4 consecutive daily fractions) followed in 6–8 weeks by definitive surgery. From 1998 to 2005, those with pathologically positive nodes received postoperative EBRT

(45 Gy in 25 fractions) with concurrent 5-FU. By ERUS and MRI, the clinical staging of the tumors were T2 ($n=3$), T3 ($n=93$), T4 ($n=4$), N0 ($n=58$), and N1–N2 ($n=42$). Ninety-six patients underwent surgery; 2 refused the operation based on a normal ERUS after treatment; 2 died before surgery, one from a stroke and the other from a myocardial infarction. Acute toxicity related to brachytherapy was limited to grade 2 proctitis in 99 patients, with 1 patient receiving grade 3 proctitis requiring transfusion. One patient who refused surgery developed mild rectal stenosis but did not require dilation. Of the group that underwent surgery, 29 % were ypT0N0-2, 34 % demonstrated residual tumor, and 37 % had micro-foci of residual disease. Only one patient had microscopic positive margins; this patient had no evidence of disease at five year follow-up. Postoperative adjuvant external beam therapy and chemotherapy were given in 27 of the 31 patients with positive nodes. The median follow-up time was 60 months. At 5 years, the actual local recurrence rate was 5 %, disease-free survival was 65 %, and the overall survival rate was 70 % [18]

- This cohort was updated in 2015; a total of 483 patients received neoadjuvant endorectal HDR brachytherapy alone; 43 received postoperative external beam radiation therapy. The complete sterilization rate was 27 % and the rate of positive nodes was 30.7 %. Median follow-up time was 63 months. Actuarial local recurrence rate was 4.8 %. Disease-free survival was 65.5 %. Overall survival rate was 72.8 % [19]

- The authors concluded that HDR endorectal brachytherapy is an effective neoadjuvant treatment for patients with resectable rectal cancer that offers excellent local control with a favorable toxicity profile [18, 19]

Ongoing Clinical Trials

- Phase I, Dose Escalation Trial of Endoluminal High-Dose Rate Brachytherapy with Concurrent Chemotherapy for Rectal or Anal Cancer in Patients with Recurrent Disease or Undergoing Nonoperative Management
  - Ongoing single-institution (MSKCC) trial involving anorectal cancer patients to determine the *maximum tolerated dose* and assess rates of acute and late toxicity after endorectal brachytherapy with concurrent capecitabine or 5-fluorouracil
  - Patients who previously received pelvic EBRT ± chemotherapy and will not undergo surgery
  - Dose escalation 1200 cGy in a systematic fashion
    - Three dose tiers
      - 1500 cGy (500 cGy per fraction)
      - 1800 cGy (600 cGy per fraction)
      - 2100 cGy (700 cGy per fraction)
  - Brachytherapy will be administered in 3 fractions, 1 fraction/week
  - Dose will be prescribed to the minimum peripheral dose, or the dose-line encompassing the tumor as contoured on the CT or MRI. In addition to brachytherapy, patients will receive concurrent capecitabine or 5-FU
  - The primary objective of this trial is to establish the maximum tolerated dose (MTD) and to determine toxicity rates of endorectal brachytherapy with concurrent 5-FU-based chemotherapy
- Phase II, Study of High-Dose Rate Endorectal Brachytherapy in the Treatment of Locally Advanced Low Rectal Cancer (Sidney Kimmel Cancer Institute — Johns Hopkins)
  - Ongoing Phase II study (but no longer recruiting participants) of locally advanced resectable rectal cancer patients (T2N1 or T3N0-1) examining *pathologic response* of neoadjuvant high-dose endorectal

brachytherapy in comparison to standard-of-care neoadjuvant chemoradiation
- Daily dose of 6.5 Gy over 4 consecutive days
- Primary Endpoint: Pathologic complete response. Secondary endpoints include biologic and radiographic predictors of response to therapy, adverse events (gastrointestinal toxicity), quality of life as measured by the QLQ-C30, and tumor regression/response
- Goal was to enroll 30 patients; will report primary outcome in 2020

- Phase II: CORRECT (Chemoradiation OR Brachytherapy for RECTal Cancer) (PI: Sidney Kimmel Cancer Institute—Johns Hopkins—Multiple institutions)
  - Ongoing Phase II study (currently recruiting participants)
  - Neoadjuvant IMRT with concurrent capecitabine vs. neoadjuvant endorectal HDR brachytherapy (6.5 Gy daily over 4 consecutive days)
  - To be followed by FOLFOX6 x 12 cycles followed by surgical resection
  - Primary outcome: pathologic complete response rate
  - Secondary outcomes: biologic and radiographic predictors of response, acute and long-term toxicity, quality of life, sphincter preservation rates, locoregional control, distant metastases, and overall survival
  - Goal enrollment 138 patients; estimated completion 2018

HDR Brachytherapy in the Management of Anal Cancer

- No reported series focusing specifically on the use of brachytherapy to treat recurrent anal cancer; however, several groups have reported their experience using

EBRT with an HDR brachytherapy boost in the upfront management of primary anal cancer

■ As one example, Oehler-Janne et al. treated 81 anal cancer patients with EBRT (45 Gy in 25 fractions) followed either immediately by an EBRT boost (14.4 Gy in 8 fractions) or 3 weeks later by an interstitial ^{192}Ir interstitial brachytherapy boost (14 Gy in 7 fractions over 3 days). There was a lower rate of acute dermatitis and hematologic toxicity in the brachytherapy group. There was no difference in other acute toxicities, late toxicity, or quality of life between the two cohorts. Chronic toxicity in the brachytherapy group consisted of grade ≥ 2 proctitis in 19 % of patients and grade 1–2 incontinence in 18 %. At 5 years, the local failure rate was 10.3 % in the brachytherapy group and 15.4 % in the EBRT group ($P = 0.5$) [20]

■ Kapp et al. treated 39 patients with T1-2N0-2M0 anal cancer with split-course EBRT (50–50.4 Gy) ± chemotherapy (5-FU and MMC) and an integrated ^{192}Ir brachytherapy boost (6 Gy) during the 1–2 week split. Patients who achieved a partial tumor response ($n = 7$) received a second ^{192}Ir brachytherapy boost (6 Gy) after a 6–8 week delay. Brachytherapy was provided with interstitial needles and/or an endorectal cylinder. Acute toxicity among brachytherapy patients was similar to that of patients receiving EBRT ± chemotherapy alone. Late complications included proctitis ($n = 2$), occasional sphincter dysfunction ($n = 1$), and circumscribed ulcers at the site of the primary tumor ($n = 7$). The rate of 5-year local control was 76 % and colostomy-free survival was 73 %. For the patients in whom the anus was conserved, full continence was recorded in 28/30 (93 %) [21]

■ These groups have demonstrated the feasibility and safety of using HDR brachytherapy to treat cancers of the anal canal

Timing for Endorectal Brachytherapy

- Definitive treatment for small rectal (T1, T2) tumor
- Neoadjuvant therapy for patients with newly diag-
  nosed rectal cancer with previous pelvic radiation
- After   EBRT ± chemotherapy,   concurrent   with
  capecitabine or 5-FU
- Medically inoperable rectal tumor
- Patients requiring an APR and refuse
- Palliative treatment for patients with Stage IV
  disease
- Salvage for small recurrent, anal cancers

Goal for Endorectal Brachytherapy
of Anorectum

- **Local control:** If patients with locally persistent or
  recurrent disease after chemoradiation decline to
  undergo an abdominoperineal resection (APR) or are
  unfit for radical surgery, endorectal brachytherapy
  may represent an option for providing local disease
  control. Brachytherapy enables delivery of high-dose
  radiation directly to a rectal tumor, with relative sparing of the surrounding normal tissues. In these patients,
  brachytherapy can be employed with the goal of
  improving complete response and avoiding radical
  resection. Given the conformal dose distribution,
  treatment may be provided in several large fractions,
  providing a radiobiological advantage over conven-
  tionally fractionated RT
- **Improved quality of life:** Endorectal brachytherapy
  can be applied to improve outcomes and individualize
  treatment of patients with rectal cancer. Given the
  morbidity of radical surgery, and its long-term impact
  on quality of life, selective nonoperative treatment
  may be an alternative in some cases. With appropriate
  use of endorectal brachytherapy, rectal surgery may be

selectively omitted from the management of some rectal cancer patients. These include individuals for whom surgery poses a prohibitive risk, or who refuse to have an APR, or whose cancers respond dramatically to chemoradiation

■ **Palliative:** Endorectal brachytherapy also serves a palliative purpose in the management of patients with metastatic disease who may benefit from local therapy, but for whom radical resection is inappropriate. With advances in treatment options for rectal cancer and continued collaboration with our colleagues across disciplines, endorectal brachytherapy provides an additional option to better tailor therapies based on patient risk factoring and tumor characteristics, taking into account the impact of treatment on each patient's quality of life

Selection Criteria for Implantation

■ Palpable or MRI-visible low-lying tumor
■ Tumor may be concentric or eccentric
■ Maximum tumor length of 7 cm at time of brachytherapy start to allow accessibility by 10 cm applicator
■ Rectal: preferably no invasion of anal canal (increased risk of anal necrosis). Invasion of anal canal permitted for recurrent anal primary

Patients Who Are Not Candidates for Endorectal Brachytherapy

■ Patients with contraindications to general anesthesia
■ Proximal rectal tumors (>10 cm from the anal verge)
■ ECOG performance status 3

Medical Operability

- Comprehensive evaluation including
  - Within 45 days of treatment start:
    - History and Physical examination
    - Performance status
    - Weight
    - Review of current medications
    - Assessment of baseline comorbidities, including baseline pain assessment
    - Imaging:
      - MRI of the pelvis with DCE and DWI series (unless contraindicated)
      - CT of the chest/abdomen/pelvis as a baseline to evaluate for systemic disease
  - Within 30 days of treatment start:
    - Quality of life assessments: EORTC QLQ-C30, EuroQol 5D-5L, and BFI assessments
    - Standard preoperative evaluation including determination of normal cardiac function
      - No active coronary artery disease
      - No New York Heart Association class II, III, or IV disease
      - No arrhythmia requiring treatment
    - Proctoscopy, with photograph of the tumor if possible
    - Anesthesia consent
  - Within 14 days of treatment start
    - Labs: CBC, PT and PTT, CMP, CEA (for rectal cancer patients only), and pregnancy test drawn within 14 days prior to procedure start
      - ANC ≥ 1.5 cells/mm^3 and PLT $\geq 100,000$/mm^3
      - Adequate Renal function: Creatinine $<1.5\times$ the upper limit of normal (ULN) or calculated creatinine clearance of ≥ 50 cc/min
      - Adequate Hepatic functions: Bilirubin less than 1.5 mg/dL; (except in patients with Gilbert's Syndrome, who must have a total

bilirubin less than 3.0 mg/dL); AST or ALT <3× ULN, or <5× ULN if known liver metastases

Applicator

- There are several options for anorectal applicators including Varian's Capri™ rectal and vaginal applicator (Varian, Palo Alto, CA, USA), the Nucletron® Intracavitary Mold Applicator Set (Elekta AB, Stockholm, Sweden), and the Anorectal (AR) applicator (Ancer Medical, Hialeah, FL, USA)

The Capri™ Applicator (Fig. 11.1)

- Allows for highly asymmetric dose distributions
- One central channel and 12 peripheral channels
- Barium sulfate to allow simple catheter detection
- Inflatable with air or saline
- Internal markers allow for identification of catheters

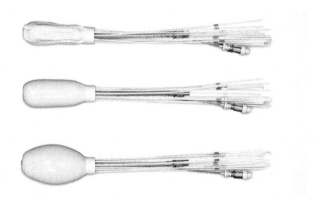

FIG. 11.1. Varian's Capri™ rectal and vaginal applicator (Used with permission of Varian, Palo Alto, CA, USA)

- Soft silicone exterior
- Single use
- CT Compatible

The Intracavitary Mold Applicator Set (IMAS) from Nucletron®

- Made of a flexible material with several channels for the radioactive source
- One central catheter and eight peripheral catheters, enabling delivery of a variety of dose patterns, limiting normal tissue toxicity, and improving dose delivery to the tumor
- Markers on the handle, the base, and one or more catheters of the device assist with positioning
- High torsional stiffness prevents twisting during placement
- Tip: A saline-inflatable balloon may help to push the applicator flush against the rectal mucosa

The Anorectal (AR) Applicator [22, 23] (Fig. 11.2)

- Multichannel applicator with two concentric balloons
- The inner balloon supports eight radially symmetric source lumens; the compliant outer balloon expands to

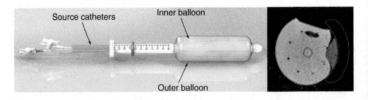

FIG. 11.2. Anorectal (AR) applicator (*left*) and phantom study to simulate a protruding tumor structure (*right*). (*Left*: Used with permission of Ancer Medical, Hialeah, FL, USA; *Right*: Used with permission from Cohen, Gilad N. et al. Evaluation of a New MRI Compatible Brachytherapy Ano-rectal Applicator. Brachytherapy 2014; 13: S48)

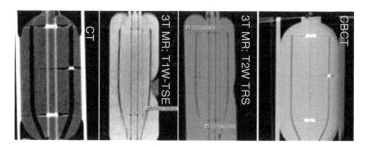

FIG. 11.3. Anorectal (AR) applicator visualized in CT, and T1 and T2 MRI sequences. (Courtesy of Gil'ad Cohen, PhD, Memorial Sloan Kettering Cancer Center, NY, NY)

separate the normal rectal mucosal wall and the source lumens yet deform around a firm, exophytic rectal mass
- The effective treatment zone of the applicator, in which the source lumens maintain the cylindrical geometry, is 10 cm long and is delineated by two central markers for positioning and treatment verification
- Single use
- Reduces the dose to the contralateral rectal wall to less than 50 % of prescription [22]
- CT and MRI compatible (Fig. 11.3)

Guidelines for Implantation

- At least 4 weeks from prior major surgery or radiotherapy (recommend waiting 4 weeks after EBRT prior to implant)
- On an outpatient basis
- MSKCC approach: In the operating room under general anesthesia
- Canadian approach: In operating or procedure room without general anesthesia
- Can be delivered once weekly for 3 consecutive weeks or a daily dose of 6.5 Gy over 4 consecutive days

Pre-procedure Advice

- Golytely prep prior to each procedure with water enema the morning of the procedure
- Semi-sterile procedure
- Antibiotics at the time of the procedure
- Exam under anesthesia prior to each procedure. Patient in dorsal lithotomy position with legs up in whole leg stirrups
- Colorectal surgeon present at first fraction to place gold fiducial markers above and below the tumor

Procedure Tips

- Identify and mark extent of tumor
- Insert and secure endorectal applicator
- In the event of circumferential narrowing that prevents insertion of the endorectal applicator, a single-channel Bougie applicator (similar to a Savary Dilator with a single internal lumen for placement of the HDR catheter) has been used

Treatment Planning

- CT and MRI will be obtained for treatment planning to develop a conformal radiation dose specific to the rectal tumor, thus minimizing the dose to the bladder and small bowel [23] (Fig. 11.4)
- Prescription dose and fractionation:
  - MSKCC approach: 3 fractions, each spaced apart by 7 days (±1 day)
    - Clinical trial for dose escalation currently ongoing to evaluate maximum tolerated dose: 12–21 Gy in 4–7 Gy per fraction

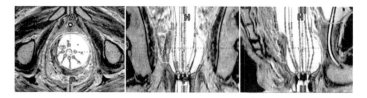

FIG. 11.4. Tumor with respect to the applicator and source lumens. Orthogonal views of an MRI with the water-filled applicator in situ. The GTV (yellow) is seen pressing into the outer baffle. (Courtesy of Gil'ad Cohen, PhD, Memorial Sloan Kettering Cancer Center, NY, NY.)

- Canadian approach: Daily dose of 6.5 Gy over 4 consecutive days
- Structures to be contoured
    - Gross tumor volume (GTV)
    - Normal rectum
    - Applicator
    - Bladder
    - Urethra
    - Bowel
- Dose constraints for organs at risk
    - Rectal surface Dmax < 15 Gy/fraction
    - Bladder Dmax < 5 Gy/fraction
    - Urethra Dmax < 4 Gy/fraction
    - Bowel < 4 Gy/fraction
- Treatment planning will be performed with computerized dosimetry. The dose will be prescribed to the isodose line that best covers the target volume, while minimizing dose to adjacent normal tissue
- A dose volume histogram (DVH) is generated and reviewed [23] (Fig. 11.5)

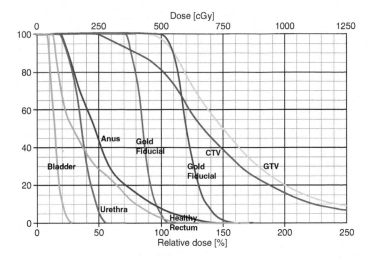

Fig. 11.5. DVH for the plan in Fig. 11.4 shows GTV (*yellow*), CTV (*magenta*, an expansion of the GTV overlapping some healthy rectal and anal muscle), anus (*blue*), healthy rectum (*cyan*), urethra (*dark green*), bladder (*light green*), and superior and inferior gold fiducial markers (*red*). (Courtesy of Gil'ad Cohen, PhD, Memorial Sloan Kettering Cancer Center, NY, NY)

Treatment Delivery

■ Prior to each treatment, fluoroscopic imaging is used to verify catheter positioning and position/rotation of the applicator and confirm the treatment geometry using rigid registration of the CBCT and planning MRI. After registration of the applicator images, positioning was evaluated based on the match of the pre-implanted gold fiducial markers [22, 23] (Figs. 11.6 and 11.7)

■ Despite nonrigid nature of the applicators and use of new applicator at each treatment session, treatment geometry should be reproducible within 2.5 mm [23]

■ HDR brachytherapy will be administered using an HDR afterloader with an ^{192}Ir source in a shielded room

■ Following treatment planning, the HDR afterloader will be attached to the applicator

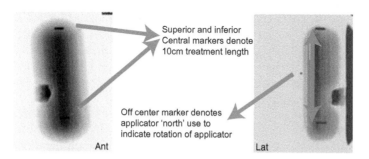

Superior and inferior
Central markers denote
10cm treatment length

Off center marker denotes
applicator 'north' use to
indicate rotation of applicator

Ant

Lat

FIG. 11.6. Pre-implanted gold fiducial markers (*blue arrows*) as seen on CT in a phantom. (Courtesy of Gil'ad Cohen, PhD, Memorial Sloan Kettering Cancer Center, NY, NY)

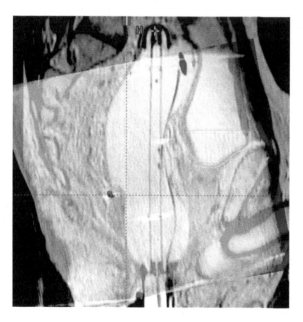

FIG. 11.7. Pretreatment verification. Planning MRI is registered to pretreatment CBCT. Built-in applicator fiducials (*green*) are matched. The quality of registration is assessed based on the match of fiducials placed in the patient (*red*). (Courtesy of Gil'ad Cohen, PhD, Memorial Sloan Kettering Cancer Center, NY, NY)

- After completion of treatment, the applicator will be removed, anesthesia will be reversed, and the patient will be extubated or monitored anesthesia care (MAC) with local anesthesia together with sedation and analgesia is completed. Epidural or local anesthesia may be appropriate in some patients
- After adequate observation (≥ 1 h) to ensure safety, the patient will be discharged home if appropriate
- If discharge is not deemed appropriate on the day of the procedure, the patient may be admitted overnight for further observation and management

Image Guidance Utilization

Use of Image Guidance Pre-procedure

- MRI of the pelvis with T1, T2, DCE and DWI series
- CT pelvis

Types of Image Guidance to Potentially Use and Pros/Cons

- Tumor is better seen on MRI
- Gold fiducials are better seen on CT; gold appears black on MRI

Use of Image Guidance During Procedure

- If MR simulator available in department, this can be utilized to evaluate placement of applicator and can be fused with CT images for contouring
- An O-arm can be used in the OR to obtain a CT scan to confirm placement of the applicator prior to delivery of treatment

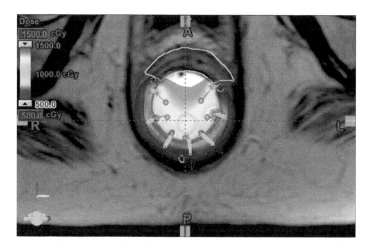

FIG. 11.8. Distribution of implant showing sparing of the contralateral rectal wall in a patient. (King, M, Cohen G, Wu, A et al. Prospective Evaluation of Endoluminal High Dose Rate Brachytherapy with Concurrent Chemotherapy for Rectal or Anal Cancer Patients: Initial Clinical Results. Brachytherapy May–June, 2016; 15,Supplement 1:S142)

Evaluation and Distribution of Implantation

- A dose volume histogram (DVH) is generated and reviewed (Fig. 11.5)
- Isodose lines are reviewed to confirm GTV coverage, identify potential hot spots, cold spots, and doses to the normal tissues [24] (Fig. 11.8)

Follow-up and Assessment of Response

- Clinical Assessment of Response: More frequent follow-up is recommended to survey for potential recurrence
    - Follow-up by Radiation Oncology and Surgery departments every 3 months for the first 6 months,

> then every 6 months until 2 years after completion of brachytherapy
>
> ■ Evaluated by proctoscopy at each of these time points to assess response
> ■ During follow-up, any nodularity, mass, ulcer, or radiographic abnormality should prompt consideration of a biopsy

■ Radiographic assessment of Tumor Response after Brachytherapy

> ■ Prior to treatment and at 3, 6, and 12 months (±3 weeks) after the completion of brachytherapy, Pelvic MRI with DCE and DWI series
> ■ At baseline and at 6, 12, and 24 months (±3 weeks) after brachytherapy, CT of the chest/abdomen/pelvis to evaluate for distant disease progression

■ Re-staging of rectal cancer patients may be difficult after RT, due to inflammation and fibrosis. Many researchers have evaluated how to accurately identify a complete tumor response to chemoradiation therapy (CRT)

> ■ Digital rectal examination (DRE) is insufficient
>
> > ■ In a prospective trial of 94 patients with T3, T4, or N1 rectal cancer who were evaluated by the same surgeon at diagnosis and preoperatively, only 21 % (3 of 14) who had a pCR were correctly identified by preoperative DRE. Furthermore, the extent of pathological downstaging was underestimated in almost 80 % of patients [25]
>
> ■ Endoscopy may be used to evaluate the rectum; however, biopsies obtained after CRT must be interpreted with caution
>
> > ■ One group found the negative predictive value of a benign biopsy after CRT to be only 21 % [26]. Furthermore, regional nodal disease may persist despite a complete response of the primary tumor. In one study, 12 % of patients with a pCR in the rectal wall had nodal metastases [27]. Therefore, additional evaluation is necessary

- ▨ Radiographic response parallels tumor regression and predicts patient outcomes [28]
- ■ ERUS and MRI may be difficult to interpret after CRT. Accuracy for T-stage has been reported as 48–72 % by ERUS and 47–52 % by standard MRI, and for N-stage as 77–80 % and 64–68 %, respectively [29–32]
- ■ Use of PET to determine response to CRT remains investigational [33, 34]. Several studies correlate the extent of metabolic tumor response on positron emission tomography (PET) with pathological response; however, the results have not been consistent
- ■ DCE-MRI: Several groups have shown that the addition of dynamic contrast enhancement (DCE) to standard MRI series increases the sensitivity and specificity for detection of tumor response. DCE-MRI quantitates the movement of injected contrast between the intracellular, extracellular/interstitial, and vascular compartments. The vascularity and cell density of tissue determine the pharmacokinetics of contrast enhancement [35, 36]
- ■ DWI-MRI: DWI-MRI reflects the microscopic motion of water molecules in tissues and thus reveals information about the tissue architecture. DWI-MRI provides a quantity, the apparent diffusion coefficient (ADC), as an indicator of water motion restriction or tissue cellularity. As a tumor becomes necrotic and cell membranes more leaky, the ADC increases. Multiple groups have shown that changes in ADC provide a more accurate indication of tumor response than conventional MRI alone [37–40]

Toxicity

- ■ Anticipated Toxicities of Anorectal Brachytherapy
  - ■ Likely
    - ▨ Proctitis, resulting in rectal bleeding, mucous discharge, tenesmus, and/or discomfort

- Urinary urgency, dysuria
- Perianal skin erythema for low-lying rectal or anal tumors
- Fatigue
- Less Likely
  - Rectal ulceration
  - Abdominal pain, cramping
  - Diarrhea
  - Decreased production of red blood cells, possibly requiring transfusion
  - Decreased production of white blood cells, possibly predisposing to infection
  - Decreased number of platelets, possibly resulting in bleeding
- Rare, but Serious
  - Severe rectal bleeding
  - Rectal fistulization
  - Large bowel obstruction
  - Urinary obstruction
  - Reaction to general anesthesia
  - Death
- Late Effects of Radiation Therapy May Include
  - Proctitis
  - Altered sphincter functioning
  - Infertility
  - Early menopause in premenopausal women who have not undergone an ovarian transposition
  - Vaginal dryness and narrowing
- Acute toxicity is defined as occurring from 0 to 90 days after brachytherapy, and late toxicity is defined as occurring from 91 days to 2 years after brachytherapy
- Management of Brachytherapy Toxicity
  - Antidiarrheals: For symptoms of diarrhea and/or abdominal cramping, patients can take loperamide. Additional antidiarrheal measures can be used at the discretion of the treating physician. Patients should be instructed to increase fluid intake to help maintain fluid and electrolyte balance during episodes of diarrhea

References

1. American Cancer Society. Cancer facts & figures 2016. Atlanta: American Cancer Society; 2016.
2. Sauer R, Becker H, Hohenberger W, et al. Preoperative versus postoperative chemoradiotherapy for rectal cancer. N Engl J Med. 2004;351(17):1731–40.
3. Bosset JF, Collette L, Calais G, et al. Chemotherapy with preoperative radiotherapy in rectal cancer. N Engl J Med. 2006; 355(11):1114–23.
4. Valenti V, Hernandez-Lizoain JL, Baixauli J, et al. Analysis of early postoperative morbidity among patients with rectal cancer treated with and without neoadjuvant chemoradiotherapy. Ann Surg Oncol. 2007;14(5):1744–51.
5. Pucciarelli S, Toppan P, Friso ML, et al. Preoperative combined radiotherapy and chemotherapy for rectal cancer does not affect early postoperative morbidity and mortality in low anterior resection. Dis Colon Rectum. 1999;42(10):1276–83, discussion 1283–4.
6. Peeters KC, van de Velde CJ, Leer JW, et al. Late side effects of short-course preoperative radiotherapy combined with total mesorectal excision for rectal cancer: increased bowel dysfunction in irradiated patients—a Dutch colorectal cancer group study. J Clin Oncol. 2005;23(25):6199–206.
7. Hendren SK, O'Connor BI, Liu M, et al. Prevalence of male and female sexual dysfunction is high following surgery for rectal cancer. Ann Surg. 2005;242(2):212–23.
8. Lange MM, den Dulk M, Bossema ER, et al. Risk factors for faecal incontinence after rectal cancer treatment. Br J Surg. 2007;94(10):1278–84.
9. Binkley GE. Radiation in the treatment of rectal cancer. Ann Surg. 1929;90(6):1000–14.
10. Binkley GE. Gold radon seeds in rectal cancer. Ann Surg. 1935;102(1):72–7.
11. Sischy B, Hinson EJ, Wilkinson DR. Definitive radiation therapy for selected cancers of the rectum. Br J Surg. 1988;75(9):901–3.
12. Gerard JP, Ayzac L, Coquard R, et al. Endocavitary irradiation for early rectal carcinomas T1 (T2). A series of 101 patients treated with the Papillon's technique. Int J Radiat Oncol Biol Phys. 1996;34(4):775–83.
13. Papillon J. Present status of radiation therapy in the conservative management of rectal cancer. Radiother Oncol. 1990;17(4):275–83.

14. Maingon P, Guerif S, Darsouni R, et al. Conservative management of rectal adenocarcinoma by radiotherapy. Int J Radiat Oncol Biol Phys. 1998;40(5):1077–85.

15. Gerard JP, Chapet O, Ramaioli A, et al. Long-term control of T2-T3 rectal adenocarcinoma with radiotherapy alone. Int J Radiat Oncol Biol Phys. 2002;54(1):142–9.

16. Aumock A, Birnbaum EH, Fleshman JW, et al. Treatment of rectal adenocarcinoma with endocavitary and external beam radiotherapy: results for 199 patients with localized tumors. Int J Radiat Oncol Biol Phys. 2001;51(2):363–70.

17. Hoskin PJ, de Canha SM, Bownes P, et al. High dose rate afterloading intraluminal brachytherapy for advanced inoperable rectal carcinoma. Radiother Oncol. 2004;73(2):195–8.

18. Vuong T, Devic S, Podgorsak E. High dose rate endorectal brachytherapy as a neoadjuvant treatment for patients with resectable rectal cancer. Clin Oncol. 2007;19(9):701–5.

19. Vuong T, Devic S. High-dose-rate pre-operative endorectal brachytherapy for patients with rectal cancer. J Contemp Brachytherapy. 2015;7(2):183–8.

20. Oehler-Janne C, Seifert B, Lutolf UM, et al. Clinical outcome after treatment with a brachytherapy boost versus external beam boost for anal carcinoma. Brachytherapy. 2007;6(3):218–26.

21. Kapp KS, Geyer E, Gebhart FH, et al. Experience with split-course external beam irradiation +/- chemotherapy and integrated Ir-192 high-dose-rate brachytherapy in the treatment of primary carcinomas of the anal canal. Int J Radiat Oncol Biol Phys. 2001;49(4):997–1005.

22. Cohen GN, et al. Evaluation of a new MRI compatible brachytherapy ano-rectal applicator. Brachytherapy. 2014;13:S48.

23. Cohen G, Goodman K. TU-AB-201-07: image guided endorectal HDR brachytherapy using a compliant balloon applicator. Med Phys. 2015;42:3595.

24. King, M, Cohen G, Wu, A, et al. Prospective evaluation of endoluminal high dose rate brachytherapy with concurrent chemotherapy for rectal or anal cancer patients: Initial clinical results. Submitted to American Brachytherapy Society Annual Meeting; 2016.

25. Guillem JG, Chessin DB, Shia J, et al. Clinical examination following preoperative chemoradiation for rectal cancer is not a reliable surrogate end point. J Clin Oncol. 2005;23(15):3475–9.

26. Perez RO, Habr-Gama A, Pereira GV, et al. Role of biopsies in patients with residual rectal cancer following neoadjuvant

chemoradiation after downsizing: can they rule out persisting cancer? Colorectal Dis. 2012;14(6):714–20.

27. Zmora O, Dasilva GM, Gurland B, et al. Does rectal wall tumor eradication with preoperative chemoradiation permit a change in the operative strategy? Dis Colon Rectum. 2004;47(10): 1607–12.

28. Patel UB, Taylor F, Blomqvist L, et al. Magnetic resonance imaging-detected tumor response for locally advanced rectal cancer predicts survival outcomes: MERCURY experience. J Clin Oncol. 2011;29(28):3753–60.

29. Maor Y, Nadler M, Barshack I, et al. Endoscopic ultrasound staging of rectal cancer: diagnostic value before and following chemoradiation. J Gastroenterol Hepatol. 2006;21(2):454–8.

30. Vanagunas A, Lin DE, Stryker SJ. Accuracy of endoscopic ultrasound for restaging rectal cancer following neoadjuvant chemoradiation therapy. Am J Gastroenterol. 2004;99(1):109–12.

31. Kuo LJ, Chern MC, Tsou MH, et al. Interpretation of magnetic resonance imaging for locally advanced rectal carcinoma after preoperative chemoradiation therapy. Dis Colon Rectum. 2005;48(1):23–8.

32. Chen CC, Lee RC, Lin JK, et al. How accurate is magnetic resonance imaging in restaging rectal cancer in patients receiving preoperative combined chemoradiotherapy? Dis Colon Rectum. 2005;48(4):722–8.

33. Capirci C, Rubello D, Chierichetti F, et al. Long-term prognostic value of 18F-FDG PET in patients with locally advanced rectal cancer previously treated with neoadjuvant radiochemotherapy. AJR Am J Roentgenol. 2006;187(2):W202–8.

34. Cascini GL, Avallone A, Delrio P, et al. 18F-FDG PET is an early predictor of pathologic tumor response to preoperative radiochemotherapy in locally advanced rectal cancer. J Nucl Med. 2006;47(8):1241–8.

35. Dinter DJ, Horisberger K, Zechmann C, et al. Can dynamic MR imaging predict response in patients with rectal cancer undergoing cetuximab-based neoadjuvant chemoradiation? Onkologie. 2009;32(3):86–93.

36. Gollub MJ, Gultekin DH, Akin O, et al. Dynamic contrast enhanced-MRI for the detection of pathological complete response to neoadjuvant chemotherapy for locally advanced rectal cancer. Eur Radiol. 2012;22(4):821–31.

37. Kim SH, Lee JM, Hong SH, et al. Locally advanced rectal cancer: added value of diffusion-weighted MR imaging in the evaluation

of tumor response to neoadjuvant chemo- and radiation therapy. Radiology. 2009;253(1):116–25.

38. Curvo-Semedo L, Lambregts DM, Maas M, et al. Rectal cancer: assessment of complete response to preoperative combined radiation therapy with chemotherapy—conventional MR volumetry versus diffusion-weighted MR imaging. Radiology. 2011;260(3):734–43.

39. Jung SH, Heo SH, Kim JW, et al. Predicting response to neoadjuvant chemoradiation therapy in locally advanced rectal cancer: diffusion-weighted 3 Tesla MR imaging. J Magn Reson Imaging. 2012;35(1):110–6.

40. Patterson DM, Padhani AR, Collins DJ. Technology insight: water diffusion MRI—a potential new biomarker of response to cancer therapy. Nat Clin Pract Oncol. 2008;5(4):220–33.

Chapter 12
MRI Image-Guided Low-Dose Rate Brachytherapy for Prostate Cancer

Amy C. Moreno, Rajat J. Kudchadker, Jihong Wang, and Steven J. Frank

Introduction

- Permanent prostate brachytherapy (PPB) has emerged as a standard of care for localized prostate cancer
- MRI provides optimal imaging of the prostate from diagnosis to treatment assessment
- This chapter will discuss the application of image-guided brachytherapy using radioactive isotopes in the treatment of prostate cancer
- Three radioactive isotopes commonly used for prostate cancer LDR brachytherapy are Iodine-125 (I-125), Palladium-103 (Pd-103), and Cesium-131 (Cs-131)

A.C. Moreno, MD • S.J. Frank, MD (✉)
Department of Radiation Oncology, University of Texas MD Anderson Cancer Center, Houston, TX, USA
e-mail: akmoreno@mdanderson.org; sjfrank@mdanderson.org

R.J. Kudchadker, PhD • J. Wang, PhD
Department of Radiation Physics, University of Texas MD Anderson Cancer Center, Houston, TX, USA
e-mail: rkudchad@mdanderson.org; Jihong.wang@mdanderson.org

© Springer International Publishing AG 2017   319
J. Mayadev et al. (eds.), *Handbook of Image-Guided Brachytherapy*, DOI 10.1007/978-3-319-44827-5_12

Rationale for MR Image-Guided Brachytherapy

- Biochemical outcomes and morbidity profiles after PPB are comparable to surgery and external beam radiation therapy (EBRT)
- With careful patient selection, pretreatment planning, implanting, and postimplant evaluation, permanent prostate brachytherapy (PPB) can be a convenient, safe, and effective method of treating prostate cancer
- MRI is the optimal imaging for prostate brachytherapy. MRI can reduce the level of target volume uncertainty as it has superior soft tissue delineation compared to ultrasound and CT [1]
- Advances in MRI, treatment planning software, and stranded seeds with positive contrast MRI markers allow for improved brachytherapy treatment plans with the goals to improve overall quality of life (QOL) and survival outcomes
- Intraoperative fluoroscopic images demonstrate the changes in technique that have occurred in brachytherapy leading to higher quality treatment with improved outcomes

Goal of Brachytherapy: Definitive

- The goal of PPB is to accurately deliver a high therapeutic radiation dose to the prostate while significantly limiting radiation exposure to nearby structures such as the external urinary sphincter, bladder, and rectum, thereby reducing treatment-associated morbidity
- PPB can be utilized as a monotherapy option for low or intermediate risk prostate cancer or as part of tri-modality therapy for high risk localized prostate cancer
- Challenges of PPB: Appropriate training is lacking and quality assurance is still a problem

- Standardization of PPB technique and evaluation is key to optimizing outcomes

Pertinent Anatomy for Brachytherapy

- Prostate anatomy as seen on ultrasound, CT, and MRI (Fig. 12.1)
- Pelvic anatomy on MRI, T2-weighted images (Fig. 12.2a–d)

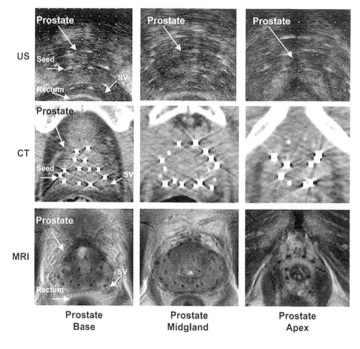

FIG. 12.1. Prostate anatomy as seen on ultrasound, CT, and MRI (Used with permission from Frank, S.J., et al., A novel MRI marker for prostate brachytherapy. Int J Radiat Oncol Biol Phys, 2008. 71(1): 5–8)

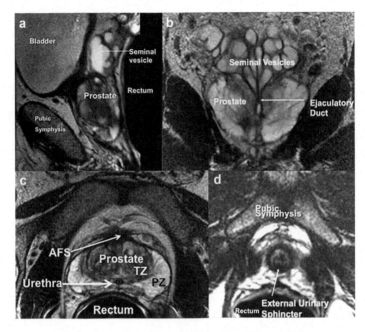

FIG. 12.2. (**a–d**) Pelvic anatomy on MRI, T2-weighted images (*AFS* anterior fibromuscular stroma, *TZ* transition zone, *PZ* peripheral zone)

Pathology

Typical Pathology

- Prostate tissue is generally acquired from a standard 12-core transrectal ultrasound-guided prostate biopsy or an MRI–ultrasound fusion-guided biopsy
- Most prostate cancers are adenocarcinomas. Other variants: Ductal (endometrioid), mucinous (colloid), signet ring cell, and pseudohyperplastic carcinomas
- The Gleason grading system is based on glandular architecture with grades ranging from 3 (moderately differentiated) to 5 (poorly differentiatcd/anaplastic). The primary and secondary grades are added together

to obtain the final Gleason score. A higher score is associated with a worse prognosis

Rationale for Brachytherapy

- The value of brachytherapy. The economic costs, complication rates, patient reported outcomes, disease control, and overall survival after LDR brachytherapy for the treatment of prostate cancer have been recently analyzed [2–4]. Brachytherapy was found to be of relative low cost compared with surgery and external beam radiation therapy, have less acute complications while providing excellent rates of disease control and survival
- See Table 12.1 for disease-free survival rates

Selection Criteria

Selection for Implantation

- Stratify patients into pretreatment risk groups low, intermediate, or high risk using NCCN or D'Amico stratification guidelines (Table 12.2)
- Ideal patients for monotherapy [5]:
  - Low or intermediate risk disease
  - Good performance status (ECOG 0–1)
  - Low urinary symptoms (IPSS <15)

TABLE 12.1 Disease-free survival rates

Risk category	5–10 Year bPFS	5–10 Year CSS
Low	87–98 %	>95 %
Intermediate	70–85 %	75–90 %
High	30–80 %	60–80 %

bPFS biochemical progression free survival, *CSS* cancer-specific survival

TABLE 12.2 NCCN and D'Amico (bold) risk stratification for clinically localized prostate cancer

Risk category	Primary tumor (T)		Gleason score		PSA (ng/ml)
Low	T1-T2a	and	≤6	and	<10
Intermediate	T2b-T2c (**T2b**)	or	7	or	10–20 (**10–19.9**)
High	T3a (**T2c-T3**)	or	8–10	or	>20 (**≥20**)

- No pubic arch interference, PAI (assess during simulation, see section in this chapter on "Image Guidance Utilization")
- Verify no evidence of gross extracapsular extension of disease or seminal vesicle involvement using endorectal MRI (see section in this chapter on "Use of Image Guidance Pre-procedure")
- Relative contraindications
  - A history of transurethral resection of prostate gland
  - Active inflammatory processes (acute prostatitis or active inflammatory bowel disease)
  - Predictive factors for acute urinary retention: IPSS >15, postvoid residual volume >100 cm^3, and median lobe hyperplasia
- A colonoscopy is recommended within 3 years prior to permanent seed implant. The colonoscopy facilitates screening for colorectal malignancies and avoids unnecessary biopsies of a treatment-related anterior rectal ulcer [6]. Unnecessary biopsies may subsequently lead to a nonhealing ulcer and fistula
- Isotope selection depends on clinician preference and experience. Our recommendations are in Table 12.3

When to Implant (Post-EBRT)

- If used as part of tri-modality therapy, PPB boost is recommended within 2–4 weeks after EBRT

TABLE 12.3 Isotope selection recommendations

Risk features	Isotope	Therapy
Low	Cs-131, I-125, Pd-103	Monotherapy
Intermediate	Cs-131, I-125, Pd-103	Monotherapy
High	I-125, Pd-103	Tri-modality (Boost)

- ADT is prescribed for a total duration of 9 months and is started 2–3 months prior to treatment

Clinical Guidelines to Judge Readiness for Implantation

- Each clinician must learn how to utilize the imaging tools (US, CT, and MRI) and apply them toward the simulation, treatment planning, and implantation processes (see section in this chapter on "Use of Image Guidance Preprocedure")
- Implantation should occur only after evaluation of diagnostic imaging, careful patient selection, and pre-planning dosimetry have been completed
- A phantom simulator training program can help improve degree of consistency between trainees to perform uniformly high-quality implants [7]

Medical Operability: Anesthesia Consent, Guidelines for CBC, Anticoagulation

- Standard preoperative clearance requirements

Image Guidance Utilization

Use of Image Guidance Preprocedure

- Evaluation process

- Become familiarized with pelvic/prostate anatomy on MRI (Fig. 12.2a–d)
- Prostate cancer in the left peripheral gland on MRI

    - T2-weighted imaging (T2-W): *hypointense* signal
    - Diffusion-weighted imaging (DWI): *hyperintense* signal
    - Apparent diffusion coefficient (ADC): *hypointense* signal

- Simulation

    - Preimplant simulation (US or MRI based) should be performed 2–4 weeks prior to implant
    - With ultrasound, key features include:

        - Identifying the prostate base on sagittal imaging and prostate apex on axial imaging
        - Obtaining the length and volume of the entire prostate
        - Performing pubic arch evaluation to verify no potential obstruction of anterior needle insertion by a narrow pubic arch

- PAI can be assessed using US, CT, or MRI-based imaging of the prostate mid-gland. For US based, patients are placed in the dorsal lithotomy position and a stylet is inserted through the template grid and held superiorly over the nailbed of the opposite hand index finger which has been placed against the perineum. Freedom from pubic bone is assessed to ensure the technical feasibility of performing a high quality implant
- Capturing the images required for treatment planning purposes, starting 0.5 cm superior to the base of the prostate and ending 0.5 cm inferior to the apex

    - With MRI planning:

        - Accurate setup is important, particularly endorectal coil placement just superior to the base of the prostate

- A traditional, inflatable balloon-type endorectal coil is associated with deformation of prostate gland if fully inflated [8]; however, a partially inflated endorectal coil is an option
- The rigid Invivo endorectal coil has the same diameter of an ultrasound probe and therefore prevents gland deformation (Fig. 12.3a–c)
- Recommended MRI sequences and protocols discussed in section in this chapter on "Recommended MRI Sequences and Protocols."
- Dicom data are transferred to an MRI-based planning software
- A virtual simulation is performed to take into consideration the anatomical differences between MRI treatment planning and intraoperative ultrasound images during implantation. MRI simulation image acquisition is obtained with the patient supine while intraoperative ultrasound imaging occurs with patients legs in the dorsal lithotomy position

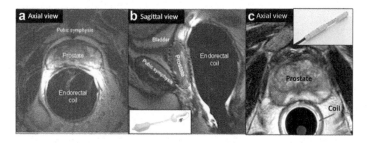

FIG. 12.3. Prostate gland deformation with traditional inflatable endorectal coil as seen on (**a**) Axial and (**b**) Sagittal T2-W imaging. There is no anatomic deformation with (**c**) The Sentinelle endorectal coil array which is the same size as the ultrasound probe and limits deformation of the prostate. (**a** and **b** used with permission from Albert, J.M., et al., Magnetic resonance imaging-based treatment planning for prostate brachytherapy. Brachytherapy, 2013. 12(1): 30–7)

- Treatment planning: Template Registration
  - Both US or MRI-based treatment planning systems (TPS) require this initial step
  - The center of the prostate gland should be placed midline in the template grid and the posterior edge of the gland between rows 1 and 2 (Fig. 12.4a)
  - For MRI-based TPS, angulate the virtual rectal probe by −5° to −10° to take into consideration the legs down during the MRI simulation versus the legs in the dorsal lithotomy position in the operating room (Fig. 12.4b). Fusion (real-time or cognitive) of the intraoperative ultrasound images and treatment planning MRI images should be performed at the time of the implant
- Treatment planning: Contouring
  - Identify the image slice with the base of the prostate and set it as reference image
  - Contour the prostate, rectum, bladder, urethra, and seminal vesicles (Fig. 12.5)

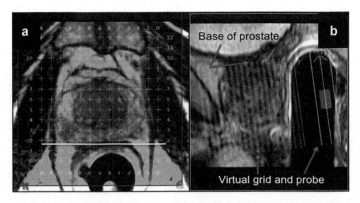

Fig. 12.4. (a) MRI-based TPS grid, *yellow line* demarcates posterior edge of prostate between rows 1 and 2; (b) MRI-based TPS orientation of virtual probe

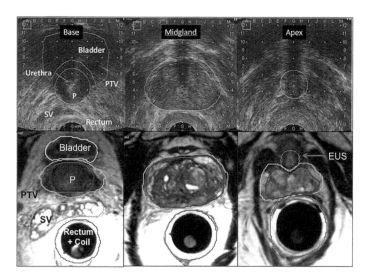

FIG. 12.5. Organ contours on US (*top row*) and MRI (*bottom row*). *EUS* external urinary sphincter, *P* prostate, *PTV* planning target volume, *SV* seminal vesicles

- If using an MRI-based TPS, contour organs on T2-W images. The external urinary sphincter (EUS) can also be visualized and contoured
- Planning Target Volume (PTV): Prostate gland with a 2–3 mm expansion superiorly, inferiorly, and laterally. The posterior margin should be 0 mm or the same as the prostate since the Denovier's fascia separates the prostate gland posteriorly from the anterior wall of the rectum
- Treatment planning: Dosimetry
  - Optimization will vary depending on the isotope used and amount of activity per seed
  - Starting on a mid-gland slice, use isotope-specific loading technique to plan seed placement to avoid excessive dose heterogeneity to the urethra and rectum

- ▪ Palladium: modified uniform loading technique
- ▪ Iodine: modified peripheral loading technique
- ▪ Cesium: modified peripheral loading with rectal modification technique

- Avoid seed placement in the external urinary sphincter at the apex which can adversely affect patients' urinary quality of life
- Avoid placing seeds superior to the urethra in the center of the template grid in order to prevent needle trauma to the penile urethra during implantation
- The planning target volume is the entire prostate gland with appropriate margin based on the risk of extracapsular extension of disease and imaging uncertainties
- Focal brachytherapy targeting the prostate cancer tumor alone is currently investigational. The value of dose escalation of the MRI dominant lesion is currently being assessed in prospective clinical trials
- PTV V200 isodose line should create an "avoidance ring" around the center of the prostate gland where urethra/EUS are located
- Review dose distribution on axial (Fig. 12.6), sagittal, and coronal views
- Optimize seed placement by using standard loaded needles (seed-marker-seed-marker, etc.) in the periphery and reserve specialized needles (customized) for the periurethral region (Fig. 12.7)
- Use activity per volume nomograms as a quality assurance indicator to confirm the amount of total activity that will be required for an implant according to prostate volume
- Suggested dosimetric parameters are presented in Table 12.4

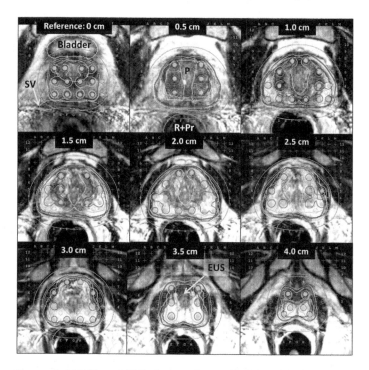

FIG. 12.6. MRI-based TPS dosimetric preplan shown in sequential axial slices (*EUS* external urinary sphincter, *SV* seminal vesicles, *P* prostate, *R+Pr* rectum with endorectal coil. Isodose lines: *Orange*—50 % prescribed dose; *Yellow*—90 %; *Thick Red*—100 %; *Light green*—150 %; *Magenta*—200 %. Note: Prostate is outlined in *dark blue* and PTV is outlined in *light blue*)

Types of Image Guidance to Potentially Use and Pros/Cons

■ See Table 12.5

Use of Image Guidance During Procedure

■ Intraoperative MRI-US fused images can be used for implantation (Fig. 12.8)

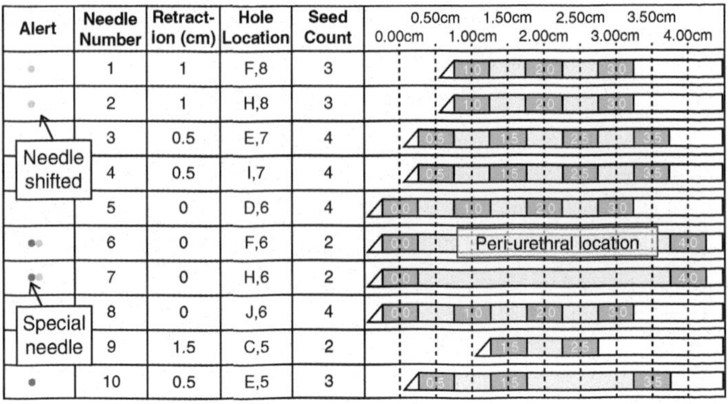

Alert	Needle Number	Retraction (cm)	Hole Location	Seed Count	0.00cm — 0.50cm — 1.00cm — 1.50cm — 2.00cm — 2.50cm — 3.00cm — 3.50cm — 4.00cm
○	1	1	F,8	3	
○	2	1	H,8	3	
Needle shifted	3	0.5	E,7	4	
	4	0.5	I,7	4	
	5	0	D,6	4	
●○	6	0	F,6	2	Peri-urethral location
●○	7	0	H,6	2	
Special needle	8	0	J,6	4	
	9	1.5	C,5	2	
●	10	0.5	E,5	3	

FIG. 12.7. Description of first ten needles used for an LDR brachytherapy case. Note that standard, preloaded needles are used in the periphery while special, customized needles are in periurethral locations

TABLE 12.4 Suggested dosimetric parameters

Parameter	I-125	Pd-103	Cs-131
Prostate V100	>95 %	>95 %	>95 %
Prostate V150	<60 %	<70 %	<50 %
Prostate V200	<20 %	<40 %	<15 %
Urethral/EUS V200	<1 %	<1 %	<1 %
Rectum V100	<1 cm³	<1 cm³	<0.5 cm³

■ Alternatively, US or MRI-based treatment plans are cognitively fused with real-time US images

Guidelines for Implantation

Preprocedure Advice

■ Common radioactive isotope strands used:
  ■ I-125, Pd-103, Cs131

TABLE 12.5 Types of image guidance to potentially use and pros/cons

Imaging	Pros	Cons
Ultrasound	Widely used for preoperative assessment of the prostate and for intraoperative seed implantation	Limited image resolution of prostate apical anatomy
CT	Widely used, quick image acquisition	Limited image resolution of prostate base and apex
		Degradation of image due to implanted metallic seeds
Endorectal MRI	Improved soft tissue delineation	Higher risk of motion artifact
	Rigid Invivo endorectal coil or deflated (30 cm^3) nonrigid coil reduces prostate anatomy deformation	Limited availability/accessibility to MRI
		Low clinician experience with MR
		Sequences can vary depending on diagnostic protocols

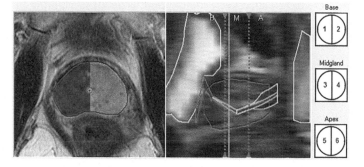

FIG. 12.8. MRI–US fusion

- Reduce implantation team intraoperative stress with preplanning
- Develop a quality and safety checklist that facilitates the quality assurance process to ensure each patient receives optimal treatment
- Simulation and implantation should be consistent in order to achieve a high quality implant
- Proper documentation of operative procedure is essential

Procedure Tips for Transperineal Permanent Prostate Brachytherapy

- On day of implant, administer antibiotics before procedure (e.g., 2 g Cefoxitin)
- After placing the patient under general anesthesia, deliver 10 mg of Decadron
- Place the patient in the dorsal lithotomy position, prep and drape the perineum
- Insert a 14-French coude catheter into the urethra/bladder and fill with 100 mL of sterile water
- Insert a nonlatex condom over an Endo P2 transrectal probe covered with KY jelly and insert into rectum
- Visualize the apex and base of the prostate using sagittal imaging and the apex using axial imaging (critical to the success of the implant to avoid implanting into the urethra or bladder)
- Visualize entirety of the prostate gland in fibromembranous segments to verify they are consistent with the preoperative treatment plan (usually 5 mm slices) and measure length of prostate
- Align US grid to be consistent with MR grid from pretreatment plan
- Perform cognitive fusion of MRI treatment plan images with real-time US images of the prostate. Software is also available for real-time ultrasound–MRI fusion

- Insert preloaded needles into the gland according to the pretreatment plan beginning anteriorly and working posteriorly. It is recommended that needles be advanced to mid gland using real-time axial images of the prostate gland and then make final advancement to the prostate base on sagittal view
- Isotope-specific peripheral loading technique is recommended. Avoid the urethra by not placing any seeds in the middle column
- Monitor the posterior row of needles in the sagittal plane with respect to the anterior rectal wall to avoid unnecessary dose to the rectum and subsequent morbidity
- Always consider where the prostate is in real time and modify the preplan as needed
- Consider performing intraoperative optimization with needle adjustments and additional seed placement by revising TPS plans in the OR if adequate dosimetry is not achieved using the preoperative treatment plan

Verification of Brachytherapy Implantation

- Upon completion of the implant, a fluoroscopic image is compared to the preplan coronal image in the operating room to verify the seed distribution is consistent
- Evaluate urine for hematuria. Postimplant cystoscopy is not routinely necessary unless there is concern for urinary trauma or seeds/strands in the urethra/bladder
- If satisfied with implant, survey the room and empty needles using a Geiger meter
  - Less than 1 mR/h at 1 m does not require radiation precautions

Evaluation of Implantation

- Postoperative dosimetry allows for evaluation of implant quality
- An immediate postimplant MRI and CT scan should be performed in order to evaluate dose distribution to ensure a high quality implant [9]
- A follow-up MRI and CT on postoperative day 30 may be appropriate to evaluate dose distribution after resolution of postimplant gland edema

Distribution of Implant

- Ultrasound-CT-based evaluation
  - Localize all seeds using US-based TPS and evaluate final dose distribution
- MRI-based evaluation (Siemens 1.5 T with Invivo endorectal coil or GE 3 T with inflatable endorectal coil filled with 30 cm³ of sterile water)
  - Contour anatomy on 3DT2-weighted images
  - Localize seeds by reference to Sirius™ MRI Markers (C4 Imaging, Bellaire, TX, USA) using MRI T1 Flash (Siemens, Munich, Germany) or GE equivalent sequences, confirming with CT as necessary (Fig. 12.9)
  - Evaluate dose distribution (Fig. 12.10)

Review Imaging Real Time or When a Change Is Needed

- In some circumstances where adequate dosimetry is not achieved, the clinician should consider intraoperative optimization of brachytherapy implant by adjusting the treatment plan in real time using the TPS in the operating room

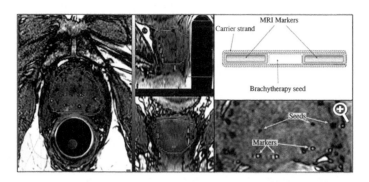

FIG. 12.9. MRI-based seed localization using 1.5 T Siemens 3D axial FLASH images. Seeds are hypointense while markers in between seeds have a hyperintense signal

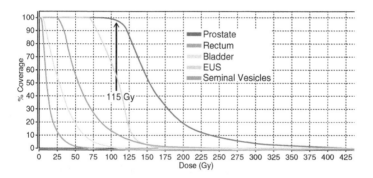

FIG. 12.10. Dose–volume histogram for a Cs-131 implant

- Postimplant dosimetric assessment should occur on day 0 (see section in this chapter on "Treatment Planning Considerations: Dose Distribution"). If there is not adequate coverage of the prostate (prostate V100 > 95 %), consideration should be made to take the patient back to the OR for additional seed implantation to optimize dosimetry and treatment

Treatment Planning Considerations

Optimal Monotherapy Brachytherapy Dose Rx

- See Table 12.6

Optimal Dose Distribution with Isodose Curves

- Dose distributions (Fig. 12.11)
- Postimplant dosimetric assessment using MRI provides the ideal quality assurance of the treatment with brachytherapy. This imaging should occur on postoperative day 0. Sirius™ MRI Markers between the seeds facilitates seed localization in order to provide a more precise postimplant dosimetric analysis and to ensure a high quality implant is performed [10, 11]
- The T1 MRI sequence is optimal for seed localization while the T2 MRI is optimal for anatomical delineation of the prostate base, apex, and external urinary sphincter. The images can be fused to provide optimal anatomical imaging with precise dosimetry and quality assurance

Table 12.6 Optimal monotherapy brachytherapy dose Rx

Isotope	Activity	Half-life	Mean energy	90 % Dose
I-125	0.391 mCi	59.4 days	28 KeV	144 Gy
	0.497 U			204 days
Pd-103	1.9 mCi	17 days	21 KeV	125 Gy
	2.457 U			58 days
Cs-131	3.135 mCi	9.7 days	30 KeV	115 Gy
	2.0 U			33 days

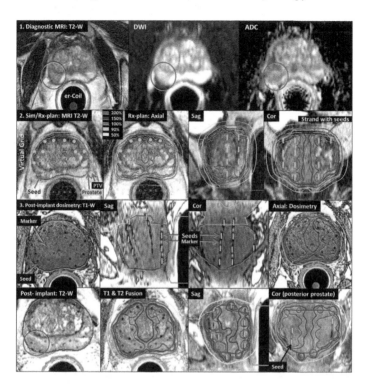

FIG. 12.11. MRI from diagnosis (row 1) to simulation and treatment planning (row 2) to postimplant assessment (rows 3 and 4). Row 1: Diagnostic MR axial images showing prostate cancer located in the right peripheral zone (*red circle*). Row 2: Simulation MR T2-W image with virtual grid in place. Prostate and PTV have been contoured. Pretreatment plan dosimetry shown in axial, sagittal, and coronal views. Row 3: Postimplant assessment. T1-W image showing seeds (hypointense) and markers (hyperintense) within the prostate. Prostate outlined in *blue*. Strand with seeds (*green*) and markers (*white*) seen on sagittal and coronal views. Row 4: Postimplant T2-W highlights prostate anatomy. Postimplant fused T1 and T2 images provide optimal anatomical information and precise dosimetry. Note: The MRI-based pretreatment plan was cognitively fused with real-time intraoperative US imaging of the prostate for implantation (US images not shown)

■ The endorectal coil provides high SNR to ensure appropriate visualization of the Sirius™ MRI Markers without prostate anatomic distortion and ensures consistent high quality prostate imaging from diagnosis, simulation, treatment planning, and postimplant assessment

Toxicity

Toxicity Side Effect Review

■ Common side effects include:
  ■ Urinary—dysuria, hematuria, polyuria, urinary retention [12]
  ■ Erectile dysfunction
■ Rare side effects include:
  ■ Rectal bleeding
  ■ Urethral stenosis or stricture
  ■ Seed migration (rare with stranded seeds)

Management of Brachytherapy Toxicity according to Disease Site

■ Prophylactic use of alpha blockers does not affect retention rates but results in faster return of IPSS to baseline
■ Postimplant, patient is discharged home with a tapering Medrol® Dosepak (Pfizer, New York, NY, USA), Flomax® (Boehringer Ingelheim Pharmaceuticals, Ingelheim am Rhein, Germany), Aleve®, Bayer, Leverkusen, Germany), ciprofloxacin, Cialis® (Eli Lilly, Indianapolis, IN, USA), and Urelle® (Azur Pharma, Dublin, Ireland) to reduce acute side effects
■ Evaluation by a urologist is recommended if there is a concern of a chronic urethral stricture

Follow-up

- Patients should be followed at regular intervals with their PSA and EPIC QOL outcomes
- PSA bounce
  - May occur in up to 40 % of hormone-naïve patients within 12–30 months after undergoing PPB
  - It does not impact long-term biochemical outcome
- For rising PSA following 30 months, MRI of the prostate is recommended to assess for recurrence as well as biopsy consideration

The Future of PPB: MRI-Assisted Radiosurgery (MARS)

- Trend toward MRI use from diagnosis to response assessment (Fig. 12.11)
  - Diagnostic MRI, MRI-guided biopsy, MRI simulation, MRI treatment planning, MRI-based implanting (US–MRI fusion or intraoperative MRI), MRI postimplant dosimetry, MRI surveillance with PSA monitoring
- The increased utilization of positive contrast MRI markers and development of automatic strand localization in the treatment planning system

Recommended MRI Sequences and Protocols

Introduction

- Two types of endorectal coil are commonly used for prostate MR imaging: the inflatable balloon disposable type (BTC) and the rigid reusable type (InVivo rigid coil)
- MR imaging protocol typically consists of a 3D Fast Gradient Echo scan which highlights the markers and

facilitates localization of the seeds, and a 3D T2-weighted anatomical scan of the prostate with identical scan location and slice thickness

Imaging Sequences and Acquisition Parameters for GE Scanners

- The inflatable BTC is used with a 3T GE Signa HDxT scanner
- The BTC is inserted into the rectum and inflated with 30 cm^3 of air instead of the typical full inflation of 60 cm^3 used for diagnostic exams
- To reduce bowel motion artifact, injection of glucagon is given immediately after coil insertion
- The imaging protocol consists of a 3D FSPGR sequence and a 3D T2-weighted FSE scan (CUBE)
- 3D axial FSPGR
  - TR = 6.18, TE = Min Full (~3.3 ms), flip angle = 20, number of excitations (NEX) = 8, field-of-view (FOV) = 14 cm, imaging matrix = 256 × 256, frequency encoding direction A/P, slice thickness = 2 mm with no gap, bandwidth (BW) = ±83.33 kHz
- 3D T2-weighted axial fast-spin-echo (3D CUBE)
  - Exactly matching slice location, orientation, and thickness, with TR = 2000, TE = ~120, NEX = 1, FOV = 14 cm, Imaging matrix = 224 × 224 (extrapolated to 512 × 512), frequency encoding direction = A/P, slice thickness = 2 mm with no gap, ETL = 74, BW = ±41.67 kHz

Imaging Sequences and Acquisition Parameters for 1.5T Siemens MAGNETOM Aera Scanners

- The InVivo rigid coil is used with the 1.5T Siemens scanner

- Coil insertion is done in the supine position and the coil is positioned against the anterior rectal wall by using a locking articulated arm attached to the table-top support with the REC coil assembly
- Injection of glucagon immediately after the insertion of the coil to suppress bowel motility
- The imaging protocol consists of a 3D axial FLASH and a 3D T2-weighted axial SPACE scan
- 3D axial FLASH
  - TR = 6, TE = 2.38, flip angle = 25, average = 3, FOV read = 150 mm, FOV phase = 100 %, imaging matrix = 256 × 256, phase encoding direction R/L (i.e., frequency encoding direction A/P), phase oversampling = 100 %, slice thickness = 1.00 – 1.5 mm, BW = 500 Hz/Pixel
- 3D T2-weighted axial SPACE
  - Exactly matching slice location, orientation and thickness, TR = 1600, TE = 87, average = 1.4, FOV read = 150 mm, FOV phase = 100 %, imaging matrix = 256 × 256, phase encoding direction = R/L, phase oversampling = 77 %, slice oversampling = 33.3 %, flip angle = 170, echo spacing = 4.38 ms, turbo factor = 80, BW = 454 Hz/Pixel

References

1. Tanderup K, et al. Magnetic resonance image guided brachytherapy. Semin Radiat Oncol. 2014;24(3):181–91.
2. Grimm P, et al. Comparative analysis of prostate-specific antigen free survival outcomes for patients with low, intermediate and high risk prostate cancer treatment by radical therapy. Results from the Prostate Cancer Results Study Group. BJU Int. 2012;109 Suppl 1:22–9.
3. Frank SJ, et al. An assessment of quality of life following radical prostatectomy, high dose external beam radiation therapy and brachytherapy iodine implantation as monotherapies for localized prostate cancer. J Urol. 2007;177(6):2151–6; discussion 2156.

4. Fisher CM, et al. Knife or needles? A cohort analysis of outcomes after radical prostatectomy or brachytherapy for men with low- or intermediate-risk adenocarcinoma of the prostate. Brachytherapy. 2012;11(6):429–34.
5. Expert Panel on Radiation et al. American College of Radiology Appropriateness Criteria permanent source brachytherapy for prostate cancer. Brachytherapy. 2011;10(5):357–62.
6. Sharp HJ, et al. Screening colonoscopy before prostate cancer treatment can detect colorectal cancers in asymptomatic patients and reduce the rate of complications after brachytherapy. Pract Radiat Oncol. 2012;2(3):e7–13.
7. Thaker NG, et al. Establishing high-quality prostate brachytherapy using a phantom simulator training program. Int J Radiat Oncol Biol Phys. 2014;90(3):579–86.
8. Albert JM, et al. Magnetic resonance imaging-based treatment planning for prostate brachytherapy. Brachytherapy. 2013;12(1):30–7.
9. Henry AM, et al. The effect of dose and quality assurance in early prostate cancer treated with low dose rate brachytherapy as monotherapy. Clin Oncol (R Coll Radiol). 2015;27(7):382–6.
10. Lim TY, et al. MRI characterization of cobalt dichloride-N-acetyl cysteine (C4) contrast agent marker for prostate brachytherapy. Phys Med Biol. 2014;59(10):2505–16.
11. Frank SJ, et al. A novel MRI marker for prostate brachytherapy. Int J Radiat Oncol Biol Phys. 2008;71(1):5–8.
12. Anderson JF, et al. Urinary side effects and complications after permanent prostate brachytherapy: the MD Anderson Cancer Center experience. Urology. 2009;74(3):601–5.

Chapter 13
High-Dose Rate Brachytherapy for Prostate Cancer and Clinical Appendix

Yao Yu, I-Chow Hsu, Mitchell Kamrava, and Albert J. Chang

Introduction

Rationale for Brachytherapy (BT)

- To conformally deliver high doses of radiation to the prostate while sparing adjacent structures
- Dose escalation, whether with LDR brachytherapy, HDR brachytherapy, or external beam radiotherapy, has been shown to improve local control and biochemical failure-free survival [1–5].
- The low α/β of prostate cancer provides a radiobiologic basis for high-dose-per-fraction treatment [6].

Y. Yu, MD • I.-C. Hsu, MD, FACR, FASTRO (✉)
A.J. Chang, MD, PhD
Department of Radiation Oncology, University of California, San Francisco, 1600 Divisadero St, Suite H1031, San Francisco, CA 94143, USA
e-mail: yao.yu@ucsf.edu; ihsu@radonc.ucsf.edu; albert.chang@ucsf.edu

M. Kamrava, MD
Ronald Reagan UCLA Medical Center, 757 Westwood Plaza, Los Angeles, CA 90095, USA
e-mail: mkamrava@mednet.ucla.edu

© Springer International Publishing AG 2017
J. Mayadev et al. (eds.), *Handbook of Image-Guided Brachytherapy*, DOI 10.1007/978-3-319-44827-5_13

Indications

- Boost
  - HDR brachytherapy was initially developed as a method of dose escalation in the era of 2D radiation planning [7]. These techniques have yielded excellent local control and improved biochemical recurrence-free survival.
  - Prospective and randomized data support the use of dose escalation using HDR brachytherapy [4, 8].
- Monotherapy
  - HDR brachytherapy as monotherapy is an established paradigm for low- and selected favorable-intermediate risk prostate cancer.
  - Investigators have evaluated this treatment strategy for unfavorable and high-risk prostate cancer; however, this remains investigational [9, 10].
- Salvage
  - HDR alone may be considered for isolated local failure after prior radiotherapy.
  - Retrospective series have yielded favorable long-term local control with moderate toxicity [11, 12].

Pertinent Anatomy for Brachytherapy

- See Fig. 13.1 for zonal anatomy of the prostate.
- See Fig. 13.2 for MRI of tumor.

Pathology

- Adenocarcinoma is the most common cancer of the prostate.
- Other histologies—including small cell, neuroendocrine, and squamous cell carcinoma—are uncommon and typically have poor prognosis.

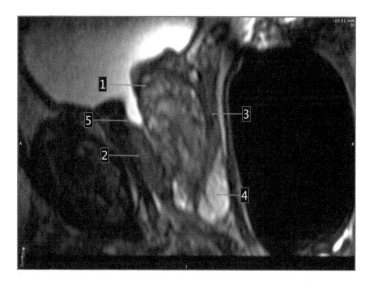

FIG. 13.1. Sagittal T2-weighted MRI with endorectal coil illustrates the zonal anatomy of the prostate. *1* transitional zone; *2* anterior fibromuscular stroma; *3* central zone; *4* peripheral zone; *5* TURP defect

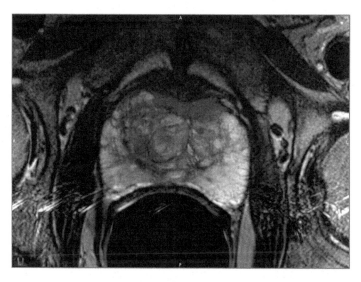

FIG. 13.2. Axial T2-weighted MRI with endorectal coil reveals T2-hypointense tumor in the anterior fibromuscular stroma

- Gleason pattern, perineural invasion, disease volume, extracapsular spread, seminal vesicle invasion, and location of disease are important pathologic risk stratification variables.

Rationale for Brachytherapy

- Local control is 85–99.7 % for most fractionation schemes
- See Table 13.1 on HDR boost outcomes.
- See Table 13.2 on HDR monotherapy outcomes.
- See Table 13.3 on HDR salvage outcomes.

Selection Criteria

Patient Selection

- Patients must be able to tolerate catheter implantation and anesthesia and should have prostate and pelvic anatomy that is amenable to adequate catheter placement.
- Prostate Size/Pubic arch interference
  - Large prostate size may preclude adequate placement and distribution of the HDR catheters, especially in combination with pubic arch interference. Prostate volume >60 cc may be difficult to implant for template-based catheter placement. In this situation, a free-hand technique (vs. template-based technique) will be the preferred method to allow for placement of catheters to ensure adequate dose coverage.
  - The authors have not adopted a strict size cutoff, provided implantation is technically feasible, as evaluated on TRUS. Additional catheters are occasionally needed to provide adequate coverage.
  - The authors have favored a freehand catheter implantation approach with inverse-planned optimization to account for unfavorable geometries.

TABLE 13.1 HDR boost outcomes: Selected studies

Study	N	Risk	Interval (mo)	bNED	bRFS	LC	Dose/Fx
Astrom 2005 [28]	214	Low–High	60	82		99	EBRT 50 Gy/25 fx HDR
		Low	60	92			20 Gy/2 fx
		Int	60	87			
		High	60	56			
Deger 2005 [29]	442	Low–High	60		65	85	40–50.4 Gy/20–28 fx HDR
		Low	60		81		18–20 Gy/2 fx
		Int	60		65		
		High	60		59		
Demanes 2005 [30]	209	Low–High	120			99.5	EBRT 36 Gy/20 fx HDR
		Low	120		90		22–24 Gy/4 fx
		Int	120		87		
		High	120		69		

(continued)

TABLE 13.1 (continued)

Study	N	Risk	Interval (mo)	bNED	bRFS	LC	Dose/Fx
Martinez 2011 [8]	472	Int–High	120	70.6		92.2	EBRT 46 Gy/23fx HDR
BED1.2 <238	167		120	56.9		85.7	BED(1.2) 92.13–243.42 Gy
BED1.2 >238	305		120	81.1		97.2	
Kaprealian 2012 [31]	165	Int–High	60	90	89.9		EBRT 45 Gy/25 fx HDR 18 Gy/3 fx–19 Gy/2 fx
Hoskin 2012 [4]	218	Int–High					EBRT 55 Gy/20 fx
RT alone	108		84		48		vs EBRT 37.75 Gy/13 fx HDR
RT + Boost	110		84		66		17 Gy/2 fx
Martinez 2016 [32]	483	High (Gs 8–10)					EBRT 36-46 Gy (in 1.8–2 Gy fx) HDR variable by institution
PSA ≤40	439		120	57.4		93.4	
PSA >40	44		120	10.3		84.0	

TABLE 13.2 HDR monotherapy outcomes: Selected studies

Study	N	Risk	Interval (mo)	bNED	LC	Dose/Fx
Demanes 2011 [33]	298	Low–Int	96	97	99	38 Gy/4 fx 42 Gy//6 fx
Prada 2012 [34]	40	Low–Int	32			19 Gy/1 fx
		Low	32	100		
		Int	32	88		
Hoskin 2012 [35]	197	Int–High	36	91-99		34 Gy/4 fx 36 Gy/4 fx
			36	99		31.5 Gy/3 fx 26 Gy/2 fx
			36	91		
Zamboglou 2013 [10]	718	Low–High	96	90		38 Gy/4 fx 38 Gy/4 fx
	395	Low	60	95		34.5 Gy/3fx
	177	Int	60	93		
	146	High	60	93		
Yoshioka 2015 [9][a]	190	Int–High			98.4	48 Gy/8 fx 54 Gy/9 fx
	79	Int	96	91		45.5 Gy/7 fx
	111	High	96	77		

(continued)

TABLE 13.2 (continued)

Study	N	Risk	Interval (mo)	bNED	LC	Dose/Fx
Hauswald 2016 [36][b]	448	Low–Int	120	97.8	99.7	42–43.5 Gy/6 fx
	288	Low	120	98.9		
	160	Int	120	95.2		

[a]73 % received ADT
[b]9 % received ADT

TABLE 13.3 HDR Salvage outcomes

Study	N	Prior RT	Interval (mo)	bNED	Dose/Fx
Lee 2007 [12]	21	EBRT	24	89	36 Gy/6 fx
Jo 2012 [37]	11	EBRT+HDR boost HDR monotherapy		64 % (crude)	22 Gy/2 fx
Chen 2013 [11]	52	EBRT	60	51	36 Gy/6 fx 50 % neoADT
Yamada 2014 [38]	42	EBRT	60	68.5	32 Gy/4 fx

- Pretreatment lower urinary tract symptoms (LUTS)/ Sexual Health Inventory
  - Obstructive urinary symptoms are the primary form of HDR brachytherapy toxicity. Excessive pretreatment LUTS may predict for increased post-treatment toxicity. Pretreatment AUA symptom score should be obtained in all patients prior to treatment. The authors do not use a strict IPSS for treatment exclusion.
  - Optimize medical management of LUTS prior to implantation. An alpha-1 receptor antagonist is recommended for patients with obstructive urinary symptoms.
  - Sexual function is an important part of counseling regarding prostate cancer. A sexual health inventory for men (SHIM) score should be obtained for all patients prior to treatment.
- Transurethral resection of prostate (TURP)
  - Prior TURP may be associated with increased risk for urinary toxicity.
  - Without adequate visualization of the TURP defect, HDR brachytherapy is contraindicated.

- Techniques to improve visualization and avoidance of the TURP defect may reduce this risk to baseline.
- HDR can be considered for patients with prior TURP, provided >6 month interval between HDR and TURP, and appropriate visualization of the TURP defect during optimization.
- Inflammatory Bowel Disease
  - Patients with inflammatory bowel disease may be at increased risk for rectal toxicity. HDR should be used with caution [14, 15].

Who Should Get HDR Brachytherapy?

- Boost
  - EBRT with HDR boost, with or without ADT can be considered for all risk groups
  - HDR boost is an effective form of dose escalation, with EQD2 ($\alpha/\beta = 1.5$) on the order of 60–70 Gy for the boost component.
  - Local control is ~95 % with adequate target coverage, regardless of risk category.
  - Boost can be delivered before or after external beam radiation.
- Monotherapy
  - HDR monotherapy has been used on trial for patients of all risk groups.
  - The most mature evidence is for patients with low- or favorable intermediate-risk disease.
  - Monotherapy has the added advantage of reducing treatment time compared with EBRT, and can be completed in a single implant, provided adequate image guidance and dosimetry are available.
- Salvage
  - Prolonged biochemical disease-free intervals have been reported for patients with isolated local recurrences, treated with salvage brachytherapy. Careful review of prior radiotherapy records, PSA,

and high-quality diagnostic imaging with TRUS, TRUS-guided biopsy, and MRI can be useful for identifying and defining recurrent disease.

- Biopsies within 2 years may be subject to high false-positive rates [16, 17].
- Short disease-free intervals and rapid doubling times may portend occult metastatic disease
- The authors have favored treatment of the whole gland during salvage
- Hemi-gland salvage radiation has been used on an experimental basis
- The benefit of neoadjuvant and adjuvant androgen deprivation remains undefined in this context.

- Medical Condition
  - Anesthesia: Catheter placement can be placed under epidural anesthesia, conscious sedation, nerve block, or general anesthesia. Patients should have appropriate anesthesia evaluation prior to treatment. Contraindications may vary depending on selected anesthesia.
  - CBC: ANC>1000 cells/μL, Platelets>60,000 cells/μL, Hgb>7 g/μL.
  - Coagulation profile: pTT, INR
  - Anticoagulation
    - Stop anticoagulants prior to treatment 5 days prior to treatment
    - Heparin bridge if patients cannot tolerate prolonged periods without anticoagulation (e.g., mechanical heart valve, history of clotting or CVA, arrhythmia).

Image Guidance Utilization

Preprocedure Image Guidance

- Transrectal Ultrasound (TRUS)
  - Essential component of pretreatment evaluation to identify the prostate, evaluate prostate size, identify

and localize targetable lesions, identify seminal vesicle invasion or extracapsular extension.

- Broad interface between a cancerous lesion and the prostate capsule predicts increased risk for extracapsular extension

■ CT Abdomen/Pelvis or Pelvic MRI
  - Consider for T3 or T4 disease, or if the estimated risk for nodal involvement exceeds 10 % (NCCN guidelines)
  - Endorectal coil MRI can improve imaging of the prostate and identify dominant intraprostatic lesions (DILs).
  - MRI can be fused with CT to assist with target delineation and planning

■ Tc99m Bone Scan/NaF PET/CT
  - Consider for:
    ▪ T1 tumors with PSA > 20
    ▪ T2 tumors with PSA > 10
    ▪ Gleason 8 or higher
    ▪ T3 or T4 disease

■ Advanced/Investigational Imaging
  - MRI with endorectal coil and MRI spectroscopy can be used to identify DILs [18].
  - ^{66}Ga-PSMA PET/CT, ^{11}C-Choline PET/CT may be more sensitive than CT or MRI for extra-prostatic disease [19].
  - Lymphotropic Superparamagnetic Nanoparticles (Combidex) may have increased sensitivity for nodal disease [20].

Equipment

- Brachytherapy catheter selection: 16-gauge 25 cm catheters
- Transrectal ultrasound with stepper/stabilizer: Ultrasound and stepper
- Template (optional): Martinez template

- Afterloader: Nucleotron 18 channel MicroSelectron
- Source Isotope: Iridium 192
- Treatment Planning Software: Oncentra

Implant Procedure

- Preprocedure instructions
    - Stop ASA, NSAIDs 1 week prior to treatment
    - Preprocedure anesthesia evaluation
    - NPO at midnight before the procedure
    - Bowel preparation: Fleets enema the morning of the procedure
- Day of procedure
    - Anesthesia
    - Positioning: Place the patient in the dorsal lithotomy position.
    - SCDs: Sequential compression devices should be used when possible to prevent clotting
    - Preprocedure antibiotics: Administer Ancef 1 g immediately prior to procedure. Patients with penicillin allergies can be given Ciprofloxacin 400 mg immediately prior to the procedure.
    - Ensure adequate bowel prep for visualization
    - Sterile Surgical Preparation: Povidone-iodine prep of the perineum, penis, inguinal regions. Draped in sterile fashion, exposing the perineum, penis and anus exposed.
    - Position the transrectal ultrasound and visualize the prostate

Image-Guided Catheter Placement

- Hollow brachytherapy catheters can be placed using either a template or freehand (preferred by the authors).
- Catheters are placed via the perineum, under real-time transrectal ultrasound guidance with visualization of urethra, periprostatic tissue, and catheters

- A Foley catheter with aerated gel can aid in visualization of the urethra
- Adequate catheter depth can be confirmed with post-procedure cystoscopy to ensure catheters are tenting, but not puncturing the bladder
- Catheters can be fixed using either a template, or with sutures and dental putty (Fig. 13.3).

Image-Guided Treatment Planning

- US, CT, or MRI can be used for image-guided treatment planning and optimization.
- Planning can be forward or inverse planned (preferred by the authors).
- Accurate catheter identification on cross-sectional imaging and correlation with afterloader channels is critical.

Guidelines for Implantation

Implantation Pattern

- Peripheral catheter placement allows more uniform distributions, improved coverage, and steeper dose gradients
  - Rule of thumb: 2/3 peripheral, 1/3 central
- We favor a 16 catheter arrangement with 4 periurethral catheters to decrease urethral dose (Figs. 13.3 and 13.4a, b).
- Placement of the 4 periurethral catheters are critical for urethral-sparing HDR brachytherapy [21].
- Placement of catheters near the rectal interface can be critical for fine tuning the rectal dose
- Additional catheters can be used for large or irregular prostate shapes. The maximum number of catheters may be determined by afterloader capacity

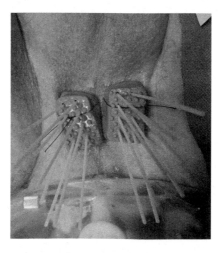

FIG. 13.3. Transverse sections of transrectal ultrasound-guided catheter placement. Catheters are placed in an anterior to posterior fashion to limit shadowing artifact

- Postimplantation cystoscopy is important for evaluating the depth of each catheter and to ensure coverage of the base of the prostate
- Isodose lines and dose–volume histograms are shown for a representative patient (Fig. 13.5a–c).

Catheter Fixation

- After all catheters are applied, they must be fixed to minimize migration between catheter placement and treatment delivery.
- For nonuniform loading, accurate catheter enumeration, delineation, and catheter migration management is particularly critical
- The authors favor use of a plastic grid, dental putty, and sutures for catheter fixation
- Repeat CT prior to each fraction can ensure adequate placement and allows room for adjustment

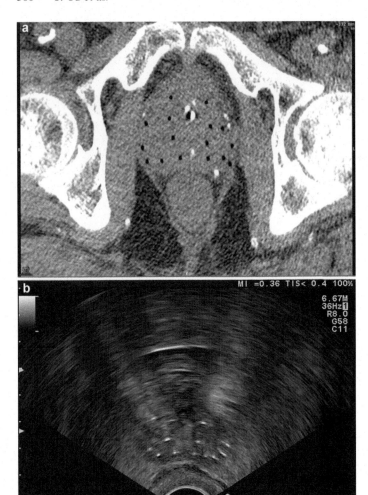

Fig. 13.4. (**a** and **b**) Postimplantation CT (**a**) and US (**b**) demonstrate catheter pattern

TURP Defect Visualization

■ If HDR in the setting of prior TURP is attempted, adequate visualization is imperative to minimize toxicity

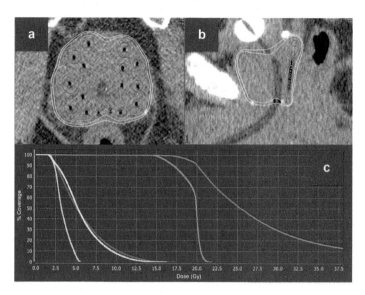

FIG. 13.5. (**a–c**) HDR dosimetry for a gentleman with cT1c, Gleason 3 + 4 prostate cancer involving 2/23 cores, PSA of <5, treated with HDR monotherapy, 19 Gy in 1 fraction. In the *top panel*, representative (**a**) axial and (**b**) sagittal images are shown with the 200 % (*red*), 120 % (*orange*), 100 % (*green*), and 90 % (*yellow*) isodose lines. The associated DVH with the bladder (*yellow*), bulb (*green*), rectum (*brown*), target (*red*), and urethra (*blue*) is shown in (**c**)

- Urethral contrast can be used to visualize the TURP defect on TRUS

Treatment Planning Considerations

Inverse Planning vs. Forward Planning

- Authors recommend inverse planning simulated annealing (IPSA) software for treatment planning optimization. Specific dose targets can be easily (and quickly) achieved

- Benefits may be greatest with difficult cases (e.g., large prostate, intraprostatic calcifications)
- Inverse planning may decrease planning time

CT vs. US-Guided Planning

- Both strategies have been used by experienced teams to achieve excellent results
- CT-based planning offers accurate catheter reconstruction
- Catheters or intraprostatic calcifications may cast "shadows" on ultrasound-based systems that obscure the catheter location.
- CT-based planning systems offer excellent delineation of critical structures, including the rectum, bladder, urethra, and urogenital diaphragm.
- The seminal vesicles are easily visualized on CT, which can allow safe implantation and accurate dosimetry
- It may be difficult to differentiate the prostate from periprostatic tissue on CT
- Intraprostatic lesions can be identified on ultrasound, and coverage can be ensured
- Ultrasound-based planning in a shielded OR can significantly speed up workflow

Dose and Fractionation

- Choice of fractionation is highly variable in the literature and dependent on multiple factors
- The authors favor single-fraction treatment to limit trauma from repeated implants; however, this requires precise delivery of conformal radiation doses and strict attention to dose constraints.
- BID fractions should be delivered with ≥ 6 h interfraction interval

- ▪ Boost
  - ▪ 15 Gy × 1 fraction in 1 implant
  - ▪ 9.5 Gy × 2 fractions in 1 implant
- ▪ Monotherapy
  - ▪ 7 Gy × 6 BID fractions in two implants, separated by 1 week
  - ▪ 9.5 Gy × 4 BID fractions in 2 implants, separated by 1 week
  - ▪ 12–13.5 Gy × 2 fractions in one implant
  - ▪ 19–21 Gy × 1 fraction (Early experience shows acceptable control and toxicity; however, follow-up remains limited.)
- ▪ Salvage
  - ▪ 6 Gy × 6 BID fractions in two implants, separated by 1 week.
  - ▪ 8 Gy × 4 fractions (over 30 h) in 1 implant

Dose Constraints

See Table 13.4 for dose constraints.

TABLE 13.4 Dose constraints

Coverage:
V100 >90 %
Normal Tissue Constraints
Urethral V125 % <1 cc[a]
Urethral V150 % =0 cc
Rectal/Bladder V75 % <1 cc

Doses are computed on a 1 mm dose grid
[a]Prostatic tissue lying between the urethra and the rectum. Necrosis of this tissue could lead to urethra-rectal fistulas

Urethral-Sparing Treatment Plans

- ■ May reduce urinary toxicity following treatment [21–23].
- ■ It may be useful in re-irradiation

Toxicity

Acute Toxicity

- ■ Pain
  - ■ Acute pain is primarily secondary to catheter trauma
  - ■ Managed with over-the-counter NSAIDs or oral narcotics.
- ■ LUTS
  - ■ Transient exacerbation of LUTS is expected
  - ■ Significantly improved by 2 weeks, with recovery of acute toxicity by 3 months
  - ■ Patients can be discharged on Flomax if pretreatment urinary symptoms are significant (IPSS > 15)
  - ■ Consider continuing Foley catheter placement for 1 week after treatment if the patient is at high risk for urinary obstruction
- ■ Hematospermia
  - ■ Generally self-limited, but can be common following catheter placement. Patients should be counseled about this possibility.
- ■ Prostatitis
  - ■ Patients with pain not adequately managed with over-the-counter NSAIDS can be considered for a short course of antibiotics
- ■ Early Urinary Obstruction
  - ■ Patients with preexisting LUTS may experience exacerbation of their lower urinary tract symptoms.

This may be particularly prominent in patients with large median lobes

- Patients should be counseled about this possibility and the possible need for temporary urinary catheter.
    - Corticosteroids and NSAIDS can be used to reduce acute inflammation.
- Hematuria/clot retention
    - Hematuria from brachytherapy catheter placement, Foley catheter placement, or cystoscopy can occasionally be seen.
- Gastrointestinal toxicity
    - GI toxicity, primarily manifested by diarrhea, is uncommon following HDR brachytherapy alone.
    - This can be managed with dietary modification (removal of high-residue foods), loperamide

Late Toxicity

- GU
    - Mild late urinary frequency and urgency common
    - Grade 3 toxicity is rare and can include stricture (~0–12 %) and hematuria (~5–10 %).
    - Long-term catheter dependence is rare
- Erectile function
    - Erectile dysfunction is multifactorial
    - Radiation-induced erectile dysfunction tends to develop as a late toxicity [24].
    - The incidence appears to be similar to or better than RP [25] and comparable to external beam radiation.
    - Use of ADT increases this risk
    - Treat with PDE inhibitors
- Infertility
    - Patients may have dry seminal fluid following radiotherapy, which can reduce fertility. Sperm banking is recommended.

- ■ Genetic Defects
  - ■ Conception may still be possible following radiation; however, there may be a risk for increased birth defects due to radiation exposure. Sperm banking is recommended.
- ■ Rectal Toxicity
  - ■ Urgency, frequency can be increased
  - ■ Intermittent rectal bleeding can be observed
  - ■ Avoid rectal biopsies, as these can lead to urethra-rectal fistula formation

Rare Toxicities

- ■ Tumor seeding
  - ■ Case reports exist of bladder or rectal wall seeding; however, these are extremely rare.
- ■ Urethro-Rectal Fistula
  - ■ Rare, associated with rectal biopsies following treatment
- ■ Secondary malignancy
  - ■ Very uncommon for prostate cancer treated with radiation (any form), <1 % [26, 27].

Appendix A

Mitchell Kamrava

Prostate Case Study 13.1: HDR Monotherapy

A 70-year-old male presented with an elevated PSA of 5.5. His previous PSAs were not elevated. He was referred to a urologist who preformed a digital rectal examination which was normal. He subsequently recommended the patient undergo a multiparametric MRI (mp-MRI) of the prostate followed by targeted and systematic biopsies. His mp-MRI showed a PI-RADS 4 lesion in the peripheral zone of the left apex (Fig. 13.6). Targeted biopsy showed Gleason score 3+4

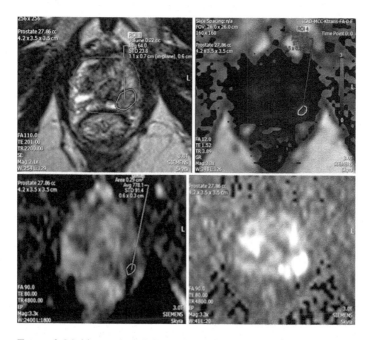

FIG. 13.6. Multiparametric MRI prostate images including T2 (*top left*) with lesion in left apex contoured in *yellow* and prostate contoured in *green*, DCE (*top right*), ADC map (*bottom left*), and DWI (*bottom right*)

disease in 2 out of 4 targeted biopsy cores and Gleason score $3+3$ disease in 2 out of 12 systematic (right base and left mid gland) biopsy cores.

The patient had a past medical history significant for some hypertension and elevated cholesterol. He had no previous history of a transurethral resection of the prostate and his International Prostate Symptom Score was 8 and his Sexual Health Inventory for Men score was 20.

Discussion: The patient was a candidate for active surveillance or definitive treatment with either surgery or radiation therapy. With regards to radiation therapy the options of standard external beam, hypofractionated external beam, stereotactic body radiation therapy, low-dose rate brachytherapy, and high-dose rate brachytherapy were discussed with the patient. The option of including a short course of androgen deprivation therapy was also discussed with the patient. After a balanced discussion the patient decided to proceed with HDR brachytherapy with no androgen deprivation therapy.

Procedure with Image Guidance: Transrectal ultrasound was used to guide the transperineal placement of brachytherapy catheters both in and around the prostate and the proximal seminal vesicles (Fig. 13.7). Following the catheter insertion a CT simulation was performed for dosimetric planning.

Treatment plan: We planned for a brachytherapy dose of 13.5 $Gy \times 2$ fractions delivered in two separate implants spaced one week apart from each other. The CTV was the prostate and the proximal seminal vesicles. Organ at risk constraints were rectal wall D0.1 $cc < 85\%$, bladder wall D0.1 $cc > 80\%$ but $< 95\%$, and urethra D0.1 $cc < 110\%$. Target coverage constraints were D90% 100–115%, V100% 97–100%, and V150% $< 35\%$. The patient's mp-MRI was

→

FIG. 13.7. (continued) catheters with respect to symmetry, straight trajectory, and adequate spacing relative to the urethra. Completed implant on the bottom with red Foley catheter, beige rectal catheter, and Kerlix™ (Covidien, Dublin, Ireland) bolster around the template sutured to the perineum

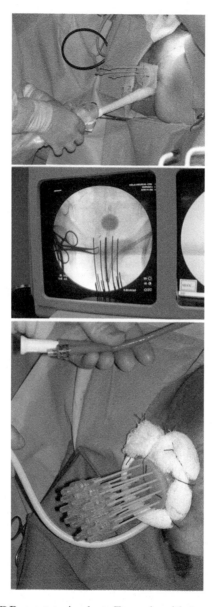

FIG. 13.7. HDR prostate implant. Example with transrectal ultrasound and template with anterior needles placed first. AP fluoroscopy (*middle*) can be used to verify the position of the anterior

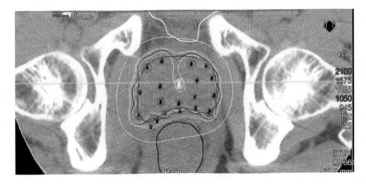

Fig. 13.8. Isodose distribution on an axial CT slice. Red contour is the prostate, yellow is the bladder, and brown is the rectum

fused with the CT simulation images to assist with accurately identifying the prostate base, apex, and index lesion identified in the left apex. The isodose curves with the CTV are shown in Fig. 13.8.

Prostate Case Study 13.2: HDR Salvage

A 72-year-old male diagnosed with prostate cancer in 2008 with clinical T2a, PSA 4.1, and Gleason score 3 + 3 disease. He was treated definitively with low-dose rate I-125 seed brachytherapy to a dose of 145 Gy in 2009 (Fig. 13.9). His PSA reached a nadir of 1 by 2011 and then gradually rose to 4.2 by 2013. At that time he had a bone scan and CT scan of the abdomen and pelvis which were negative for metastatic disease. He had a multiparametric MRI performed showing a 1.1 cm lesion in the left seminal vesicle (Fig. 13.10). He then had a targeted and systematic prostate biopsy showing 2/12 cores positive (both in the left base) for Gleason score 4 + 4 disease. He was started on Lupron® (AbbVie Inc, North Chicago, IL, USA) and then sent for consultation for possible salvage brachytherapy.

The patient had a past medical history significant for diabetes, hypertension, and hyperlipidemia. He had no previous

Isodose Legend Gy [% of Prescription Dose]	290.00 [200,00%]	145.00 [100,00%]
	217.50 [150,00%]	130.50 [90,00%]
	174.00 [120,00%]	72.50 [50,00%]

Anatomy/Landmark Legend	Prostate	Rectum

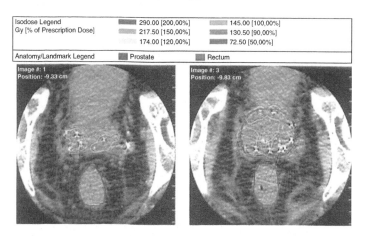

FIG. 13.9. Axial CT images near the prostate base from the I-125 LDR prostate implant showing the distribution of the seeds and isodose lines

history of a transurethral resection of the prostate and his International Prostate Symptom Score was 12 and his Sexual Health Inventory for Men score was 14 (this was measured after the patient had started Lupron®).

Discussion: The patient was a candidate for multiple treatments including observation, androgen deprivation alone, surgery, cryotherapy, high-intensity frequency ultrasound, whole gland high-dose rate brachytherapy, and partial gland high-dose rate brachytherapy. After a balanced discussion the patient decided to proceed with HDR partial gland salvage brachytherapy with 6 months of androgen deprivation therapy.

Procedure with Image Guidance: The procedure was performed using transrectal ultrasound guidance to assist in the placement of catheters to cover the left prostate hemi-gland with the urethra serving as the division between the right and left prostate.

Treatment plan: We planned for a brachytherapy dose of 6 Gy × 6 fractions to the left hemi-prostate and the left seminal vesicle delivered in two separate implants spaced one

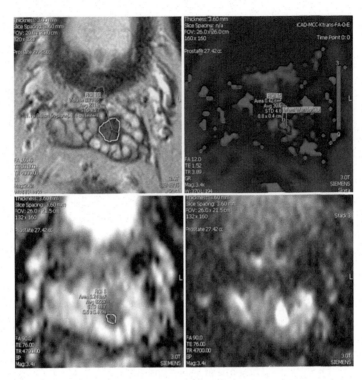

FIG. 13.10. Multiparametric MRI findings demonstrating disease in the left seminal vesicle. T2 image *top left*, DCE imaging *top right*, ADC map *bottom left*, and DWI imaging *bottom right*

week apart from each other. Organ at risk constraints were rectal wall D0.1 cc < 85 %, bladder wall D0.1 cc > 80 % but < 95 %, and urethra D0.1 cc < 110 %. Target coverage constraints were D90% 100–115 %, V100% 97–100 %, and V150% < 35 %. The patient's mp-MRI was fused with the CT simulation images to assist with accurately identifying the prostate base, apex, and disease in the left seminal vesicle. The isodose curves with the CTV are shown in Fig. 13.11.

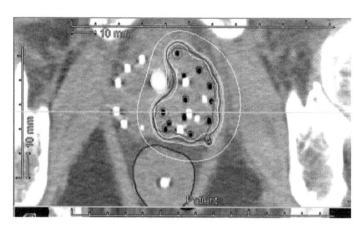

FIG. 13.11. Axial CT slice showing distribution of HDR catheters in a hemi-gland distribution and the corresponding isodose lines. The *red* contour represents the CTV. The *blue* isodose line is the 100 % isodose line and the *white line* is the 50 % isodose line

Appendix B: Prostate HDR

This appendix includes forms developed and in clinical use by the Brachytherapy Division at the University of California Los Angeles. It includes contributions from multiple team members including doctors (Mitchell Kamrava, D. Jeffrey Demanes), nurse (Kayla Kafka), physician assistant (Lalaine Zaide), therapist (Tom Wong), and physicist (Sang-June Park).

Appendix Form 13.1. Operative report.
PROSTATE HDR BRACHYTHERAPY PROCEDURE REPORT

DATE	IMPLANT #

Radiation Oncologist:

Urologist:

PREOPERATIVE DIAGNOSIS: Prostate Adenocarcinoma
T___ PSA___ Gleason___

POSTOPERATIVE DIAGNOSIS: same

ANESTHESIA:

COMPLICATIONS: None   ESTIMATED BLOOD LOSS: Minimal

PROCEDURES:

1. Examination under anesthesia
2. Proctosigmoidoscopy
3. Cystoscopy
4. Transrectal ultrasound for interstitial brachytherapy guidance.
5. Complex interstitial brachytherapy prostate
6. Fiducial marker insertion procedure
7. Fluoroscopy

1. Examination under Anesthesia
   The patient was placed under spinal anesthesia and placed in the lithotomy position.
   Perineal examination: no findings that preclude proceeding with brachytherapy. Digital examination findings:

2.Proctosigmoidoscopy:

After negative digital rectal examination, a 25 cm rigid sig-moidoscope with obturator was inserted into the rectum. It was advanced to a depth of _____cm under direct visual-ization with insufflation and suction performed as needed. Findings:

3.Cystoscopy:

The operative field was prepared and draped. The flexible cystoscopy was performed before and during the brachyther-apy procedure. The scope was utilized during the implant to ensure that there were no catheters in the lumen of the ure-thra at the completion of brachytherapy procedure. Findings:

4.Transrectal ultrasound guidance and prostate volume analysis

A multiplane real-time ultrasound scanner with biplane probe was inserted into the rectum. The transverse and longitudinal pelvic images were generated. Prostate, blad-der, and seminal vesicle anatomy was studied and the pros-tate volumes were recorded. The ultrasound was utilized throughout the implant procedure to guide the brachy-therapy applicator placement. Findings:

5.Complex interstitial brachytherapy applicator placement prostate: (Transrectal ultrasound, fluoroscopic and cystos-copy guidance).

The patient was placed in the lithotomy position, prepared and draped for the procedure. An 18-French, 5cc radi-opaque Council type urinary catheter was inserted into the bladder and the balloon was inflated with 10 cc of diluted (1:4) Hypaque contrast material. The catheter plug was inserted after the bladder was partially emptied to allow optimal visualization of the prostate and bladder.

A template guide was placed on the perineum and used to direct the brachytherapy catheter insertion. A double-glove technique (with digital rectal palpation of the pros-tate) was utilized to place the two brachytherapy catheters anterior (beneath the pubic arch) and two lateral to the prostate capsule.

A transverse ultrasound image of the prostate was obtained. The four initial brachytherapy catheters were visualized and adjusted for optimal position. The catheters were guided into the tissues by adjusting the position of the template and applying pressure on the catheters as they were advanced. Two more catheters were placed between the anterior and the lateral ones (on either side of midline) to complete the anterior portion of the implant.

Additional brachytherapy catheters were then inserted around the lateral prostate capsule and through the substance of the prostate. The sequence of brachytherapy catheter insertion was first anterior, second lateral, third into the substance of the prostate. The posterior plane was inserted last. The position of each catheter was adjusted with the aid of the ultrasound probe and variable angle fluoroscopy. Penetration of the urethra or the rectum was avoided. The posterior implant catheters were located just within the prostate capsule above the anterior rectal wall. The medial parts of the seminal vesicles were implanted along with the posterior row of catheters.

Total number of catheters:

The template was sutured to the perineum. A roll of sterile surgical gauze was fashioned into a bolster and sutured at 5 points to the perineum with 1-0 silk. The template was snugly tied to the bolster and the bolster was wrapped and tied around the template to firmly fix the template on the perineum and to protect the scrotum. A 22-gauge Foley catheter was inserted into the rectum with the 30 cc balloon inflated with diluted contrast. The urinary catheter placed to gravity and the rectal catheter was plugged.

6.Fiducial marker insertion procedure:

The platinum marker seeds were used to delineate the base and apex of the prostate. They were implanted prior to completion of the brachytherapy catheter placement in order to make use of the central template guides. The anatomic sites that required marking were determined based upon clinical and radiological data. The relationship of tumor to normal tissue was taken into consideration in selection of locations for marker insertion. A 17-gauge needle with funnel attachment applicator was used for placement of the marker seeds. Placement was guided with clinical information, fluoroscopy, and ultrasound. Traction was applied to the tissues when possible during the insertion process. The applicator needle was inserted into the tissue and positioned in relation to the target treatment volume. The stylette was removed and the marker seed was loaded into the funnel portion of the needle. The fiducial marker was then inserted into the tissue by fully inserting the stylette into the needle applicator until the stylette fully contacted the funnel portion of the applicator. This process was repeated serially for each marker and tissue location. Hemostasis at the marker insertion sites was achieved by direct pressure. The procedure was completed by radiological confirmation of marker number, position, and tissue relationships. Total fiducial markers:

7.Fluoroscopy:

Fluoroscopy was performed in anterior–posterior and lateral projections. The distributions of the brachytherapy catheters, marker seeds, bones, and the urinary and rectal catheter were identified. Implant adjustments were made throughout the procedure. The catheter and anatomic relationships were determined. Final brachytherapy catheter adjustments were made based upon lateral fluoroscopy.

DISPOSTION:

The patient completed the procedure in good condition. Simulation radiography, computerized dosimetry, and HDR brachytherapy were scheduled to follow in sequence.

Appendix Form 13.2. Post-operative orders.
POSTOPERATIVE ORDERS:
Template Brachytherapy Implants

1.Admit to: ___23 hour Observation ___ Regular Ward ___ICU
2.NO RADIATION PRECAUTIONS REQUIRED
3.Patient under (Radiation/Oncology Service)
4.Activity: BEDREST. Patient to remain on gurney. Turn Q2hrs while awake.
5.Supine with 2 pillows under knees, lateral with 2 pillows between knees, head <20 degrees and foot of bed flat.
6.Diet: ___NPO ___Clear liquid ___Low Residue (soft diet)
7.IV: D5 ½ NS with 20mEq KCL at _____ ml/hr
8.Incentive Spirometry: Q2hrs
9.Foley Catheter: Foley to closed gravity drainage. Irrigate foley cath with Normal Saline PRN
10.Call Physician PRN: Excessive bleeding or pain
11.Input/ Output: Q shift
12.Sequential Compression Device for DVT prophylaxis:
13.Medications:

a. PAIN:	___PCA (see order sheet)
b. SLEEP:	___Ambien 10mg PO at bedtime PRN
c. ANXIETY:	___Ativan 1 mg po q 2hrs PRN
d. NAUSEA:	___Zofran 4 mg q 6hrs IV PRN
e. TEMPERATURE	___Tylenol 500mg PO Q4hrs PRN
f. ANTIBIOTICS:	___Cefotetan 1gm IV Q12hrs
	___Levaquin 500mg IV Q24hrs
	___Cleocin 600mg IV Q8hrs

Appendix Form 13.3. Prostate HDR template diagram.

PROSTATE HDR TEMPLATE DIAGRAM

DATE:_____ IMPLANT #:___/___   MD:_____

Protocol: ☐ HDR Monotherapy   ☐ HDR Focal ☐ HDR + EBRT

TRUS Length:_____cm, Vol _____cc   TURP: ☐ YES   ☐ NO

Template: ☐ Custom   ☐ Syed   ☐ CET   ☐ Liberty   ☐ Nucletron

Appendix Form 13.4. HDR written directive.

UCLA Department of Radiation Oncology
HDR Brachytherapy Written Directive

Patient Name: _____   Date of Birth: _____

Patient ID Number: _____

Treatment Site: _____   Applicator: __Interstitial__

Rx Dose per Faction (Gy): _____   Isotope: __Ir-192__

Total # of Fractions: _____   Step size (mm): _____

Total Rx Dose (Gy): _____

Prescription to : __Prostate CTV__

Attending Radiation Oncologist: _____
   (authorized user physician)

Appendix Form 13.5. HDR plan summary.

UCLA Department of Radiation Oncology
HDR Brachytherapy Plan Summary

Patient Name: _____   Date of Birth: _____

Patient ID Number: _____

Treatment Site: _____   Applicator: Interstitial
                                           (applicator/implant diagram attached)

Rx Dose per Faction (Gy): _____   Isotope: Ir-192

# of Fractions: _____   Step size (mm): _____

Total Rx Dose (Gy): _____

Prescription to : Prostate CTV

Attending Radiation Oncologist: _____
(authorized user physician)

Fx #	Plan Date	# Ch	# Dwells	Air Kerma (mGy m^2/h)	Plan Tx Time (sec)	mGy @ 1m	Rx / Fx (Gy)	Planner	Checker

Fx #	Tx Date	Elapsed Days	Rx / Fx (Gy)	Air Kerma (mGy m^2/h)	Tx Time (sec)	mGy @ 1m	Cumulative Dose (Gy)	Physicist (AMP)	Physician (AU)

Final Check:

Total HDR Dose: [   ] (Gy)

Appendix Form 13.6. HDR special physics consult and dosimetry.

UCLA Department of Radiation Oncology
Special Physics Consultation &
HDR Final Dosimetry Endpoints

Patient Name: _____   ID: _____
Treatment Site: _____ Prostate (Interstitial) _____
Plan Date: _____
Rx (Gy)/fx: _____
Fraction #: _____

	Dose (Gy)/fx	Total # of fx's	Total (Gy)
Rx Dose (Gy):			
Previous External:			

		Clinical Range (%)	cc
D90% Target:	100%-115%		
V100% Target:	97% - 100%		
V150% Target:	< 25% -35%		
V100% Total:			
Target Volume:			

Rectal Wall:	D0.1cc < 85%	D1.0cc	D2.0cc	
%of Rx				%
Gy				Gy

Bladder Wall:	80% < D0.1cc < 95%	D1.0cc	D2.0cc	
%of Rx				%
Gy				Gy

Bladder Balloon:	60% < D0.1cc < 80%	D1.0cc	D2.0cc	
%of Rx				%
Gy				Gy

*Urethra:	D0.1cc < 110%	D1.0cc < 105%	D2.0cc	
%of Rx				%
Gy				Gy

*for TURP: 105%
*for Monotherapy: 110% and D1.0cc < 105%
*for Combotherapy: 120% and D1.0cc < 115%

Small Bowel:	D0.1cc < 85%	D1.0cc	D2.0cc	
%of Rx				%
Gy				Gy

I requested this consult to the qualified medical physicist for special consultative dosimetry report.
Please evaluate target coverage (CTV V100 and V150) and dose to critical structures (D0.1cc, D1.cc,
and D2cc) based upon high-dose-rate brachytherapy dosimetry constraints. I reviewed results of the
consult.

Attending physician (authorized user)

Appendix Form 13.7. Pre- and postpatient treatment survey.

UCLA Department of Radiation Oncology
Pre & Post-Treatment Patient Survey

Pre-treatment Check:
(Check the following items using written directive, plan report, & pre-tx record.)

Patient Name: _____ [ ] Date of Birth: _____ [ ]
Patient ID: _____ [ ]
Treatment Date: _____ [ ]
Rx / fx (Gy): _____ [ ] Tx site: **Prostate** [ ]
Fraction #: _____ [ ]

Patient Name & ID check: [ ] Daily QA completed: [ ]
Written Directive completed: [ ] Emergency Instructions / Equipment [ ]
Check dose from TPS vs. 2nd Calc using TG-43: [ ] HDR Suite Video Monitor / Intercom: [ ]
Tube connection check with implant diagram: [ ] Inspect guide tubes: [ ]

Plan Name & version check: [ ] Indexer length check: [ ]
Total channel # check: [ ] Step size check: [ ]

          mGym^2/h sec mGy @ 1m
Plan AK (mGy m^2/h) x Tx time (sec) / 3600 = [ ] [ ] [ ]
Current AK (mGy m^2/h) x Tx time (sec) / 3600 = [ ] [ ] [ ] [ ]

Pre-treatment Patient Survey (mR/hr)
Background: _____
Patient: _____
Afterloader Surface: _____

Authorized User Physician: _____

During treatment Check:
Console source location indicator: [ ]
Console power status indicator: [ ]
Door radiation warning light: [ ]
Radiation area monitor in the control room: [ ]

Post-treatment Patient Survey (mR/hr)
Background: _____
Patient: _____
Afterloader Surface: _____

Survey Instrument
Monitor 4/4EC (Scale x1.0) or Fluke Biomedical 451P (see Daily QA form)
If other survey meter used, record maker, model, & S/N.

Authorized Medical Physicist: _____

Appendix Form 13.8. Sample home care instructions.

HOME CARE INSTRUCTIONS AFTER HIGH-DOSE RATE BRACHYTHERAPY

Please keep your postoperative appointment: _____

_____

Diet: Begin with liquids such as soup and progress to regular diet as tolerated.

Medications: Please call the office for questions about medications, allergies, and reactions.

- Usual Prescriptions—Please resume all of your usual medications unless otherwise instructed.
- Pain—You may experience discomfort for several days after the procedure. It is typically relieved by Tylenol (acetaminophen) but may require the prescription given to you at your preoperative visit (typically Vicodin). Take ½ tab to 1 tab every 4-6 hours as needed.
- Constipation—Narcotic pain medications may cause constipation. It is important that you do not get constipated. Drink plenty of fluids and ensure you are taking a stool softener, such as Colace (docusate sodium) or drink prune juice if you are taking narcotic pain medication. If you experience constipation, you will likely need a laxative, such as senokot or milk of magnesia.
- Difficult urination—If you experience burning while urinating, you may take Pyridium. Make sure you also drink plenty of water, decrease acidic food/drink intake, and take warm water (sitz) baths. Do not use bath salts or soaps.
- Antibiotics—Preventative antibiotics (Cipro, Bactrim) are usually prescribed by your physician. Take your antibiotic twice per day for three days after your implant is removed. Begin taking your antibiotic ____

_____ .

Activities:

- Avoid heavy lifting (>10 lbs) and strenuous activities for the first few weeks.
- Do not drink alcohol or drive for 24 hours after your release from the hospital OR while you are taking narcotic pain medication.
- Keep the perineum area (bottom) as clean and dry as possible.
- You may shower. Just do not rub perineum harshly or use irritating soaps.
- A sitz bath taken 2-3 times per day (especially after bowel movements) may provide comfort.
- Be patient with urination. Do not strain. Drink plenty of water and take sitz baths to relax urinary sphincter/bladder.

CALL OUR DOCTORS OR GO TO THE EMERGENCY ROOM IF:

- You are actively bleeding.
- You have pain not relieved by prescribed pain medication or if pain is increasing in severity.
- You have a temperature over 101 degrees Fahrenheit
- You develop excessive drainage, or drainage appears cloudy or contains pus
- You are unable to empty your bladder or it is causing significant pain.

IF YOU ARE IN DOUBT ABOUT WHAT TO DO OR IF YOUR SYMPTOMS ARE URGENT OR CONCERNING, GO TO YOUR NEAREST EMERGENCY ROOM. AFTER YOUR ER VISIT, PLEAS BE SURE TO LET US KNOW YOU HAVE BEEN TO THE HOSPITAL. AFTER HOURS CONTACT INFORMATION:

- Call the hospital page operator and ask them to page your doctor.

Appendix Form 13.9. Sample notice to patients.

IMPORTANT NOTICE
TO
PROSTATE PATIENTS

Please call and speak to us about symptoms or a rising PSA and especially any proposed pelvic procedures (i.e. cystoscopy, TUR-P, dilation, sigmoidoscopy, colonoscopy) **BEFORE** those are performed. This notification and our involvement will help avoid post radiation urinary and rectal complications.

Appendix Form 13.10. Nursing notes.

<u>HDR Brachytherapy</u> for <u>Prostate Cancer Nursing Notes</u>

We perform both HDR monotherapy and HDR combination therapy for prostate cancer at UCLA. Prostate implants are placed under spinal anesthesia in our Brachytherapy Suite as well as the outpatient surgery center. Patients with higher anesthesia risk may have their implant placed in the main OR in Ronald Reagan.

Patients undergoing implant placement in the brachytherapy suite will remain in the department from the time of admission through discharge (pre-op, intra-op, and post-op). If the procedure is done in the outpatient surgery center, the patient is recovered in surgery center until they have been released from anesthesia (typically one hour). Nursing report is obtained and patient is transported to the department of Radiation Oncology by gurney. If patient's treatment planning will be CT based, the CT simulation will occur at this time.

Activity Restrictions

Patients with prostate brachytherapy implants are on strict flat bed rest. They are not to flex in the midsection as this can move or damage the implant. These patients and their visitors require thorough education to be compliant with movement restrictions. Patients may be turned from side to side with nursing assistance but are not allowed to sit up (refer to "How to turn a patient with a prostate brachytherapy implant"). If patient needs their head raised for swallowing, hygiene, or emergency situations, the patient may be placed in the reverse Trendelenburg position. This raises the head above the rest of the body without bending patient in the midsection. Patients may find that they are most comfortable eating and swallowing while lying on their side with two pillows under their head.

Patients with prostate brachytherapy implants remain on the gurney throughout their stay. The gurney mattress is firmer than that of a hospital bed, which makes it less likely that the patient's body weight will push the implant down into the mattress. The implant is checked periodically to ensure nothing is putting force on the implant.

Flow for Prostate Brachytherapy Patient

After CT simulation, implant measurements are taken by the brachytherapists. The treatment plan is then created by the physicists and approved by the radiation oncologist. The process from CT simulation to treatment start is approximately 2 hours, but can be longer if there is difficult anatomy to contour around, history of previous radiation, artifact from hip prosthesis, etc. During this time, the patient remains in the brachytherapy suite. They are able to eat and spend time with visitors during this time. Once the radiation treatment plan approved, the patient is taken for HDR treatment.

The number of treatments these patients receive typically varies between 1 and 3 per implant. If they are only to receive one treatment, implant removal will follow the initial HDR treatment. If they are to receive 2–3 treatments, they will stay overnight in the ambulatory surgery center after their initial HDR treatment. The following morning they will be brought back to the brachytherapy suite for their next CT scan and HDR treatment.

Prostate patients will either have HDR monotherapy or combination therapy. Monotherapy is brachytherapy only, with no external beam radiation therapy before or after. Combination therapy is brachytherapy plus external beam treatment. Patients with higher risk prostate cancer usually receive combination therapy, with or without androgen deprivation (ADT).

Most patients have two implants one week apart for HDR monotherapy, and a single implant for HDR combination therapy.

Pain Control

There are several ways to manage pain in the prostate brachytherapy patient. Patient-controlled analgesia (PCA) is the pain control method of choice for patients receiving multiple fractions requiring overnight admission. To minimize side effects, pain control is achieved by also utilizing nonnarcotic pain medications such as acetaminophen, ketorolac, etc. These medications will typically be ordered as standard PRN medications. By utilizing small doses of different categories of pain medication, it is easier to avoid significant side effects from large doses of narcotics that would occur in narcotics used alone. It also facilitates the discharge process as patients will be less likely to be dizzy, nauseated, etc.

If the patient is receiving only one fraction per implant and will be discharged the same day, a PCA is typically not warranted as very little of it will be used prior to discharge. For these patients, PRN IV and oral pain medications will be ordered.

All prostate brachytherapy patients will also receive spinal anesthesia at the time of implant insertion, which provides pain control as well. For patients who are not able to receive spinal anesthesia due to difficult anatomy or contraindication, general anesthesia may then be initiated.

Discharge

The patient is able to be discharged once the implant is removed, they are deemed stable by the MD, they are steady on their feet and have urinated a sufficient amount on their own. It is important to encourage hydration in these patients during their stay. It not only helps them urinate prior to discharge, but also helps clear any hematuria, clots, or sediment that often develops in the urine while this type of implant is in place.

At this time of discharge we given them verbal and written discharge instructions, contact information, and arrange for them to be taken to the car of whoever is driving them home. Please refer to "Discharging a Patient after Prostate Implant Removal."

Follow-Up

Patients are seen one week after final implant removal for post-op visit. For patients who are from far away, they have a phone post-op appointment and see their regular doctor in one week after removal.

Patients then follow-up in clinic every 3 months and have their PSA levels checked every three months for 2 years, then less frequently after that.

Nursing-Specific Care for Patient with a Prostate Brachytherapy Implant

Patients with prostate brachytherapy implants spend some time waiting in Radiation Oncology while their treatment plan is being created, and if they have multiple fractions, in between treatments. During this time they will require bedside nursing, pain management, hygiene, turning, etc.

The following is required for caring for these patients:

- Vital signs q 2-4 hours, per nursing discretion
- Reposition patient every 2 hours (see "how to turn a patient with a prostate implant")
- Pain management

- Intake and Output
- Encourage hydration and have water within reach
- Encourage nutrition by ordering food for patient (low fiber diet)
- If patient is on PCA, hourly documentation of PCA usage
- Sequential compression device for DVT prophylaxis
- Patient education during treatments and at time of discharge
- Bladder irrigation (manual or continuous, depending on needs)

The majority of patients with prostate brachytherapy implants remain outpatient. However, these patients are may be admitted to the inpatient unit if they have significant comorbidities that place them at a higher risk, or if they develop complications during their outpatient stay that require transfer to inpatient care (hematuria, hypotension, etc.).

How to Turn a Patient with a Prostate Brachytherapy Implant

1. Have patient bed both knees and plant their feet on the bed
2. Place a pillow between the patient's thighs, making sure it is not touching the implant (Photo 1)

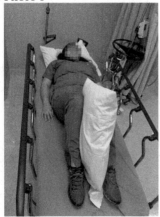

3. Patient slowly turns themselves to the desired side, making sure shoulders, hips, and knees turn in unison. This motion prevents twisting in the midsection. Patient may turn all the way on their side if they desire. (Photos 2 and 3)

Photo 2

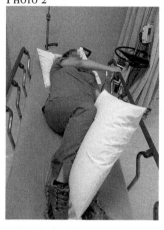

Photo 3

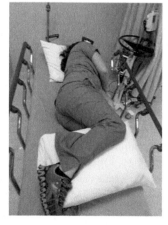

4. Ensure implant is free floating and that nothing is pushing on it. The pillow is to remain between the patient's legs. An additional pillow behind the back may provide comfort.

Prostate Implant Removal

Once the final HDR treatment is complete, it is time for implant removal. The implant is removed in the brachytherapy suite by the MD or PA and the RN. The nursing staff assists with all removals and are ready to intervene if complications develop.

The following supplies are needed for prostate implant removal:

- Large chux (pad) under the patient
- 2 packs of sterile 4 × 4 gauze, open and placed near the implant
- Scissors
- Hemostat
- Sharps container at the foot of bed
- Garbage can within reach
- 1 liter sterile normal saline for irrigation
- Foley catheter irrigation tray
- continuous bladder irrigation supplies (in room, just in case severe hematuria develops)
- cystoscopy irrigation tubing
- 3L bag of normal saline
- IV pole
- 3-way Foley catheter with 30 cc balloon

A timeout is always performed prior to the implant removal to ensure correct patient, correct number of treatments given, and that the implant is to be removed. This timeout is documented in the patient's medical record.

During the removal, the color of the urine is monitored closely. Patients are at risk of developing hematuria during or after implant removal. If hematuria develops, the Foley catheter is manually irrigated. If hematuria is severe or does not clear with manual irrigation, continuous bladder irrigation is initiated.

There is typically little pain reported with prostate implant removals, but many of these patients are nervous about the removal and a little bit of reassurance helps.

After the implant is removed, pressure is held to the site until all bleeding has stopped. At this time, the patient may be sat up in bed and PCA/IV fluids are discontinued. It is important that the patient is sat up gradually to avoid sudden dizziness, nausea, or drop in blood pressure. The IV saline lock is left in place until the moment of discharge.

Over the next 15 minutes, the urine output is closely observed to monitor for delayed hematuria. If hematuria develops, the Foley catheter is irrigated with sterile normal saline. If no hematuria develops, the Foley catheter is irrigated with 200cc sterile normal saline to ensure there is no sediment or clots. The bladder is then filled with 150-200cc sterile normal saline and is capped to ensure the saline doesn't drain out. The catheter is then removed and the patient is given a urinal and privacy and asked to urinate.

Patients must urinate at least 100cc prior to discharge. If they are unable to urinate, the MD is notified. Some patients just need more time before they are able to urinate, some patients need to hydrate more, and some need to go home with a Foley catheter reinserted. This is handled on a case-by-case basis.

If the patient did develop severe hematuria that required continuous bladder irrigation, the patient will often need to remain admitted with the catheter in place until the hematuria has resolved. This can take a matter of hours up to a few days.

The implant removal is documented in the patient's medical record. A thorough patient assessment is documented at this time as well.

Discharging Patient after Prostate Implant Removal:

Patients with prostate brachytherapy implants are technically considered outpatients as they stay in the brachytherapy suite or ambulatory surgery center. This means that once the implant is removed, they are discharged directly from the Radiation Oncology Department. (If the prostate patient is a higher risk and is a hospital inpatient on the surgical unit, this does not apply—they will be discharged from the hospital unit.)

394   Y. Yu et al.

Once patient is dressed they ambulate with nursing assistance. If the patient reports feeling dizzy or lightheaded, the MD/PA may order a 0.9 % NaCl IV fluid bolus. They may also order a 0.9 NaCl IV bolus of 250 or 500cc if the patient has had low urine output during their stay or if they are having difficulty urinating after the Foley catheter is removed.

Once the patient has urinated a sufficient amount (>100cc), is steady on their feet, has vital signs within normal limits, and is feeling ready to leave, they are given their discharge instructions. These patients will all be scheduled for a one-week post-op appointment. For the patients that live out of town, this appointment may be done over the phone, as long as they are checked out by their local doctor in one week to ensure they are healing.

Please see the next page for current discharge instructions for prostate brachytherapy patients.

Patients are given a blue seat cushion and a clean urinal for the ride home. They are not required to use the cushion, but many patients find it to be helpful. They may also use a pillow, if they choose.

Once the discharge instructions have been given to the patient (both verbally and as a printed copy), all questions have been answered, and the patient is steady on their feet, the IV is removed. The MD comes to see the patient and the patient is then allowed to be discharged. Prostate brachytherapy patients are NOT allowed to drive themselves home. Patients are made aware of this prior to their day of surgery and are to have a responsible adult present with them to drive them home.

References

1. Beckendorf V, Guerif S, Le Prisé E, et al. 70 Gy versus 80 Gy in localized prostate cancer: 5-year results of GETUG 06 randomized trial. Int J Radiat Oncol Biol Phys. 2011;80:1056–63.
2. Dearnaley DP, Jovic G, Syndikus I, et al. Escalated-dose versus control-dose conformal radiotherapy for prostate cancer: long-term results from the MRC RT01 randomised controlled trial. Lancet Oncol. 2014;15:464–73.

3. Pollack A, Zagars GK, Starkschall G, et al. Prostate cancer radiation dose response: results of the M. D. Anderson phase III randomized trial. Int J Radiat Oncol Biol Phys. 2002;53:1097–105.

4. Hoskin PJ, Rojas AM, Bownes PJ, et al. Randomised trial of external beam radiotherapy alone or combined with high-dose-rate brachytherapy boost for localised prostate cancer. Radiother Oncol. 2012;103:217–22.

5. Peeters STH, Heemsbergen WD, Koper PCM, et al. Dose-response in radiotherapy for localized prostate cancer: results of the Dutch multicenter randomized phase III trial comparing 68 Gy of radiotherapy with 78 Gy. J Clin Oncol. 2006;24:1990–6.

6. Brenner DJ, Hall EJ. Fractionation and protraction for radiotherapy of prostate carcinoma. Int J Radiat Oncol Biol Phys. 1999;43:1095–101.

7. Stromberg J, Martinez A, Gonzalez J, et al. Ultrasound-guided high dose rate conformal brachytherapy boost in prostate cancer: treatment description and preliminary results of a phase I/II clinical trial. Int J Radiat Oncol Biol Phys. 1995;33:161–71.

8. Martinez AA, Gonzalez J, Ye H, et al. Dose escalation improves cancer-related events at 10 years for intermediate- and high-risk prostate cancer patients treated with hypofractionated high-dose-rate boost and external beam radiotherapy. Int J Radiat Oncol Biol Phys. 2011;79:363–70.

9. Yoshioka Y, Suzuki O, Isohashi F, et al. High-dose-rate brachytherapy as monotherapy for intermediate- and high-risk prostate cancer: clinical results for a median 8-year follow-up. Int J Radiat Oncol Biol Phys. 2016;94(4):675–82.

10. Zamboglou N, Tselis N, Baltas D, et al. High-dose-rate interstitial brachytherapy as monotherapy for clinically localized prostate cancer: treatment evolution and mature results. Int J Radiat Oncol Biol Phys. 2013;85:672–8.

11. Chen CP, Weinberg V, Shinohara K, et al. Salvage HDR brachytherapy for recurrent prostate cancer after previous definitive radiation therapy: 5-year outcomes. Int J Radiat Oncol Biol Phys. 2013;86:324–9.

12. Lee B, Shinohara K, Weinberg V, et al. Feasibility of high-dose-rate brachytherapy salvage for local prostate cancer recurrence after radiotherapy: the University of California-San Francisco experience. Int J Radiat Oncol Biol Phys. 2007;67:1106–12.

13. Whittington R, Broderick GA, Arger P, et al. The effect of androgen deprivation on the early changes in prostate volume

following transperineal ultrasound guided interstitial therapy for localized carcinoma of the prostate. Int J Radiat Oncol Biol Phys. 1999;44:1107–10.

14. Song DY, Lawrie WT, Abrams RA, et al. Acute and late radiotherapy toxicity in patients with inflammatory bowel disease. Int J Radiat Oncol Biol Phys. 2001;51:455–9.

15. Tromp D, Christie DRH. Acute and late bowel toxicity in radiotherapy patients with inflammatory bowel disease: a systematic review. Clin Oncol (R Coll Radiol). 2015;27:536–41.

16. Crook JM, Bahadur YA, Robertson SJ, et al. Evaluation of radiation effect, tumor differentiation, and prostate specific antigen staining in sequential prostate biopsies after external beam radiotherapy for patients with prostate carcinoma. Cancer. 1997;79:81–9.

17. Crook JM, Perry GA, Robertson S, et al. Routine prostate biopsies following radiotherapy for prostate cancer: results for 226 patients. Urology. 1995;45:624–31. discussion 631–2.

18. Reed G, Cunha JA, Noworolski S, et al. Interactive, multimodality image registrations for combined MRI/MRSI-planned HDR prostate brachytherapy. J Contemp Brachytherapy. 2011;3:26–31.

19. Eiber M, Maurer T, Souvatzoglou M, et al. Evaluation of hybrid ^{68}Ga-PSMA ligand PET/CT in 248 patients with biochemical recurrence after radical prostatectomy. J Nucl Med. 2015;56:668–74.

20. Harisinghani MG, Barentsz J, Hahn PF, et al. Noninvasive detection of clinically occult lymph-node metastases in prostate cancer. N Engl J Med. 2003;348:2491–9.

21. Cunha JAM, Pouliot J, Weinberg V, et al. Urethra low-dose tunnels: validation of and class solution for generating urethra-sparing dose plans using inverse planning simulated annealing for prostate high-dose-rate brachytherapy. Brachytherapy. 2012;11:348–53.

22. Hsu IC, Bae K, Shinohara K, et al. Phase II trial of combined high-dose-rate brachytherapy and external beam radiotherapy for adenocarcinoma of the prostate: preliminary results of RTOG 0321. Int J Radiat Oncol Biol Phys. 2010;78:751–8.

23. Hsu IC, Hunt D, Straube W, et al. Dosimetric analysis of radiation therapy oncology group 0321: the importance of urethral dose. Pract Radiat Oncol. 2014;4:27–34.

24. Sanda MG, Dunn RL, Michalski J, et al. Quality of life and satisfaction with outcome among prostate-cancer survivors. N Engl J Med. 2008;358:1250–61.
25. Jo Y, Junichi H, Tomohiro F, et al. Radical prostatectomy versus high-dose rate brachytherapy for prostate cancer: effects on health-related quality of life. BJU Int. 2005;96:43–7.
26. Murray L, Henry A, Hoskin P, et al. Second primary cancers after radiation for prostate cancer: a systematic review of the clinical data and impact of treatment technique. Radiother Oncol. 2014;110:213–28.
27. Wiltink LM, Nout RA, Fiocco M, et al. No increased risk of second cancer after radiotherapy in patients treated for rectal or endometrial cancer in the randomized TME, PORTEC-1, and PORTEC-2 trials. J Clin Oncol. 2015;33:1640–6.
28. Aström L, Pedersen D, Mercke C, et al. Long-term outcome of high dose rate brachytherapy in radiotherapy of localised prostate cancer. Radiother Oncol. 2005;74:157–61.
29. Deger S, Boehmer D, Roigas J, et al. High dose rate (HDR) brachytherapy with conformal radiation therapy for localized prostate cancer. Eur Urol. 2005;47:441–8.
30. Demanes DJ, Rodriguez RR, Schour L, et al. High-dose-rate intensity-modulated brachytherapy with external beam radiotherapy for prostate cancer: California endocurietherapy's 10-year results. Int J Radiat Oncol Biol Phys. 2005;61:1306–16.
31. Kaprealian T, Weinberg V, Speight JL, et al. High-dose-rate brachytherapy boost for prostate cancer: comparison of two different fractionation schemes. Int J Radiat Oncol Biol Phys. 2012;82:222–7.
32. Martinez AA, Shah C, Mohammed N, et al. Ten-year outcomes for prostate cancer patients with Gleason 8 through 10 treated with external beam radiation and high-dose-rate brachytherapy boost in the PSA era. J Radiat Oncol. 2016;5:87–93.
33. Demanes DJ, Martinez AA, Ghilezan M, et al. High-dose-rate monotherapy: safe and effective brachytherapy for patients with localized prostate cancer. Int J Radiat Oncol Biol Phys. 2011;81:1286–92.
34. Prada PJ, Jiménez I, Gonzalez-Suarez H, et al. High-dose-rate interstitial brachytherapy as monotherapy in one fraction and transperineal hyaluronic acid injection into the perirectal fat for the treatment of favorable stage prostate cancer: treatment description and preliminary results. Brachytherapy. 2012;11:105–10.

35. Hoskin P, Rojas A, Lowe G, et al. High-dose-rate brachytherapy alone for localized prostate cancer in patients at moderate or high risk of biochemical recurrence. Int J Radiat Oncol Biol Phys. 2012;82:1376–84.
36. Hauswald H, Kamrava MR, Fallon JM, et al. High-dose-rate monotherapy for localized prostate cancer: 10-year results. Int J Radiat Oncol Biol Phys. 2016;94:667–74.
37. Jo Y, Fujii T, Hara R, et al. Salvage high-dose-rate brachytherapy for local prostate cancer recurrence after radiotherapy - preliminary results. BJU Int. 2012;109:835–9.
38. Yamada Y, Kollmeier MA, Pei X, et al. A phase II study of salvage high-dose-rate brachytherapy for the treatment of locally recurrent prostate cancer after definitive external beam radiotherapy. Brachytherapy. 2014;13:111–6.

Chapter 14

Gynecologic Cancer and High-Dose Rate Brachytherapy: Cervical, Endometrial, Vaginal, Vulva and Clinical Appendix

Jyoti Mayadev and Sushil Beriwal

Introduction

Rationale for Brachytherapy (BT)

- To allow for definitive doses after pelvic chemoradiation (CRT) or radiation (RT) in cervical cancer
- BT has been shown to improve local control, DFS, and OS for cervical cancer, and OS for vaginal cancer compared to those who do not get BT [1–3]

J. Mayadev, MD (✉)
Department of Radiation Oncology, UC Davis Comprehensive Cancer Center, University of California Davis Medical Center, 4501 X Street, G0140, Sacramento, CA 95817, USA
e-mail: jmayadev@ucdavis.edu

S. Beriwal, MD
Department of Radiation Oncology, University of Pittsburgh School of Medicine, Magee-Women's Hospital, Pittsburgh, PA, USA
e-mail: beriwals@upmc.edu

© Springer International Publishing AG 2017
J. Mayadev et al. (eds.), *Handbook of Image-Guided Brachytherapy*, DOI 10.1007/978-3-319-44827-5_14

- BT decreases local recurrence in early stage high inter-mediate risk endometrial cancer
- BT with or without pelvic RT is a curable option for patients with medically inoperable endometrial cancer
- Organ preservation in vaginal cancer
- Dose escalation and organ preservation in vulvar cancer

Goal of Brachytherapy: Definitive, Adjuvant

Cervix, Vagina

- Definitive treatment sequenced toward the terminal portion of pelvic RT or CRT
- Adjuvant/salvage — vaginal brachytherapy or interstitial brachytherapy depending on if there is residual disease, sequenced with or without radiation ± chemotherapy

Uterus

- Postoperative adjuvant treatment — vaginal BT
- Medically inoperable — to control symptoms and cure (NCDB, SEER) data
- Salvage or Recurrence — BT used in combination with external beam RT (EBRT) to definitively treat iso-lated vaginal recurrences

Vulva

- Definitive dose after CRT for organ preservation with disease extending to vagina, periurethra, or perineum

Timing Post-EBRT or Postdebulking of the Tumor

- To decrease the implant size, dose to critical surround-ing structures, sequence the brachytherapy toward the end of EBRT or after completion of EBRT maintain-ing appropriate treatment timeliness. Avoid BT on chemotherapy infusion days

Pertinent Anatomy for Brachytherapy

- See Fig. 14.1a: T2-weighted sagittal MRI showing the posterior extent of a locally advanced cervical cancer. Usually the size will likely decrease by 50 % with CRT, therefore this patient was deemed to need an interstitial BT implant upfront

Pathology

Typical Path for Cervix, Uterus, Vagina, Vulva

- Cervix, Vagina, Vulva—squamous cell, adenocarcinoma, adenosquamous; rare—small cell, melanoma
- Human Papilloma Virus (HPV) is one of the most well-established risk factors for cervical, vaginal, and vulvar cancer
- Uterus—adenocarcinoma, clear cell carcinoma, papillary serous carcinoma, carcinosarcoma, leiomyosarcoma

Cervix

Selection Criteria

Implantation and Applicator Selection

- Definitive: after optimal tumor debulking with RT or CRT
- Applicator selection determined by clinical exam pre-EBRT and post-EBRT, preprocedural imaging, response to RT or CRT
- Clinical assessment: size of the tumor for applicator selection, topography of the response, vaginal involvement upfront and residual, urethral involvement upfront or residual

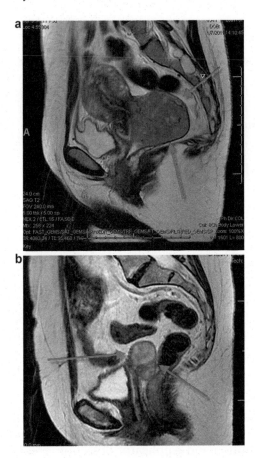

FIG. 14.1. (**a**) T2 weighted sagittal MRI showing the posterior extent of a locally advanced cervical cancer. Usually the size will likely decrease by 50% with CRT, therefore this patient was deemed to need an interstitial BT implant upfront. (**b**) T2 weighted sagittal MRI showing a primary vaginal cancer after a previous hysterectomy with the posterior extension of disease. Vaginal jelly was placed for better delineation of vaginal extension and visualization of the vaginal mucosa

- Applicator: three categories—standard intracavitary, hybrid intracavitary and interstitial, interstitial standard vs. custom applicator
- Consider tandem and ring for fixed geometry and ease of use
- Consider tandem and ovoid for tumor with lateral extension or if narrow vagina limits optimal ring placement
- Standard intracavitary tandem and ring/ovoid—if tumor size less than 4 cm, limited to the cervix
- Standard tandem and cylinder or use of a tandem with a multichannel cylinder—if minimal disease upfront in the vagina that shows a response of clinical mucosa irregularity without depth >0.5 cm and minimal parametrial (PM) disease
- Hybrid intracavitary with supplemental needles (Vienna applicator (ring based), Utrecht applicator (ovoid based), freehand needles in a standard tandem and ring)—tumor with greater than 4 cm extent or if critical organs dose high with standard tandem and ring/ovoid applicator
- Hybrid approach—Needles will allow for lateral 15 mm extension at point A level; or if tumor residual is a bulky posterior mass consider freehand approach. For this approach, start with placing needles about 1–1.5 cm lateral to the tandem in the inner ring or lateral to the ovoids. Insert the needles about 2–2.5 cm or based on your image guidance. Stabilize the needles to the tandem using elastic bands and measure the needles relative to the tandem for quality assurance to be alerted to unintentional movement
- Tandem and cylinder with lateral needles or multichannel cylinder—to help with the anterior and posterior dose distribution, changes the shape from a circle to a more ovoid distribution to decrease the rectal and bladder dose

- Interstitial—larger than 4 cm mass, distal vaginal extension, irregular anatomy, lateral PM residual disease, postsupracervical hysterectomy, vesicovaginal, or recto vaginal fistula
- If patient presents with any fistula, do not underdose the tumor. If vesicovaginal fistula, consider diverting nephrostomy tubes and if a candidate, loop ileostomy after complete response and biopsy confirmation. If patient presents with rectovaginal fistula, perform a diversion prior to starting RT

When to Perform BT (Post-EBRT, During EBRT)

- Consider BT during the EBRT (week 3 onward) for those with small tumors
- Otherwise implant starting the end of week 4 or week 5 to finish all treatment within 8 weeks

Clinical Guidelines to Judge Readiness for Implantation

- Laboratory values: Hct >25; platelets >50 for standard intracavitary applicator, >100 for interstitial with epidural or spinal use (may vary from institutional guidelines) (>50 if not using epidural or spinal)
- Anticoagulation aPTT, INR
- Type of sedation: Oral pain medications, local sedation, conscious sedation, deep sedation monitored by an anesthesiologist, neuroaxial anesthesia with a spinal, epidural, or combination, or general anesthesia
  - Determine medical comorbidity such as CHF, sleep apnea, respiratory risk
  - Determine the Mallampati airway risks and American Society of Anaesthesiologists (ASA) classification
- Fasting guidelines: NPO at midnight for conscious sedation or deep sedation

- Interstitial bowel prep: clear liquid diet in the afternoon prior to procedure, 500 ml of go lightly prep in the late afternoon, 2 docusate at noon day prior
- STOP the following medication/supplements 5 days prior to the procedure:
  - NSAIDs, Aspirin
  - If on coumadin, need to bridge days prior with low molecular weight heparin. This low molecular weight heparin is usually held 24 h prior to the procedure

Consent for Brachytherapy

- Include risks for GI, GU, Gyn, and Sexual health

Image Guidance Utilization

Preprocedure: Within 1 Week of Brachytherapy

- MRI—T2-weighted image to define the residual disease for applicator selection and superior extent into the uterus

Use of Image Guidance during Procedure

- Transabdominal US: to guide tandem placement, prevent perforation of uterine fundus or lower uterine segment, appreciate position of uterus anteverted, neutral, retroverted; uterus direction can change during EBRT or BT
- Transrectal US: to guide position of the tandem, to place needles during the procedure real time, to help create a tandem track with cervical os obliteration or those with exophytic tumors with loss of cervix integrity

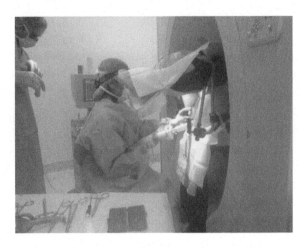

Fig. 14.2. Real time use of transrectal probe for interstitial BT

- CT: provide a 3D image for tandem or needle movement and applicator adjustment under epidural analgesia
- See Fig. 14.2 for real time use of transrectal probe for interstitial BT

Image Guidance for Planning

- 3D treatment planning is superior to 2D treatment planning in DFS outcomes and morbidities [4]
- GEC_ESTRO guidelines for planning to allow for dose escalation, superior outcomes, creation of the GTV, HR-CTV, and an expansion for the IR-CTV
- MRI with applicator—allows for soft tissue delineation and definition of the GTV
- CT with applicator—target volumes overestimate the volume, no difference in D90 doses between the MRI preprocedure and during procedure
- Allows for organs at risk to be constrained [5]

- According to a 2014 ABS survey, 95 % use CT and 35 % use MRI in BT
- MRI guidance for BT is useful prior to implantation to visualize superior or lateral PM extension
- Controversy exists on the additive benefit of using an MRI at every BT procedure, atleast consider MRI on first fraction

Guidelines for Implantation

- Preprocedure advice: exam findings, procedural positioning, exam assessment
- Exam: assess PM or vaginal extension to determine if supplemental needles are needed
- Position the patient at the end of the gynecology procedure table to allow movement of the speculum and transrectal ultrasound as needed

Procedure Tips

- If no cervical os, start central of the tumor for the best dose distribution and using ultrasound guidance, create a track for the tandem
- In patients with exophytic tumors, a false track can easily be made posterior to the endocervical canal and would need to be adjusted to avoid increasing rectal dose
- The implant may need to be adjusted during the procedure
- If the vaginal is too narrow for a standard applicator, you can switch to a tandem and cylinder with needles, or a custom made cylinder with needles made with dental putty
- If retroverted uterus—place the tandem in retroverted and then rotate the tandem to be anteverted; when

you rotate the tandem it will want to rotate back to the retroverted position, so hold the external portion of the tandem when placing the ring or ovoids to avoid perforation (use sonogram guidance to decrease risk of perforation)

■ For patients with uterine extension, you can use a longer tandem with a cylinder

■ If the vagina is very long and you cannot reach it, use an extra long speculum and pull down the cervix with a tenaculum carefully!

■ If the vaginal walls collapse in the field, cover the end of the speculum with a glove to keep the walls on the side of the vagina

■ You can use a cervical local anesthesia block with 1 % lidocaine with epi 1:100,000. Use about 15 cc, in clock face in the cervix, avoidance of the uterine arteries at 3 o'clock and 9 o'clock

■ If the tandem perforates the uterus on transabdominal ultrasound, reposition the tandem and proceed with the procedure—DO NOT ABANDON the procedure and consider IV antibiotics to be given after the procedure

■ If there is anterior vaginal extension and you cannot use an interstitial technique, perform a combination of tandem and ring and tandem and cylinder implantations

■ If on examination you feel a lot of cervical bulk, place two needles in the ring for posterior supplementation for a hybrid technique

■ Pack the vagina anteriorly for bladder neck, urethral, and vaginal mucosa doses using vaginal packing soaked with a combination of sterile water and lubrication jelly or balloon packing

■ Pack the vagina posteriorly for rectal dose sparing if you don't have a rectal retractor

■ Distal vaginal packing for applicator stability

■ Use an external fixation device or perineal bar to ensure less movement of the applicator, see Fig. 14.3

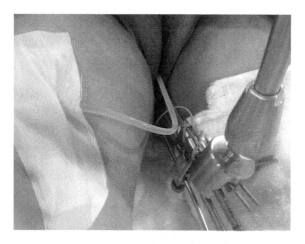

FIG. 14.3. Use of the external fixation clamp on a hybrid tandem and ring with two interstitial needles secured with elastic bands

Evaluation of Implantation

Distribution of Implant

- Verification of the BT implant real time or in the CT simulator and adjust as needed
- For a tandem and ring case: tandem should be placed in the cervix and uterus; ring should be flushed against the cervical os, packing should not displace the ring or applicator. The tandem ideally on a sagittal view is roughly 1/3 distance to the symphysis and 2/3 from the sacrum. However, in a native retroverted uterus, the tandem is closer to the sacrum
- For a tandem and ovoid: The tandem should bisect the ovoids, packing should not displace the ovoids
- If an interstitial case, adjust the needles by the needed mm according to the image review for the target volume, bladder, rectum, or sigmoid
- Use 2 mm slice thickness for accurate needle registration for planning
- Tandem in the uterus and the critical structures shielded by the depth of the myometrium

- Appreciate the location of the bowel and if anteriorly can fill bladder to push the bowel away from the implant high dose regions

Treatment Planning Considerations

Contouring

- Use of image guidance for target volume delineation
- GTV (Gross tumor volume) — if MRI-based planning
- HR-CTV (High-risk clinical target volume) — GTV plus cervix and any extension beyond the cervix into the parametria
- IR-CTV (Intermediate risk clinical target volume) — 1 cm margin on the HR-CTV for disease regression or microscopic spread. The IR-CTV contour is often used in some eurpoean center
- Vagina
- Normal tissues — Sigmoid, Bowel, Rectum, Bladder, and urethra (for vaginal extension)
- See Fig. 14.4: Axial MRI T2 weighted contours with Vienna; red arrows pointing to needle supplementation, green contour GTV, red contour HR-CTV
- See Fig. 14.5: HR-CTV Axial CT of a large cervical tumor

Optimal Brachytherapy Dose Rx with EQD2 and EBRT Doses to Create an Equivalent Dose in 2 Gy Table from the HDR Fractionation Equation

- The American Brachytherapy Society provides an online Excel format for users: https://www.american-brachytherapy.org/guidelines/LQ_spreadsheet.xls:

$BED = nd(1 + (d/(a/b)))$: n = fraction #, d = dose/fraction, a/b:3 normal tissues, 10 tumor, vagina

Deq(Effective dose equivalent 2 Gy/fx); $Deq = BED/(1 + (dref/(a/b)))$, dref = 2 Gy/fx

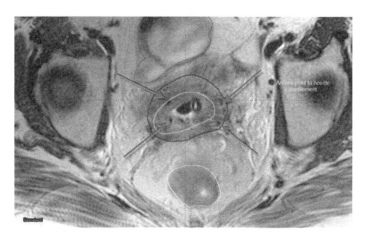

FIG. 14.4. Axial MRI T2 weighted contours with Vienna Applicator; *red arrows* pointing to needle supplementation, *green contour* GTV, *red contour* HR-CTV

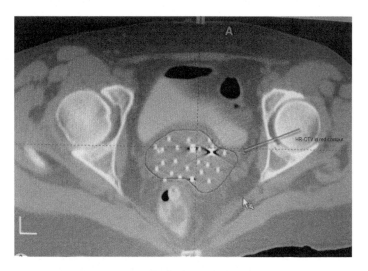

FIG. 14.5. HR-CTV axial CT of a large cervical tumor

Dose and Fractionation

- If limited to the cervix without vaginal extension, consider 5.5–6 Gy×5 (based on response and residual disease), 7 Gy×4 for intracavitary or interstitial implantations. For patients with vaginal extension, consider dose regions with a lower dose to the vaginal extension, such as 4.5 Gy×5
- Allow 48 h between output BT or at least 6 h between treatment delivery
- Be careful of the doses to the rectum for posterior vaginal extension
- If performing an interstitial implant even for a posterior vaginal tumor, do not place a needle in the rectovaginal septum, but instead treat with dose from the vaginal portion

Planning Dosimetry Goals

- HR-CTV D90-dose to cover 90 % volume at risk is 80–90 Gy. Dose based on response to EBRT. Higher dose may benefit large volume residual disease or stage III patients, 87Gy in definitive cervix
- Rectum, Sigmoid, Bowel: D2cc (dose to 2 cc volume): <EQD2 70Gy (published data show risk of grade 3 more than 10 % when above 75 Gy) [5]. Sigmoid dose may reflect worse case scenerio as moves fraction to fraction. Similarly try to reduce dose to small bowel by changing bladder filling
- Bladder D2cc: <90Gy [5] (Retro EMBRACE data suggest may be 80 Gy to limit grade 2 morbidity)
- To keep the V150 and V200 away from the vaginal mucosa on interstitial implantations
- To keep .1 cc urethra less than prescription dose and no hot spot abutting urethra
- Newer data suggest keep rectovaginal point dose to EQ 65 Gy or below to reduce vaginal moebidity

Optimization of Target Volume: Point Based, Volume Based

- Generally, the tandem will have the most dose in the central portion of the implant
- The dose is to cover the HR-CTV
- Trend to not cover the entirety of the uterus due to normal tissue constraints unless there was potential for uterine extension
- Standard intracavitary implant: normalize to pt A
  - Manually adjust (avoid graphical optimization) the dwell weight positions to decrease the dose to surrounding structures
  - Look at the D90 and D2cc, and D.1 cc of the critical structures on the DVH for feedback
- Hybrid : Intracavitary with supplemental needles
  - Considering planning as above to Pt A, and then visualize and calculate DVH on normal tissues with manually loading the needle weights to 10–20 % of tandem weight to avoid large hot spots directly in paravaginal or parametrial tissue
  - Manually achieve the optimal dose distribution with isodose curves
- Interstitial brachytherapy
  - Pt A will not be used
  - After contouring, consider manual loading vs. optimization using a treatment planning software
  - Manual: set dose constraints with either manually loading the tandem about 7–10 times the needle
  - Inverse planning technique — IPSA for Nucletron or Varian volume optimization
  - Manually achieve the optimal dose distribution with isodose curves taking with into consideration the normal tissue constraints, and the distance away from the normal tissues like the vagina from the applicator
  - Always weight the tandem the most for the implant as this is usually surrounded by a plastic obturator to hold most of the high dose region, or in the uterus

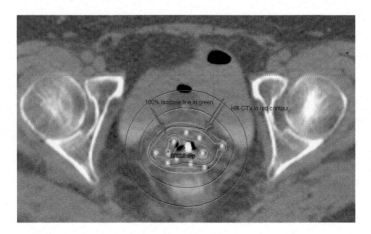

Fɪɢ. 14.6. HR-CTV of the cervical mass in red with isodose curves shown

which has a higher dose tolerance than sigmoid or surrounding structures
- See Fig. 14.6: HR-CTV of the cervical mass in red with isodose curves shown

Rationale for BT

- Local recurrence: cervical cancer with HDR brachytherapy (Table 14.1)

Toxicity

- Toxicity side effect review—common, rare
- Most rectal and bladder side effects occur within 3 years after BT, have a mean duration of 20 months, and resolve 60–80 % within 3 years [6]

TABLE 14.1 Prospective outcomes for Cervical Cancer and HDR brachytherapy

Author	No pts	Phase	Arms	Stage	WPRT	PM boost	HDR dose/fx	Fx #	total HDR	HDR Rx	HDR f/u	median f/u mo	Pelvic control (RT)	Pelvic Control (CRT)	DFS (RT)	DFS (CRT)	OS (RT)	OS (CRT)
Pearcey (2002)	259	3	RT vs. CRT (cis)	Ib–Iva	45		8	3	24	A	82	36		65	65	68	66	69
Lorvidhaya (2003, 2000)	926	3	RT vs. RT (MMC 5FU) 4 arms, reporting 2	2B–4a	50	10–16	7–7.5	4	28	A	89	60	57	86	60	70	58	62
												60	75		48	65	71	83
Garipagaoglu (2004)	44	3	RT vs. CRT (cis)	2b–3b	46–50		10	2	20	A	40	60	69	64	67	59	52	49
Lanciano (2005)	316	3	CRT (cis) vs. CRT (5Fu)	2b–4a	45	4–9	6	5	30	A	40	48				57		64
Yoon (2006)	43	1, 3	CRT (cis and 5FU) (RT 6 days/week)	1b–3b	45	5.4	4	6	24	A	37	36		88		85		75
Kim (2005, 2008)	158	3	CRT (week cis) vs. CRT (cis 5FU month)	2B–4a	40–50		5	6–7	30–35	A	39	48		87		66		67

(continued)

TABLE 14.1 (continued)

Author	No pts	Phase	Arms	Stage	WPRT	PM boost	HDR dose/fx	Fx #	total HDR	HDR Rx	median f/u	f/u mo	Pelvic control (RT)	Pelvic Control (CRT)	DFS (RT)	DFS (CRT)	OS (RT)	OS (CRT)
Toita (2012)	72	2		3–4a	30–40.1		5.5–6	2	11	A	28	24		73		70		90
Huang (2013)	267	3	CRT 2 HDR fx schema	Ib–4a	39.6–45		4.5–6	4–6	24	A	57	60		80				66
Kato (2013, 2010)	120	2		2b–3b	30–40	10	6–7	4	24–28	A	64	60		77				55
Zuliani (2014, 2010)	147	3	RT vs. CRT	3b	45					A	43	36					64	68
												60			49	54	54	56
Hareyama (2002)	151	3	RT LDR vs. RT HDR	2–3b	30–50		5.8	5	29	A		60	89		69			
							5.75–7.6	3, 4	23				69		51			
							8.65–5.76	2, 3	17.5									
Potter (2011, 2006, 2007, 2000)	156	2	RT HDR plus CT		45–50.4		7	4	28	IGBT	42	36		91	74			68

Lertsanguansinchai (2004)	112	3	Rt (LDR vs. HDR)	1b1–3b	45–50	4–9	7.5	3	22.5	A	37	36	86	70	68
Nam (2004)	46	3	HDR fx schema	1b1–4a	45		8.3 / 3 / 5	2 / 10 / 5	16.6 / 30 / 25	A	46	36		88	76
Kim (2005, 2008)	61	3	CRT 5FU cis vs. CRT cis	2b–41	41.4–50.4		6 / 7	5 / 5	30 / 35	A / A	44	48	89	59	70
Sharma (2011)	42	2	CRT (interstitial)	2b–4a	40		10	2	20	CT	23	36	62	55	47
Huang (2013)	267	3	HDR fx schema (CRT and RT)	1b–4a	39.6	5.4	6	4	24	A	57	60	80		65

Common

- Nausea, abdominal discomfort, abdominal pain, loose stools, blood in the stool, rectal urgency, decreased blood counts, loose stools, diarrhea, bladder irritation causing urgency, frequency, burning with urination, blood in the urine, vaginal irritation, vaginal bleeding, vaginal discharge, vaginal narrowing, vaginal shortening, vaginal dryness, pain with intercourse, vaginal bleeding and spotting, vaginal bleeding after intercourse, skin redness, skin tanning, skin breakdown, skin itching, skin irritation, tenderness, pain, swelling, loss of public hair, fatigue

Less Common

- GI: rectal bleeding, rectal narrowing, rectal ulcer, rectal fistula requiring surgery; bowel obstruction requiring surgery or hospitalization
- GU: ureteral stricture, risk of bladder infection, bladder inflammation, urinary urgency, hematuria, bladder contracture, decreased bladder capacity, urethral stricture, urinary incontinence, fistula requiring surgery, hemorrhagic cystitis
- GYN: vaginal tissue necrosis, vaginal ulceration, vaginal fistula requiring surgery
- MSK: lumbosacral neuropathy, pelvic insufficiency fractures, leg swelling known as lymphedema
- Radiation can also cause the formation of a secondary cancer in the field of radiation several years after the treatment

Toxicity

- See Table 14.2: reporting acute toxicity in CTCAE v. 3 or 4; late toxicity in RTOG/CTCAE v3., LENT/SOMA, EORTC

TABLE 14.2 Toxicity table (Reporting acute toxicity in CTCAE v. 3 or 4; late toxicity in RTOG/CTCAE v3., LENT/SOMA, EORTC.) NS- data not sufficient in the literature

Acute toxicity grade	GI (RT)	GI (CRT)	GU (RT)	GU (CRT)	GYN (RT)	GYN (CRT)
2	15–48 %	5–62 %	1–54 %	2–53 %	NS	NS
3	3–11 %	1–25 %	1–3 %	1–3 %	NS	NS
4	5 %	1–2 %	0 %	0 %	NS	NS
Late toxicity grade	GI (RT)	GI (CRT)	GU (RT)	GU (CRT)	GYN (RT)	GYN (CRT)
2	4–6 %	1–13 %	3–8 %	2–7 %	2–23 %	29–61 %
3	2–11 %	1–4 %	1–5 %	1–14 %	1–10 %	3–7 %
4	0–11 %	1–5 %	2–5 %	0–11 %	0–6 %	3 %

Uterus (Adjuvant Postoperative/Recurrent/ Medically Inoperable)

Adjuvant Postoperative

Selection Criteria

- Stage 1 endometrial cancer: adjuvant EBRT or vaginal brachytherapy (VB) to a hysterectomy for high intermediate risk features based on the PORTEC 1, GOG-99, and PORTEC 2 [7–9], per the ASTRO guidelines [10]
- Stage 2 endometrial cancer—pelvic EBRT +/– VB [10]
- Decision factor for adjuvant radiation is to determine if the patient needs VB with or without chemotherapy, pelvic radiation [10]
- Stage 3—consider the addition of VB after consolidative pelvic radiation for high-risk features such as

LVSI, positive margin, or high grade histology, although the absolute benefit is controversial [10]

When to Implant (Post-EBRT, During EBRT)

- After adequate healing time postsurgery. Vaginal brachytherapy to commence between 4 and 9 weeks (up to 12 weeks per traditional GOG studies) postoperative based on cuff healing [11]. Take extra precaution after laparoscopic surgery as increased risk of cuff dehiscence
- If giving a vaginal brachytherapy boost after EBRT for stage 2 or 3, start brachytherapy within 2 weeks of finishing EBRT
- Preoperative for clinical stage II and stage IIIB endometrial cancer

Clinical Guidelines to Judge Readiness for Implantation

- After adequate healing time postsurgery. Perform a clinical examination of the vaginal cuff for adequate healing.
- Patients after a laparoscopic hysterectomy require more healing time due to the closure of the vaginal cuff
- Definitive/preoperative—perform a clinical examination and focus on extension to the cervix, disease extension to the vagina
- Review the anesthesia consent, guidelines for CBC, anticoagulation

Image Guidance Utilization

Use of Image Guidance Preprocedure

- Imaging is required for adjuvant therapy if there is concern for residual disease after surgery
- Ideal brachytherapy alone candidates will have grade 1 or 2 disease confined to the endometrial cavity or superficial myometrium. If deep myometrial extension or no MRI is possible, treat with EBRT and BT

Use of Image Guidance During Procedure

- Use of ultrasound to place the applicator, avoid normal structures, and optimize applicator adjustments
- Use of 3D image guidance CT or MRI scan to determine needle and applicator adjustments and placement

Guidelines for Implantation

Preprocedure Advice: Exam Findings, Procedural Positioning, Exam Assessment

- Determine the distended vaginal length
- Decide the treatment length that needs to be treated, usually upper 3–5 cm of vagina
- Size the patient with a cylinder diameter that corresponds with the applicator available

Procedure Tips

- Ensure the vaginal cylinder is the largest diameter for the pt
- Obtain a verification sim or CT image to verify that the applicator is at the dome of the vaginal cuff
- Use an external device to make sure the applicator stays in place
- In patients with redundant vaginal folds, ensure the cylinder is at the cuff and not in a vaginal mucosal fold

Verification of Brachytherapy with Visual and Imaging

- Verify the applicator is flush to the vaginal cuff, note air gaps and fitting of the applicator
- Verify the vaginal length from previous measurements in clinic

Evaluation of Implantation

Distribution of Implant

- Implant distribution will be a dome shape with or without interstitial needle supplemental dose

- Properly fitted brachytherapy applicator should be selected
- Conforms to the vaginal apex and achieves mucosal contact with optimal tumor and normal tissue
- Review Imaging Real Time or When a Change Is Needed

Treatment Planning Considerations

Optimal Brachytherapy Dose Rx Table with EQD2 and EBRT Doses

- Determine the length of the vagina to treat after measuring the patient in the clinic
- The length varies, treat 3–5 cm or 50–67 % of the distended vaginal length
- Various dose and fractionation schedules with varying EQD2 at the vaginal surface
- Dose options: 7 Gy to 0.5 cm depth × 3 fractions [9]; 4 Gy to surface × 6 fractions (Dana Farber) or 6 Gy × 5 to surface (consider prescribing to surface for smaller diameter cylinder) (2.5 cm or below) to reduce surface dose and vaginal toxicity
- If given an adjuvant brachytherapy boost for stage 2 endometrial cancer, dose options after 45Gy EBRT, target dose is 60–70Gy EQD2: 4Gy to 0.5 cm depth × 3 fractions; 6Gy to surface × 2 or 3 fractions (RTOG and GOG)

Use of Image Guidance for Target Volume Delineation

- Consider use of CT or MRI-based planning

Optimization of Target Volume: Point Based, Volume Based

- Place optimization points on the lateral, curved, and apical portion of the cylinder for the dose distribution
- Source anisotropy can produce a lower dose at the vaginal apex and isotropic dose calculation model can result in as much as 30 % under dosage at the vaginal apex

- Implant distribution will be a dome shape
- Keep the dose of the surface and the depth of 0.5 cm recorded

Outcomes with BT

- High intermediate risk patients have a local recurrence advantage with radiation vs. observation [7, 8]
- GOG 99-EBRT reduces the risk of recurrence by 58 % vs. observation arm [8]
- PORTEC 2—vaginal brachytherapy vs. pelvic radiation: 5 years vaginal recurrence rates 1.8 % VBT vs. 1.6 % EBRT; locoregional relapse 5.1 % VBT vs. 2.1 % EBRT [9]

Uterus Recurrent

Selection Criteria

- Depending on the location of the tumor, can be a candidate for pelvic radiation followed by brachytherapy implantation
- If recurrence is grossly palpable after EBRT, need a form of interstitial implantation
- If the disease becomes submucosal only with vaginal mucosal changes and residual thickness 5 mm, consider vaginal cylinder (single channel or multichannel) boost after salvage EBRT

When to Implant (Post-EBRT, During EBRT)

- After EBRT and adequate size reduction
- Treat the entire length of the vagina with EBRT for any vaginal recurrence due to the risk of submucosal spread

Clinical Guidelines to Judge Readiness for Implantation

- Determine the location of the recurrence in the vagina—apical lesions are often more extensive than clinical exam can detect superiorly

- There can also be submucosal spread or vaginal disease
- Treat the entire vagina in cases of recurrence or gross disease in the vagina then implant the area of gross disease to definitive doses with brachytherapy
- Consider chemotherapy concurrently with EBRT for large lesions to help decrease the bulk or decrease the extension to normal tissues prior to brachytherapy

Image Guidance Utilization

- If apical lesions or recurrence that had potential invasion into the bladder or rectum, obtain an MRI pre-EBRT
- Determine the extent of disease into the paravaginal tissues, superior extension, or normal tissue invasion

Use of Image Guidance During Procedure

- Use of ultrasound to place the applicator, avoid normal structures, and optimize applicator adjustments
- Use of transrectal US to visualize bowel or rectum proximally from the needles to avoid placing the needles into the bowel
- Use of 3D image guidance CT or MRI scan to determine needle and applicator adjustments and placement

Guidelines for Implantation

- Determine the extent of recurrence disease, location in the pelvis or vagina, thickness
- Monitor treatment response during EBRT
- Target volume will be the tumor regression and the remainder of the gross disease
- If the vaginal recurrence is still palpable on examination and thicker than 5 mm, an interstitial supplementation is needed. Monitor response to treatment to determine the proportion of brachytherapy that will require interstitial supplemental dose

Procedure Tips

- Determine how much circumference and length of the vagina to treat after EBRT based on physical examination with estimation of response and location of initial tumor or mark prior to treatment with EBRT
- Determine the extension of disease and place a marker or stitch with a radiopaque tie in the area of gross disease
- Place two sutures in the vagina to hold the applicator in place
- Construct a vaginal obturator with needles surrounded by a sleeve or packing to separate the needles from the vaginal mucosal surface
- If using a template for an interstitial implantation, suture the template to the vulva
- If using a freehand technique, secure the needles to the obturator to prevent movement

Verification of Brachytherapy with Visual and Imaging

- If a stitch was placed or marker was placed in the recurrence, verify the applicator positioning
- Consider using a shielded cylinder or multicatheter cylinder if the disease is localized to a portion of the vagina
- Place a marker at the introitus and the urethra—a BB or wire w tape
- Place bladder contrast solution (5 cc omnipaque and 25 cc of saline) and 15 cc of barium in the anus for planning contrast of normal tissue doses if using CT scan for planning

Evaluation of Implantation

- Determine an area of high risk and intermediate or low risk with corresponding dose distributions
- Evaluate the dose distribution at the residual disease

- Be aware of the V150 and V200 close to the vaginal surface and ensure there is minimal confluence of the V150 and V200

Treatment Planning Considerations

Optimal Brachytherapy Dose Rx Table with EQD2 and EBRT Doses

- After 45–50 Gy EBRT, consider the location, depth, and extent of the vagina to be treated
- Limit dose to the urethra, anterior rectal wall, and posterior bladder, superiorly the bowel
- Target dose is 70–80 Gy based on location, response to EBRT, and critical organ dosimetry
- After 45 Gy EBRT give BT: 4.5 Gy to 5.5 Gy×5 fractions

Use of Image Guidance for Target Volume Delineation

- MRI for tumor and GTV extension to the vagina, superiorly, and paravaginal tissue

Optimization of Target Volume: Point Based, Volume Based

- Determine an area of high risk (gross residual disease after EBRT) and intermediate (defined at the initial physical examination or response on imaging of the tumor, microscopic extension which can be marked by clips prior to EBRT) or low risk (concern for submucosal spread) with corresponding dose distributions
- Evaluate the dose distribution at the residual disease
- Be aware of the V150 and V200 close to the vaginal surface

Outcomes with BT

- Endometrial recurrences can be salvaged with treatment, with local control in modern series of image based brachytherapy more than 85–90%

Medically Inoperable Endometrial Cancer

Selection Criteria

- BT alone can be considered in clinical Stage I with no LN involvement and no evidence of deep myometrial invasion on MRI [11]. In the absence of an MRI, use a combination of EBRT and BT [11]

When to Implant (Post-EBRT, During EBRT)

- After EBRT in patients with medically inoperable endometrial cancer

Clinical Guidelines to Judge Readiness for Implantation

- Coordination with anesthesia or preoperative clinic for any anticoagulation requirements, and medical comorbid decisions
- Patients may not be able to under sedation, in which case patient can be offered minimal medications in the clinic with a cervical lidocaine block for cervical dilation and instrument insertion

Image Guidance Utilization

Use of Image Guidance Preprocedure

- Obtain a baseline MRI and MRI before EBRT to determine the extent of disease, define a GTV and CTV, type of applicator, and suitability of brachytherapy alone [11]

Types of Image Guidance to Potentially Use, Pro/Cons

- Use of transrectal and transabominal US during the procedure for entry into the endometrial canal and positioning of the tandems into the uterus for a "Y" distribution

Use of Image Guidance During Procedure

- Use of ultrasound to place the applicator, avoid normal structures, and optimize applicator adjustments
- Use of 3D image guidance CT or MRI scan to determine needle and applicator adjustments and placement

Guidelines for Implantation

- Perform a serial dilation of the cervical os to be larger than the two tandem applicator
- In patients with a small uterus, a tandem and cylinder or tandem and ring may suffice, with uterine width <4 cm
- In patients with uterine width >4 to 5 cm, place a Rotte "Y" double tandem applicator, or insert a third tandem to help with the dose distribution between the tandem separation
- Place both tandems in the os in the uterus neutral position
- Slightly rotate each tandem in serial to achieve a "Y" distribution of the applicator
- Place an obturator (split sleeve) with packing

Procedure Tips

- Place both tandems in the os in the uterus neutral position
- Slightly rotate each tandem in serial to achieve a "Y" distribution of the applicator
- The ideal dose distribution will be obtained with the tandems in the bilateral cornu
- Place an obturator (split sleeve) with packing

Verification of Brachytherapy with Visual and Imaging

- Use of transabdominal or transrectal ultrasound for sounding the uterus for the appropriate tandem length, dilatation of the os

- Ensure that the tandems are in the uterus and have distance between the cranial extent of the tandems in a "Y" distribution
- Make sure the obturator is flush to the cervix
- Place an external clamp for reproducibility between simulation and treatment

Evaluation of Implantation

Distribution of Implant

- See a "Y" formation distribution
- Consideration of further rotation of the tandems as needed from the CT image

Treatment Planning Considerations

Optimal Brachytherapy Dose Rx Table with EQD2 and EBRT Doses

- Use of an MRI to guide target volumes of GTV—gross tumor seen on MRI, and CTV—entire uterus, cervix, and upper 1–2 cm of the vagina [11]
- In combination with EBRT 45Gy: give 5.2Gy × 4 fractions, 4Gy × 5 fractions, 6.3Gy × 3 fractions [11]
- Without EBRT: 8.5Gy × 4 fractions, 7.3Gy × 5 fractions, 6.4Gy × 6 fractions [11]. If MRI-based plan GTV 80–90 Gy and CTV 65–75 Gy [11]

Use of Image Guidance for Target Volume Delineation

- MRI to tumor extension into the myometrium, extension into the serosa, determine the bulk of disease in the uterus

Optimization of Target Volume: Point Based, Volume Based

- Weight the tandems relative to normal tissue tolerances
- There will be a high dose gradient between the tandems
- Target for the HR-CTV to be covered by the 100 % isodose line
- Figure 14.7: Dose distribution of medically inoperable endometrial cancer with CT-based planning

Outcomes with BT

- Curative intent, multiple series show 5 years DFS: 83–85 %

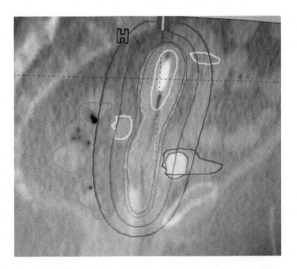

FIG. 14.7. Dose distribution of medically inoperable endometrial cancer with CT-based planning

Vagina

Selection Criteria

Selection for Implantation

- All vaginal stages for consideration of organ preservation, BT shown to increase OS [3]

When to Implant (Post-EBRT, During EBRT)

- Combine with EBRT and potentially chemotherapy if bulky disease or Stage II or above
- Implant after regression of the gross tumor with EBRT and chemotherapy in the week 4 or 5
- Avoid delay after EBRT for brachytherapy procedure

Image Guidance Utilization

Use of Image Guidance Preprocedure

- MRI preprocedure to determine the extent of disease, superior extension, and paravaginal disease

Types of Image Guidance to Potentially Use and Pros/ Cons

- Transrectal US to visualize bowel or rectum proximally from the needles to avoid placing the needles into the bowel

Use of Image Guidance During Procedure

- Use of ultrasound to place the applicator, avoid normal structures, and optimize applicator adjustments

- Use of 3D image guidance CT scan to determine needle and applicator adjustments and placement

Guidelines for Implantation

- Preprocedure advice: exam findings, procedural positioning, exam assessment
- Determine the extent of recurrence disease, location in the pelvis or vagina, thickness
- If vaginal area is irregular, can consider constructing a putty mold and making a custom applicator
- HR-CTV will include the initial disease areas of regression and microscopic spread and include the remainder of the gross disease
- If the vaginal recurrence is still palpable on examination, an interstitial supplementation is needed, generally if >0.5 cm thick on examination
- Monitor response to treatment to determine the proportion of brachytherapy that will require interstitial supplemental dose

Procedure Tips

- Determine how much circumference and length of the vagina to treat after EBRT
- Determine the extension of disease and place a marker or stitch with a radiopaque tie in the area of gross disease
- Place two sutures in the vagina to hold the applicator in place
- Construct a vaginal obturator with needles surrounded by a sleeve or packing to separate the needles from the vaginal mucosal surface
- If using a template-based approach, space the needles about 1 cm apart

Evaluation of Implantation

Distribution of Implant

- Check the dose distribution to limit the dose to the rectum, bladder, and bowel
- Implant distribution will be a dome shape with or without interstitial needle supplemental dose
- Properly fitted brachytherapy applicator should be selected
- Conforms to the vaginal apex and achieves mucosal contact with optimal tumor and normal tissue
- Review imaging real time or when a change is needed
- Make adjustments of the interstitial coverage or supplement with additional needles at the time of simulation

Treatment Planning Considerations

- See section on recurrent endometrial cancer

Use of Image Guidance for Target Volume Delineation

- Draw in a high risk, intermediate risk, or low risk vagina with varying doses
- Target volume should be encompassed with a 1-cm margin beyond the residual gross disease in the lateral, inferior, and superior margins
- If arising from area of diffuse vaginal intraepithelial neoplasia, consider target dose of an intermediate risk vagina to be a greater percentage or entire vagina to an EQD2 of 60 Gy, with higher target doses of 70–80 Gy to the gross residual tumor plus margin

Optimization of Target Volume: Point Based, Volume Based

- See section on recurrent endometrial cancer

Optimal Dose Distribution with Isodose Curves

- The volume of tissues receiving more than 150 % of the prescription dose is limited to the area adjacent to the individual needles or is contained within the vaginal obturator
- Figure 14.8: HR-CTV vagina with isodose curves on a CT-based plan

Rationale for Brachytherapy

- Vienna Series, Mock et al. [12]: The 5-year recurrence-free survival rates—100 %, 77 %, 50 %, 23 %, and 0 % for Stages 0, I, II, III, and IV, respectively. Lieskovsky et al. [13]: mean follow-up of 45 months, the crude LC rate was 87 % (47/54) Beriwal et al.: 13 pts, LC 100 % 2 years [14], ABS consensus guidelines is also a resource [13]

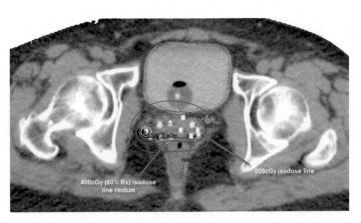

Fig. 14.8. HR-CTV vagina with isodose curves on a CT-based plan

Vulva

Selection Criteria

- Consider BT for vulva lesions with vaginal infiltration, or bulky disease on examination that is limited in extent
- Limited data exist for perineal vulvar brachytherapy with limited experience
- Caution required as skin tolerance may be low leading to higher risk of necrosis
- Caution of the movement of the superficial implantation on the vulvar surface
- Caution with air gaps on the surface and dose heterogeneity of the BT, consider custom mold applicator

When to Implant

- Implant after EBRT ± chemotherapy
- Consider BT boost in patients with gross disease vaginal extension after surgery
- Clinical guidelines to judge readiness for implantation
- On vaginal examination, determine the extent of disease prior to EBRT and the regression with EBRT
- If the lesion is discrete on the vulva and not infiltrative, consider interstitial brachytherapy boost

Image Guidance Utilization

- Image guidance to use during the procedure transvaginal ultrasound
- Most of the implant is performed with direct visualization and palpation

Guidelines for Implantation

Preprocedure Advice: Exam Findings, Procedural Positioning, Exam Assessment

- The main concern for vulvar interstitial brachytherapy is exceeding the dose tolerance of the vulva and skin tolerance, try to minimize dose on skin to EQD2 of 70–75 Gy
- Must stabilize the implant to minimize interstitial needle movement which can create a high dose region on the skin
- Secure the implant with a aquaplast mask or needle rubber grommets
- Consider a needle the in AP direction to supplement dose on the distal end of the implant with a flexible catheter
- Consider a mold or bolus on the surface of the skin to supplement dose externally
- Use a radiopaque vessel loop sutured to the clinical target area to visualize during treatment planning
- Place a metal BB on the posterior fourchette and the urethra
- Figure 14.9: vulvar interstitial BT implant

Evaluation of Implantation

Distribution of Implant

- Construct the dose positions to be 5 mm from the skin surface
- Load the applicator in the area of the most distance or packing form the mucosal surfaces

Treatment Planning Considerations

- Optimal brachytherapy dose Rx table with EQD2 and EBRT doses after 45 Gy EBRT, consider 6 Gy × 3 fractions, 3.75 Gy × 5 fractions

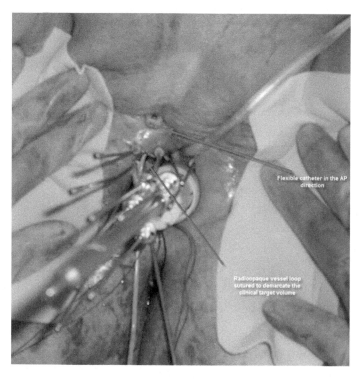

FIG. 14.9. Vulvar interstitial BT implant

Management of Gynecologic Brachytherapy Toxicity

- GI: Use of imodium, tincture of opium for diarrhea, scheduled time for a bowel movement to train the bowels
- Rectal bleeding—occurs in the first 2 years after brachytherapy due to rectal proctitis, given steroid enemas, consider argon plasma coagulation
- Inform GI doctors to not take biopsies of the mucosal changes as this can lead to an ulceration and fistula

- GU: Is mild bleeding, self resolves. If hemorrhagic cystitis—admit for bladder irrigation
- For deceased bladder capacity encourage pelvic exercises and scheduled bladder release
- GYN: Vaginal stenosis—teach to use a vaginal dilator starting one month after treatment, usually to use 1–2 times per week for at least 2 years, then based on clinical examination and discretion
- Vaginal dryness—use daily vaginal moisturizer
- Consider pelvic floor physical therapy

Appendix A

Jyoti Mayadev

Gynecologic Case Study 14.1: Intracavitary Brachytherapy for Cervical Cancer

A 30-year-old female with stage 1B2 invasive squamous cell carcinoma cervix. On initial speculum exam, the cervix and cervical os was obliterated by a 5 cm fungating ulcerative mass without vaginal extension. Rectovaginal examination was unremarkable for parametrial involvement. PET showed hypermetabolic activity in the cervix with SUV 12, and T2-weighted MRI showed gross disease as illustrated in Fig. 14.10

Discussion: She was a candidate for chemoradiation with weekly cisplatin chemotherapy and concurrent whole pelvic radiation followed by intracavitary brachytherapy. She was treated with 5 cycles of cisplatin and 45 Gy to the pelvis with external beam. She started her brachytherapy at the end of week 4

Procedure with Image Guidance: We performed intracavitary brachytherapy using a tandem and ring applicator. We sounded the uterus and placed the tandem using transabdominal and transrectal ultrasound in the procedure room under conscious sedation

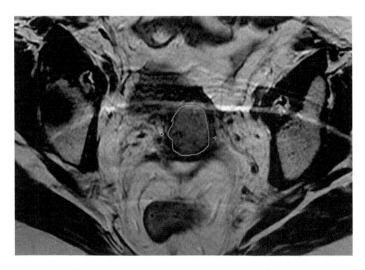

FIG. 14.10. The GTV outlined in *red* on the initial T2 weighted MRI scan

Treatment plan: We planned for a brachytherapy dose of 700 cGy HDR times 4

The organs at risk were drawn, such as the rectum, sigmoid, and bladder. The HR-CTV was constructed with visual verification of the initial MRI image, which is shown on the CT planning scan in Fig. 14.11. Using a standard loading pattern of 2:1 on the tandem and ring, the plan was generated. Then, the physician used manual optimization to decrease the dose to the organs at risk. The equivalent dose was calculated using the DVH for the D90 to the HR-CTV, and organs at risk. The isodose curves with the HR-CTV on the CT planning brachytherapy image are shown in Fig. 14.12

TREATMENT PLAN:

HR-CTV Rx dose: 700 cGy

Average point A dose: 600 cGy

ICRU Bladder point: 243 cGy

ICRU Rectal point: 235 cGy

D90 HR-CTV : 1130 cGy

D2cc Rectum: 270 cGy

D2cc Bladder: 440 cGy

D2cc Sigmoid: 440 cGy

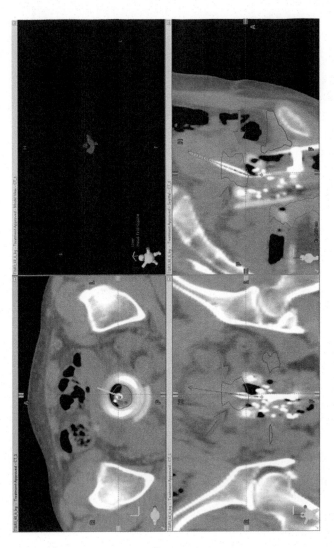

FIG. 14.11. The HR-CTV contour as depicted in *red* and with the *red arrows* on the CT planning scan

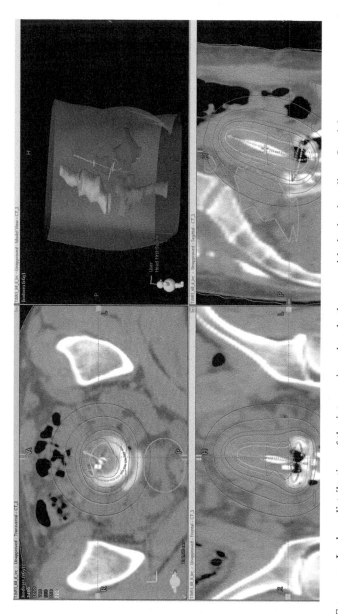

FIG. 14.12. Isodose distribution of the intracavitary brachytherapy with the isodose lines. Spatial geometry seen on the *upper right figure* with the HR-CTV, applicator, bladder, sigmoid, and rectum

Right vaginal mucosa: 1060 cGy
Left vaginal mucosa: 1015 cGy

Gynecologic Case Study 14.2: Interstitial Brachytherapy for Primary Vaginal Cancer

A 75-year-old postvaginal hysterectomy with Stage II invasive squamous cell vaginal cancer. Pelvic examination showed the vagina to be foreshortened and stenotic. There was tumor nodularity 1 cm proximal to the vaginal introitus beginning at 4 o'clock and extending to 12 o'clock position in the entirety of the vagina. There was no urethral nodularity or palpable mucosal extension of disease on the urethra. There was disease at the vaginal apex. On rectovaginal exam there is right paravaginal extension without fixation. Her pretreatment T2-weighted MRI axial image is shown in Fig. 14.13 with the GTV outlined. PET confirmed the primary vaginal mass without lymph node suspicion

Discussion: She was a candidate for chemoradiaiton with weekly cisplatin chemotherapy and concurrent whole pelvic radiation with inguinal LN radiation followed by interstitial brachytherapy. She was treated with 5 cycles of cisplatin and 45 Gy to the pelvis with external beam. She started her brachytherapy at the end of her external beam radiation

Procedure with Image Guidance: We performed interstitial brachytherapy with local sedation consisting of lidocaine jelly, superficial and deep lidocaine injections, and minimal oral narcotic pain medications. Based on her initial examination and the vaginal examination at the time of brachytherapy, we proceeded with a custom cylinder with a central and five surrounding titanium needles. Vaginal packing was wrapped around the cylinder with needles allowing the superior portion to be free of packing to advance the needles through the apex. Then, one flexible interstitial needle was placed at the 9 o'clock position freehand, 1 cm lateral to the vaginal cylinder in the perineal tissue. We used the transrectal ultrasound when placing the lateral vaginal needles. We also depended on manual palpation of the vaginal disease to determine the ideal location of these needles in the procedure room.

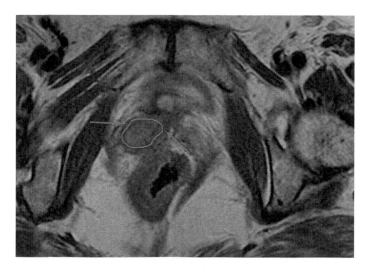

FIG. 14.13. T2 weighted MRI axial image with the vaginal GTV outlined

Treatment plan: We planned for a brachytherapy dose of 450 cGy HDR times 5

The organs at risk were drawn, such as the rectum, sigmoid, and bladder. The HR-CTV was constructed with visual verification of the initial MRI image, initial physical examination, and vaginal examination at the time of brachytherapy, which is shown on the CT planning scan in Fig. 14.14. The HR-CTV was given in two risk stratification: disease at the time of brachytherapy and initial disease or microscopic vaginal extension. Using a volumetric optimization, the plan was generated. Then, the physician used graphical optimization throughout the plan to decrease the dose to the organs at risk, or specified vaginal tissue. The equivalent dose was calculated using the DVH for the D90 to the HR-CTV, and organs at risk. The isodose curves with the HR-CTV on the CT planning brachytherapy image are shown in Fig. 14.15.

TREATMENT PLAN:

HR-CTV Rx dose: 450 cGy

D90 HR-CTV : 400 cGy

D2cc Rectum: 330 cGy

D2cc Bladder: 290 cGy

D2cc Sigmoid:98 cGy

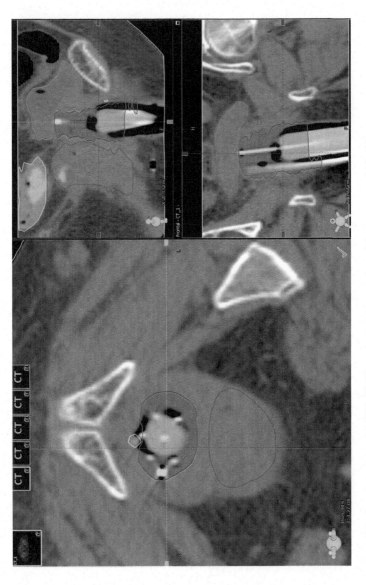

Fɪɢ. 14.14. CT planning scan with HR-CTV vaginal contour, sigmoid, rectum, and bladder

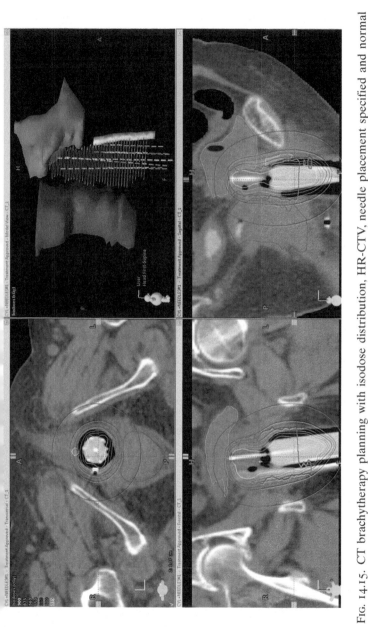

FIG. 14.15. CT brachytherapy planning with isodose distribution, HR-CTV, needle placement specified and normal structures such as the bladder, urethra, rectum

Appendix B: Gynecological Brachytherapy Procedure Checklists

Jyoti Mayadev, Sonja Dieterich, Robin Stern, Stanley Benedict

Tandem and Ring ☐   **Interstitial** ☐

BRACHYTHERAPY INTAKE FORM
Department of Radiation Oncology

┌─────────────────────────┐
│ PATIENT LABEL   │   TREATMENT ____ OF _____
│   │
│   │
└─────────────────────────┘

Radiation Oncologist:_____ Anesthesiologist:_____ Pager # _____

Pt. Phone #: _____

Tentative Treatment Day/s_____

Scheduled in EPIC YES ☐ **NO** ☐ by MOSC _____

Contact OR Scheduler @ 4-7824   SNAPBOARD OR schedule confirmed: YES ☐ **NO** ☐
Type of Anesthesia: Epidural **YES** ☐ **NO** ☐ PCA **YES** ☐ **NO** ☐ Moderate Sedation **YES** ☐ **NO** ☐

Brachytherapy Nurse: _____   **Brachytherapist** _____

I. Day before Procedure

1. Consent papers ready **YES** ☐ **NO** ☐
2. Labs checked (BMP, CBC, Coagulation Studies) **YES** ☐ **NO**☐. If out of range MD notified
    YES ☐ **NO** ☐ Date notified: _____ Time notified: _____
    For outside lab: Facility name: _____ **Contact number** _____
3. *By 3 PM* Medication orders checked in EMR **YES** ☐ **NO** ☐
4. *By 4 PM* Telephone encounter sent to Cancer Center Infusion Pharmacy with date and time of
    procedure and name of antibiotic medication **YES** ☐ **NO** ☐
5. Request for HAR sent **YES** ☐ **NO** ☐
6. Equipment : SIGMA pump **YES** ☐ **NO** ☐ Epidural pump **YES** ☐ **NO** ☐
    PCA pump **YES** ☐ **NO** ☐Alternating Limb Pump (ALP) **YES** ☐ **NO** ☐ Propaq **YES** ☐ **NO** ☐
    Anesthesia Cart checked **YES** ☐ **NO** ☐ Foley Insertion tray **YES** ☐ **NO** ☐
    Instruments prepared by Brachytherapist YES ☐ **NO** ☐

II. Day of Procedure

1. Call Pavilion Pharmacy @ **3-6102** by 0730 to confirm medication pick up **YES** ☐ **NO** ☐

2. Call Action Nurse @ **4-0775 YES** ☐ **NO** ☐ Action Nurse _____

┌───┐
│ Notes: │
│   │
│   │
│   │
│   │
└───┘

Interstitial GYN Patient Instruction Sheet

Your appointments are:

Date: _____
Time: _____
Date: _____
Time: _____

Location of procedure:

To prepare for your procedure:

- Go to the Pre-Op Anesthesia Clinic. It is a drop in Clinic and you do not need an appointment.
- Have labs drawn no later than 2 days before your procedure.
- Pick up prescriptions for antibiotics at your preferred pharmacy. You will take these after each of your procedures.
- 3 days or more before your procedure do not take any of the following: Ibuprofen (advil,motrin), Naprosyn (Aleve), aspirin (Ecotrin,Bayer,Excedrine,Bufferin,Alka seltzer, or any product containing aspirin-check the label)Echinacea,garlic capsules,ginko,ginseng,kava,St.John's Wart, Valarian, or Vitamin E, warfarin, coumadin. (Lovenox and fragmin do not take the day before your procedure)
- You may take Tylenol (Acetaminophen) for pain.
- Okay to take regular medications 2 hours before your procedure with a small sip of water.
- Clear Liquids ONLY the day before your procedure: Water,tea,coffee(without milk products),apple juice,cranberry juice,(no juice with pupl),7-up,broth (chicken,beef,veg.),jello without fruit, NO RED JELLO. No alcohol. Drink as much of these items as you can.
- Nothing to eat or drink for 8 hours before your procedure including chewing gum or hard candy.
- Start your bowel prep at 4:00PM the day before your procedure.
- Take a bath or shower on the morning of your procedure and wear clean casual, loose clothing to your procedure.
- Nail polish and lotion should not be worn.
- You must have a responsible adult to provide a ride home from discharge.
- If you any questions please call the nurse at _____.

Gynecology Interstitial Implantation

Discharge Instructions

- Please do a sitz bath twice daily for 2 days after the implant. Sitz bath is a solution of warm water, 1 tablespoon of salt, 1 tablespoon of baking soda and you place your perineum in this solution for 15 minutes.
- Please use "Butt Balm Cream" three times per day for 7 days. This has been prescribed by your radiation oncologist.
- Sit on a bag of ice twice per day for 3 days to help with labia swelling.
- Please call the radiation oncology nurse, physician, or on call doctor. The on call doctor can be reached by calling _____ and asking for the radiation doctor on call, if you have the following:

Fever greater than 100.5F

Severe vaginal bleeding

Severe burning with urination

Lower pelvic pain

Sharp abdominal pain

Expected/Common side effects:

Mild urinary burning for 2-3 days after the implant. Increasing your fluid intake may help.

Loose bowel movements

Increased number of bowel movements

Vaginal discharge or cramping

Vaginal tenderness or itching

Sore perineum or labia

Fatigue

Sexual Activity may be resumed when comfortable (usually 1 month)

Follow up

Follow up appointment with radiation oncologist

GYN BRACHYTHERAPY PROCEDURE SCHEDULING FORM
Physician:
Resident:

Date of consult:_____

Vaginal Brachytherapy Cylinder

Date range of implant #1:_____
Number of implants: 1   2   3   4   5   6
Range of dates between implants:_____

Custom planning on implant: Y   N
Conscious sedation needed: Y   N

Size of cylinder   2   2.5   3   3.5
Active length:_____
Dosimetry preplan library template available:

Tandem and Ring Brachytherapy

Date range of implant #1:_____
Number of implants: 1   2   3   4   5   6
Range of dates between implants:_____

Conscious sedation needed: Y   N
Anesthesia needed: Y   N

Interstitial Brachytherapy

Date range of implant #1:
Number of implants: 1   2   3   4   5   6
Number of fractions per implant: 1   2   3   4
Range of dates between implants:

Department of Radiation Oncology
HDR Gynecological Cylinder Simulation

1. GammaMed HDR cylindrical cylinders consist of a front segment or dome, cylindrical segments, a clamping segment, a guide tube, and a flexible probe. Single segment solid cylinders are also available. There are different cylindrical segments for each diameter (2.0, 2.5, 3.0, and 3.5 cm); the clamping segment, guide tube, and flexible probe are the same for all diameters.

2. Unless otherwise specified in the MOSAIQ prescription, the segmented cylinders will be assembled with all four cylindrical segments of the specified diameter.

3. The MOSAIQ prescription will specify the cylinder diameter, active length and treatment distance. The active length is specified by the treating physician based on clinical characteristics of the tumor, and the patient's physical vaginal length. The active length is not the same as and is not specifically related to the physical length of the cylinder.

4. Treatment flow:
    a. The physician will determine the active length and diameter of the cylinder at the clinical visit, prior to the first verification sim.
    b. The patient will receive a verification sim before every treatment/fraction.
    c. At the time of the verification sim, the attending physician will verify the physical placement of the cylinder. A radiopaque BB will be placed at the introitus. Dummy verification seeds will be placed in the cylinder. An external elastic or metal clamp fixation device will be placed on the patient to hold the cylinder apparatus in position. A series of anterior-posterior and lateral scout films will be obtained. The attending physician will verify the physical length of the vagina and placement of the vaginal cylinder at the time of the verification sim.
    d. The patient will then be transported to the HDR treatment room for treatment.

Department of Radiation Oncology
Policy and Procedures

Policy Section: Clinical Practice > HDR Brachytherapy

Title: GammaMed HDR Planning Procedure for Tandem & Ring Applicator

Author:

Effective Dates:

Introduction

Inaccuracies in the dwell positions within the ring have been reported by Varian (Product Notification Letters PNL-VS/GM-CR-30271 and PNL-GM-CR-30271 (2)). These inaccuracies have been measured and documented for the two UCD Ring and Tandem Applicator sets (See GammaMed HDR Ring Positioning Accuracy Report). The following procedure, based on the recommendation in PNL-VS/GM-CR-30271 and using the UCD-measured shift value, should be used for treatment planning in Brachyvision. Because the UCD-measured shift of 0.3 cm measured with respect to planned dwell positions is distal and not proximal, this correction method is valid.

Procedure

1. Do not use dummy markers during imaging unless requested by the physician or treatment planner to aid visualization
2. All other aspects of treatment planning for the tandem are unchanged. There is no dwell position shift or adjustment for the tandem.
3. Within Brachyvision:
   3.1. use the line density tool to find the tip of the hardware ring on the CT scan.
   3.2. Define the tip of the software ring applicator 0.3 cm beyond the inside tip of the hardware ring on the images (see figure below). If the inside tip is not distinguishable, measure 0.2 cm outward from the outside tip.
   3.3. Define the rest of the software ring applicator to lie within the inner lumen of the imaged ring.
4. In the Brachyvision Focus window,
   4.1. right click on the ring applicator and select *Properties*.
   4.2. Set *First Source Position* to 0.3 cm. Leave *Step Size* at 0.5 cm.
   4.3. The location of the dwell positions in the plan will now correspond to the actual treatment dwell positions.
5. In the ring, **use only dwell positions 121.7 – 129.2 cm** in steps of 0.5 cm. All others must be undefined or have dwell times set to 0.0 sec.
6. In the completed plan, all dwell position should end in either .2 or .7 cm.
7. A sample plan (created on a plane film) is shown in Figure 1.

Sample plan showing definition of software ring and applicator properties in Brachyvision.

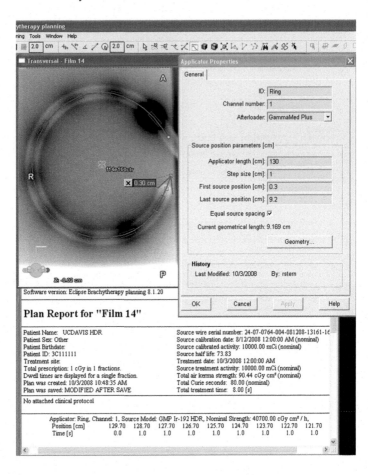

Gynecologic Interstitial High Dose Rate Implantation
Needles Verification

Date of Simulation: _____

PT Label here

Physician: Jyoti Mayadev

| Central Needle | Y | N |
| Central Tandem | Y | N |

Number of 250 mm needles inserted: _____
Number of 200 mm needles inserted: _____

Verification Length (+/- 1mm) = proximal end of needle to proximal end of button

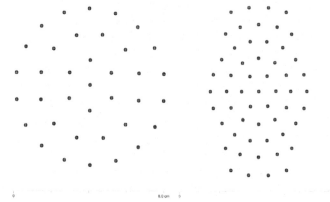

Simulation Verifications				Treatment Verifications					
Needle Number	Needle Length	Verification Length*	Therapist Initials	Treatment 1 Verif. Date	Therapist Initials	Treatment 2 Verif. Date	Therapist Initials	Treatment 3 Verif. Date	Therapist Initials
1									
2									
3									
4									
5									
6									
7									
8									
9									
10									
11									
12									
13									
14									
15									
16									
17									
18									
19									
20									
21									
22									
23									
24									

MR#: ☐☐☐☐☐☐
Name of Patient:
Date of Birth:
        Place Label Here

HDR Instrument and Workflow Checklist

Implant #: _____   Date: _____

Implant Type: _____   CT Study ID: _____

                                          # of Slices: _____   Slice Thickness:_____

Instruments:	Inserted	Removed	Inserted	Removed

Additional Planning Information

_____

_____

        Please initial each step

Post-Treatment: *(Not needed for Standard Cylinders or Tandem & Ring Procedures)*

        Removal of all instrument/applicators confirmed & vaginal check complete. _____ (MD initials)

Simulation:

_____ SIM completed, Dosimetry notified & BrachyTherapy Checklist transferred at _____ (enter time).

Dosimetry:

_____ Dosimetry notified Physician that plan is ready for MD review at _____ (enter time).
_____ Physician starts to review plan _____ (enter time).
_____ Physician notified Dosimetry that the plan is ready for physics check at _____ (enter time).
_____ Dosimetry notified Physics of that the plan is ready for physics check_____ (enter time).
_____ Physics starts to review plan _____ (enter time).

Physics:

_____ Physics notified simulation and dosimetry that 2nd check is complete at _____ (enter time).

Simulation:

_____ Sim notified Nursing that 2nd check is complete at _____ (enter time).

References

1. Hanks GE, Herring DF, Kramer S. Patterns of care outcome studies. Results of the national practice in cancer of the cervix. Cancer. 1983;51(5):959–67.
2. Han K, Milosevic M, Fyles A, Pintilie M, Viswanathan AN. Trends in the utilization of brachytherapy in cervical cancer in the United States. Int J Radiat Oncol Biol Phys. 2013;87(1):111–9.
3. Orton A, Boothe D, Williams N, et al. Brachytherapy improves survival in primary vaginal cancer. Gynecol Oncol. 2016;141(3):501–6.
4. Charra-Brunaud C, Harter V, Delannes M, et al. Impact of 3D image-based PDR brachytherapy on outcome of patients treated for cervix carcinoma in France: results of the French STIC prospective study. Radiother Oncol. 2012;103(3):305–13.
5. Potter R, Haie-Meder C, Van Limbergen E, et al. Recommendations from gynaecological (GYN) GEC ESTRO working group (II): concepts and terms in 3D image-based treatment planning in cervix cancer brachytherapy-3D dose volume parameters and aspects of 3D image-based anatomy, radiation physics, radiobiology. Radiother Oncol. 2006;78(1):67–77.
6. Georg P, Boni A, Ghabuous A, et al. Time course of late rectal- and urinary bladder side effects after MRI-guided adaptive brachytherapy for cervical cancer. Strahlenther Onkol. 2013;189(7):535–40.
7. Creutzberg CL, van Putten WL, Koper PC, et al. Surgery and postoperative radiotherapy versus surgery alone for patients with stage-1 endometrial carcinoma: multicentre randomised trial. PORTEC Study Group. Post Operative Radiation Therapy in Endometrial Carcinoma. Lancet. 2000;355(9213):1404–11.
8. Keys HM, Roberts JA, Brunetto VL, et al. A phase III trial of surgery with or without adjunctive external pelvic radiation therapy in intermediate risk endometrial adenocarcinoma: a Gynecologic Oncology Group study. Gynecol Oncol. 2004;92(3):744–51.
9. Nout RA, Smit VT, Putter H, et al. Vaginal brachytherapy versus pelvic external beam radiotherapy for patients with endometrial cancer of high-intermediate risk (PORTEC-2): an open-label, non-inferiority, randomised trial. Lancet. 2010;375(9717):816–23.

10. Klopp A, Smith BD, Alektiar K, et al. The role of postoperative radiation therapy for endometrial cancer: executive summary of an American Society for Radiation Oncology evidence-based guideline. Pract Radiat Oncol. 2014;4(3):137–44.
11. Cattaneo 2nd R, Hanna RK, Jacobsen G, Elshaikh MA. Interval between hysterectomy and start of radiation treatment is predictive of recurrence in patients with endometrial carcinoma. Int J Radiat Oncol Biol Phys. 2014;88(4):866–71.
12. Mock U, Kucera H, Fellner C, Knocke TH, Potter R. High-dose-rate (HDR) brachytherapy with or without external beam radiotherapy in the treatment of primary vaginal carcinoma: long-term results and side effects. Int J Radiat Oncol Biol Phys. 2003; 56(4):950–7.
13. Beriwal S, Demanes DJ, Erickson B, et al. American Brachytherapy Society consensus guidelines for interstitial brachytherapy for vaginal cancer. Brachytherapy. 2012;11(1):68–75.
14. Beriwal S, Kannan N, Kim H, et al. Three-dimensional high dose rate intracavitary image-guided brachytherapy for the treatment of cervical cancer using a hybrid magnetic resonance imaging/computed tomography approach: feasibility and early results. Clin Oncol. 2011;23(10):685–90.

Chapter 15
Skin Brachytherapy

Anna Likhacheva

Introduction

- Skin cancer is the most common malignancy in the United States. Nearly, three million new cases of skin cancer are diagnosed annually. This translates to 20 % lifetime risk of developing skin cancer in the United States [1]
- Incidence of both melanoma and nonmelanoma skin cancers is rising [2, 3]
- The vast majority of cutaneous malignancies are made up of BCC and SCC, collectively referred to as non-melanoma skin cancer (NMSC). Other histologic sub-types of skin cancer include melanoma, adnexal carcinomas, Merkel cell carcinoma, cutaneous lymphoma, and sarcoma
- BCC makes up approximately 80 % of NMSC and carries a better prognosis than SCC [4]
- SCC has more aggressive behavior with greater potential for local and distant recurrence [5]
- Melanoma is an aggressive malignancy responsible for >75 % of skin cancer deaths [3]. It's not typically treated with skin brachytherapy

A. Likhacheva, MD, MPH (✉)
Department of Radiation Oncology, Banner MD Anderson Cancer Center, 2946 E Banner Gateway Dr, Gilbert, AZ 85234, USA
e-mail: Anna.likhacheva@bannerhealth.com

© Springer International Publishing AG 2017
J. Mayadev et al. (eds.), *Handbook of Image-Guided Brachytherapy*, DOI 10.1007/978-3-319-44827-5_15

457

- Risk factors for NMSC are fair complexion, a history of excessive UV exposure, immune suppression, inherited disorders, and a history of skin cancer
- 25 % of skin cancers on the face are located on the nose [6]

Rationale for Brachytherapy

- Definitive management of NMSC can employ a multitude of treatment modalities, including surgical excision, topical therapies, electrocautery, cryotherapy, and radiation therapy. Treatment choice should be guided by size, location, patient fitness, and expectation for cosmetic outcomes
- Skin surface brachytherapy allows superficial dose deposition of a homogenous dose even on curved surfaces [7]. Brachytherapy offers dosimetric advantages over electron beam therapy for treatment of challenging anatomic sites such as nose, eyelids, lips, fingers, and ears [7]
- Dosimetric properties of skin surface brachytherapy allow for high dose deposition to skin surface while sparing underlying connective tissue. This enables treatment using a hypofractionated schedule
- Shorter treatment course permitted by skin brachytherapy increases access to care
- Although LDR skin brachytherapy has been utilized using radioisotope-impregnated resin, this chapter will be limited to the more common and widely practiced HDR technique

Goal of Brachytherapy

- Goal of skin surface brachytherapy is to achieve good local control with excellent cosmetic outcome in fewer fractions than with external beam radiation therapy

Pertinent Anatomy for Brachytherapy

- Epidermis and dermis are thinner on the face than other parts of the body. Epidermis is 0.04–1.5 mm and dermis is 1–4 mm thick depending on location. The dermis contains blood and lymphatic vessels, hair follicles, sweat glands, sebaceous glands, nerve endings, collagen, and elastin. Subcutis contains fat and superficial fascia. See Fig. 15.1 for normal cutaneous anatomy
- Location on the face is an important predictor of recurrence risk. H zone contains embryonal fusion planes and is more conducive to local spread (Fig. 15.2)

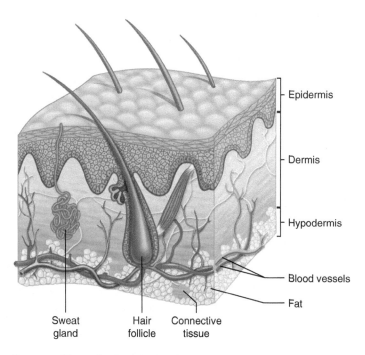

FIG. 15.1. Normal cutaneous anatomy

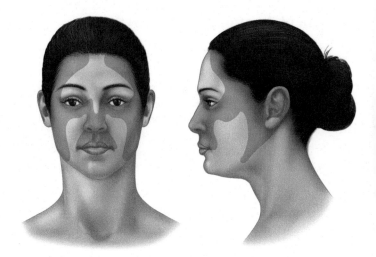

Fig. 15.2. H zone of the face

Pathology

BCC

- BCC are typically indolent tumors of the skin, arising in sun-exposed head, neck, and distal extremities.
- BCC can be divided into several distinct variants:
    - Nodular is the most common. It appears as a pearly nodule with central umbilication and telangiectasias
    - Superficial appears as red, scaly macules with indistinct margins
    - Morpheaform (sclerosing) is an aggressive variant. It appears as single flat indurated macules. PNI is common
    - Infiltrative is another aggressive variant, which appears as opaque yellowish plaques that blend with the surrounding skin
- BCC is more radiosensitive than SCC [8]
- Rate of regional and distant metastases is only 0.01 % [9].

SCC

- SCC is graded into well-, moderately-, and poorly differentiated histological subtypes
- SCC can also be categorized as superficial or infiltrative:
  - Superficial SCC manifests as a scaly, crusted plaque, or ulcer
  - Infiltrative SCC appears as a firm, indurated mass
- SCC typically has a higher local recurrence rate than BCC [10]. Metastases are usually first seen in regional nodes, followed by lung and liver
- Factors associated with regional spread are tumor site, PNI, LVSI, host immunosuppression, poor differentiation, size (>2 cm), and depth of invasion (>6 mm) [11, 12]

Other

- Cutaneous lymphoma is a radiosensitive entity. B-cell and T-cell lymphomas can be treated in definitive and palliative settings with skin brachytherapy
- Kaposi Sarcoma, a spindle cell tumor arising from endothelial cells, is typically associated with AIDS or immunosuppression although sporadic variant can be seen especially in equatorial Africa. It's amenable to radiation therapy for local control and palliation

Efficacy

- Refer to Table 15.1 to see published experience in skin surface brachytherapy

TABLE 15.1 Highlights of published experience in skin surface brachytherapy

Study	Tumor location	Patients	Treatment	Follow-up	Local control	Dose/fractions
Arenas et al. [16]	Face	134	Leipzig applicator Iridium 192	Median of 33 months	95.1 % for BCC; 93.4 % for SCC	45–57 Gy in 3 Gy fractions
Ballester-Sanchez et al. [17]	Mostly head and neck	40	Electronic brachytherapy	Unknown	90 % for 36.6 Gy/6fx; 95 % for 42 Gy/7fx	36.6 Gy in 6 fractions; 42 Gy in 7 fractions
Bhatnagar [18]	Various	122	Electronic brachytherapy	Mean of 10 months	100 %	40 Gy in 8 fractions
Debois et al. [19]	Nose	370	Custom mold applicator Cesium 137	2 years	97 % if primary treatment; 94 % if recurrence	24 Gy over 48 h
Delishaj et al. [20]	Mostly head and neck	39	Valencia applicator Iridium 192	Median of 12 months	96.25 %	40 Gy in 8 fractions; 50 Gy in 10 fractions
Guix et al. [21]	Face	136	Custom mold applicator Iridium 192	5 years	99 % if primary treatment; 87 % if recurrence	60–65 Gy in 33–36 fractions

Study	Site	n	Technique	Follow-up	Control	Dose
Gauden et al. [22]	Mostly head and neck	200	Leipzig applicator Iridium 192	Median 66 months	98 %	36 Gy in 12 fractions
Kohler-Brock et al. [23]	Various	520	Leipzig applicator Iridium 192	10 year experience	91 %	30–40 Gy in 3–10 fractions
Paravati et al. [24]	Head and neck	127	Electronic brachytherapy	Median of 16.1 months	98.7 %	40 Gy in 8 fractions
Sedda et al. [25]	Various	53	Custom mold applicator Rhenium 188 resin	Minimum 20 months	100 %	40–60 Gy
Schulte	Head and neck	1267	Soft X-rays	Mean 77 months	94.9 %	45–55 Gy in 5 Gy fractions for BCC; 60–70 Gy in 5 Gy fractions for SCC
Svoboda et al. [26]	Various	106	Custom mold applicator	Mean 9.6 months	96 %	12–50 Gy in 1–15 fractions

Selection Criteria

- Thorough physical exam of the skin and draining lymphatics should be performed at initial evaluation. Clinical photography is very useful for subsequent localization, treatment, and follow-up. Symptoms suggestive of perineural invasion (tingling, formication, etc.) should be evaluated further with imaging and correlated with pathological evaluation

- Optimal patient selection is yet to be refined. Ideal patients for definitive skin surface brachytherapy should be older adults with cutaneous malignancies that are at low risk for regional spread. Our practice uses the following exclusion criteria:
  - T2 > 4 cm, T3–T4, N1
  - Histopathologic Grade 3 (poorly differentiated)
  - Target area is adjacent to a burn scar
  - Target area is on the lip
  - Patient < 50 years of age
  - Perineural invasion
  - Lesion depth > 4 mm on clinical assessment or as assessed by ultrasound or CT
  - Prior radiation therapy to this specific anatomic location
  - Genetic disorders predisposing to skin cancers or radiation sensitivity
  - Concurrent chemotherapy or other pharmacologic agent(s) at or around the time of the radiation therapy that is/are known to produce skin reactions

Image Guidance Utilization

- Because dose deposition is superficial with skin surface brachytherapy, it is important to verify depth of invasion [13]
- When clinical exam is insufficient, ultrasound of the skin can be a useful modality to estimate depth (Fig. 15.3a, b)

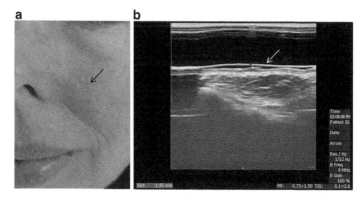

FIG. 15.3. An example of image-guidance utilization that shows the usefulness of ultrasound (**b**) of the skin to estimate depth when the clinical exam (**a**) is insufficient

- ■ CT planning performed for molds and flaps can aid in delineating the gross disease

Simulation Guidelines

The following steps are performed during simulation:
- ■ Target delineation—GTV, CTV, PTV margins, depth assessment
  - ■ CTV margins are variable (usually 4–10 mm) depending on size and histology
  - ■ Maximum recommended depth is 4 mm for skin surface brachytherapy
    <u>Applicator selection</u>
- ■ Applicators with fixed geometry
  - ■ Flat, well-circumscribed, small lesions are easily treated with shielded applicators via either remote-afterloading HDR radionuclide or electronic brachytherapy. Nucletron® (Elekta, Stockholm, Sweden) supplies cup-shaped applicators with and without a flattening filter (Valencia and Leipzig, respectively). The flattening filter improves the

homogeneity of dose-depth profile (Fig. 15.4). An outline of workflow and planning is published by Sayler et al. [14]

■ Electronic brachytherapy uses a miniature HDR X-ray source that emits photons with a maximum energy of 50 keV from the tip of a catheter. Depending on the manufacturer, applicator sizes accommodate targets up to 5 cm in diameter. Because a radionuclide is not involved, shielded vault are not required for treatment delivery

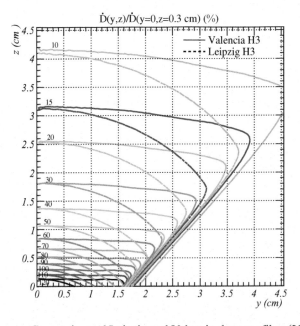

FIG. 15.4. Comparison of Leipzig and Valencia dose profiles. (Used with permission of Elekta Brachytherapy and courtesy of J. Pérez-Calatayud from Clinical Guide to Surface Treatment of Skin Cancer with Brachytherapy. Nucletron® training materials. Elekta, Stockholm, Sweden; also with permission from Granero D, Pérez-Calatayud J, Gimeno J, Ballester F, Casal E. Design and evaluation of a HDR skin applicator with flattening filter. Med Phys 2008 35(2): 495–503)

- Custom flaps and molds
  - Larger lesions over curved or irregular areas can be treated using a custom flap or mold
  - A prefabricated multi-lumen catheter flap such as the Freiburg Flap (Nucletron®, Elekta, Stockholm, Sweden) and Harrison-Anderson-Mick (H.A.M.) applicator (Mick Radio-Nuclear Instruments, Inc., Mt Vernon, NY, USA). As opposed to standard applicators, these flaps do not provide the integrated shielding of a surface applicator
  - Thermoplastic material with integrated afterloading catheters can be custom fabricated to fit the skin target. This is employed for especially challenging sites where the plasticity of a prefabricated multi-lumen catheter flap is insufficient
- Immobilization
  - Thermoplastic masks are helpful for all types of applicators to ensure constant target coverage and skin-source distance during a potentially long treatment time. Area over the target is cut out to allow access for bell-shaped applicators. Alternatively, the mask material over the target can be used to secure a custom mold or flap
- Applicator assembly
  - Bell-shaped applicators require little to no assembly. They are secured to a stable clamp, for which optimal position should be determined
  - Custom flap and molds are unique to each clinical situation, and thus require a much more involved simulation. We like to use the lattice of the thermoplastic mask to secure flaps and molds
    - CTV borders should be transposed to the mask
    - Catheters are then secured to the mask. For optimal dose coverage, lateral most catheters should be outside the CTV by at least 10 mm
    - Thin radio-opaque marking wires are placed on the skin to outline the CTV
    - Catheters are then numbered, and markers are placed in each catheter

- CT slice thickness of at least 1.5 mm allows accurate catheter reconstruction and planning
- Shielding
  - Shielding of adjacent skin and other structures is especially important when using custom molds and flaps, as they do not have integrated shielding of bell-shaped applicators. Adjacent uninvolved skin may receive a high dose from the isotropy of the nearby dwell positions
  - A small amount of scatter is present even with tungsten-shielded applicators, so that it is our practice to routinely put lead shielding over the eyes
  - Intranasal lead shielding protects the septum, posterior nasal passage, and contralateral ala when treating the nose

Evaluation of Implantation

- Treatment with skin surface brachytherapy requires thorough documentation including clinical photography of setup. This is important for reproducible setup during each fraction
- When using skin flaps and molds, a CT verification simulation may be appropriate to verify consistency of applicator position

Treatment Planning Considerations

- Optimal Brachytherapy Dose
  - Optimal dose and fractionation for skin surface brachytherapy is yet to be defined. Common regimens are listed in Table 15.2
- Optimization of Target Volume and Dose Distribution
  - Current calculations of the treatment time for surface applicators are based on the nomograms and TG-43 formalism. The prescription to depth of 3 mm results in ~138 % delivered to the skin surface

TABLE 15.2 Common prescriptions for definitive treatment of superficial nonmelanoma skin cancers (EQD2 is based on alpha/beta of 8.5)

Total dose (Gy)	Number of fractions	Dose per fraction	Treatment schedule	EQD2 (Gy)
40	8	5	2–3 times a week	51.4
42	6	7	2–3 times a week	58
42	7	6	2–3 times a week	62
45	10	4.5	2–3 times a week	55.7

- For CT planning, CTV is contoured. Ideally, D_{min} should be >95 % and D_{max} <135 %. Care should be taken to distribute dwell times as evenly as possible

Toxicity

Acute Toxicity

- Definitive treatment typically produces moist desquamation. Unlike with standard fractionation, acute toxicity peaks approximately 2 weeks after a hypofractionated course
- Radiation toxicity is more severe and time of onset is earlier in the treatment of sensitive anatomic sites, such as pretibial skin
- Treatment on or near the nose can cause acute mucositis, dryness, and epistaxis
- Treatment of periocular structures can cause conjunctivitis and permanent loss of eyelashes and eyebrows

Late Toxicity

Excellent cosmetic outcome has been reported in 85–95 % of patients treated with hypofractionated skin surface brachytherapy [15]. Common late toxicities include:

- Hypopigmentation
- Telangiectasia
- Skin atrophy
- Permanent hair loss in the treatment field

Management of Brachytherapy Toxicity

- Bland emollient should be applied daily to the treatment site
- For moist desquamation, a sterile nonadherent dressing will help keep the treatment site clean and moist, thereby promoting faster healing
- Patients should be educated to protect the irradiated skin from further tissue injury from temperature extremes, friction, sun exposure, and disinfectants

Appendix

Skin Cancer Case Study 15.1: Leipzig Applicator (Elekta, Nucletron®, Stockholm, Sweden)

A 61-year-old female presented to the attention of her dermatologist with complaints of a slowly enlarging pearly skin lesion on the left nasal ala (Fig. 15.5). Lesion size at the time of biopsy was 8 mm in greatest dimension. She was averse to having surgical intervention and was treated with definitive radiation therapy

She received skin surface radionuclide-based brachytherapy using a Leipzig applicator (Fig. 15.6). A thermoplastic mask was used to immobilize the patient during treatment. Lead shielding was using to protect the eyes, the upper lip,

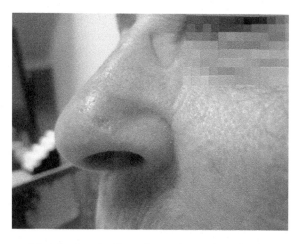

FIG. 15.5. Nodular basal cell carcinoma located on the left nasal ala in a 61-year-old woman. Central crater is the result of a shave biopsy

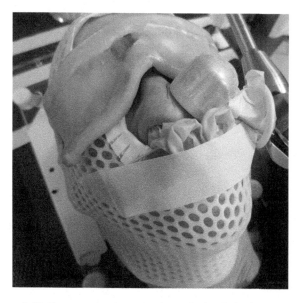

FIG. 15.6. Daily treatment setup showed the Leipzig Applicator (Elekta, Nucletron®, Stockholm, Sweden), lead shielding, and thermoplastic mask with a cutout for the nose

472   A. Likhacheva

and nasal septum from scattered radiation. She was treated to
a total of 40 Gy in 8 fractions, delivered twice a week, at least
72 h apart. The dose was prescribed to 3 mm (Fig. 15.7)

She tolerated treatment well. She developed erythema, dry
desquamation, and skin edema as the result of treatment
(Fig. 15.8). She also complained of two episodes of self-
limited nosebleeds

At 4-month follow-up, there was no evidence of residual
or recurrent disease (Fig 15.9). There was mild hypopigmentation in the treated area. She was very pleased with the
cosmetic outcome

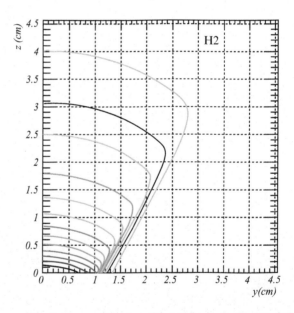

Fig. 15.7. Depth-dose profile for a 2 cm Leipzig Applicator (Elekta,
Nucletron®, Stockholm, Sweden). (Used with permission from
Pérez-Calatayud J, Granero D, Baleester F, Puchades V, Casal E,
Soriano A, Crispin V. A dosimetric study of Leipzig applicators.
International Journal of Radiation Oncology* Biology* Physics.
2005 June 1; 62(2):579–584)

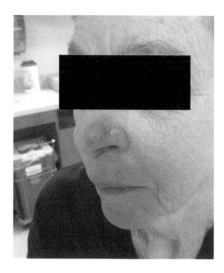

FIG. 15.8. Appearance of treatment site on the last day of treatment

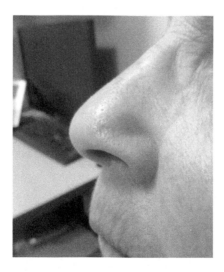

FIG. 15.9. Appearance of treatment site on the last day of treatment at 4 months after RT course

Skin Cancer Case Study 15.2: Freiburg Flap (Elekta, Nucletron®, Stockholm, Sweden)

A 61-year-old male with long-standing history of ultraviolet exposure and multiple diagnoses of nonmelanoma skin cancers. Biopsies of bilateral ala revealed well-differentiated squamous cell carcinoma (Fig. 15.10)

The patient received 40 Gy in 8 fractions on a twice-a-week basis using a Freiburg flap (Elekta, Nucletron®, Stockholm, Sweden). A thermoplastic mask was used to immobilize the patient during treatment. The flap was sewn to the matrix of the Freiburg flap (Elekta, Nucletron®, Stockholm, Sweden). Lead shielding was used to protect the cheeks, eyes, and the upper lip (Fig. 15.11). The dose was prescribed to 3 mm depth (Fig. 15.12)

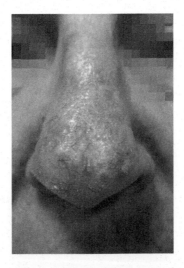

FIG. 15.10. Superficial well-differentiated squamous cell carcinoma affecting the tip of the nose and extending onto bilateral nasal ala

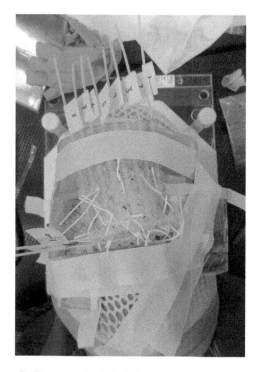

Fɪɢ. 15.11. Daily setup included thermoplastic mask, to which a Freiberg flap (Elekta, Nucletron®, Stockholm, Sweden) was sewn. Lead shielding was used to protect uninvolved surrounding structures from scattered dose

The patient developed erythema and dry desquamation at the end of his treatment course (Fig. 15.13)

At 10 months after RT, there was no evidence of residual disease (Fig. 15.14)

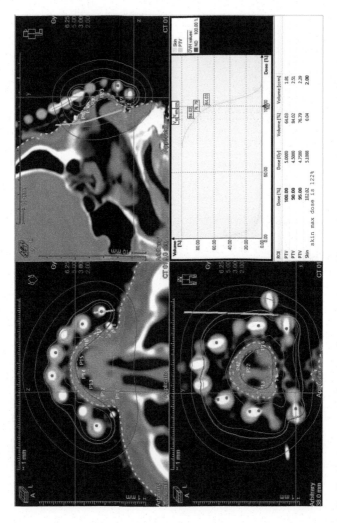

FIG. 15.12. Radiation treatment plan showing catheter reconstruction and expected dose distribution

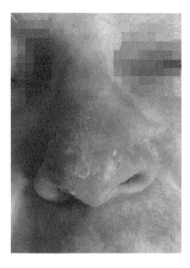

FIG. 15.13. Clinical appearance of the skin after on the last treatment day

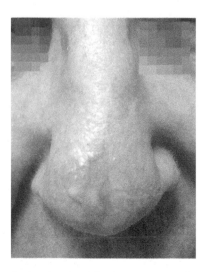

FIG. 15.14. At 10 months after RT, there was no evidence of disease. Mild hypopigmentation in the treated area

References

1. Stern RS. Prevalence of a history of skin cancer in 2007: results of an incidence-based model. Arch Dermatol. 2010;146(3):279–82.
2. Lansbury L, Bath-Hextall F, Perkins W, Stanton W, Leonardi-Bee J. Interventions for non-metastatic squamous cell carcinoma of the skin: systematic review and pooled analysis of observational studies. BMJ. 2013;347:f6153–3.
3. Siegel RL, Miller KD, Jemal A. Cancer statistics, 2016. CA Cancer J Clin. 2016;66(1):7–30.
4. Rogers HW, Weinstock MA, Harris AR, Hinckley MR, Feldman SR, Fleischer AB, et al. Incidence estimate of nonmelanoma skin cancer in the United States, 2006. Arch Dermatol. 2010;146(3):283–7.
5. Silva JJ, Tsang RW, Panzarella T, Levin W, Wells W. Results of radiotherapy for epithelial skin cancer of the pinna: the Princess Margaret Hospital experience, 1982-1993. Int J Radiat Oncol Biol Phys. 2000;47(2):451–9.
6. Koplin L, Zarem HA. Recurrent basal cell carcinoma: a review concerning the incidence, behavior, and management of recurrent basal cell carcinoma, with emphasis on the incompletely excised lesion. Plast Reconstr Surg. 1980;65(5):656.
7. Hwang IM, Leung HWC. Dosimetry characteristics of Leipzig applicators. In: Mould RF, Gurtler MW, editors. Proceedings of the 1st far east radiotherapy treatment planning workshop. Veenendaal: Nucletron-Oldelft; 1996. p. 88–9.
8. Kwan W, Wilson D, Moravan V. Radiotherapy for locally advanced basal cell and squamous cell carcinomas of the skin. Int J Radiat Oncol Biol Phys. 2004;60(2):406–11.
9. Lo JS, Snow SN, Reizner GT, Mohs FE, Larson PO, Hruza GJ. Metastatic basal cell carcinoma: report of twelve cases with a review of the literature. J Am Acad Dermatol. 1991;24(5):715–9.
10. Locke J, Karimpour S, Young G, Lockett MA, Perez CA. Radiotherapy for epithelial skin cancer. Int J Radiat Oncol Biol Phys. 2001;51(3):748–55.
11. Brantsch KD, Meisner C, Schönfisch B, Trilling B, Wehner-Caroli J, Röcken M, et al. Analysis of risk factors determining prognosis of cutaneous squamous-cell carcinoma: a prospective study. Lancet Oncol. 2008;9(8):713–20.
12. Lansbury L, Leonardi-Bee J, Perkins W, Goodacre T, Tweed JA, Bath Hextall FJ. Interventions for non-metastatic squamous cell

carcinoma of the skin. In: Lansbury L, editor. Cochrane database of systematic review. Chicheste: Wiley; 2010;(4). p. CD007869.

13. Goyal U, Kim Y, Tiwari HA, Witte R, Stea B. A pilot study of ultrasound-guided electronic brachytherapy for skin cancer. J Contemb Brachytherapy. 2015;7(5):374–80.

14. Sayler E, Eldredge-Hindy H, Dinome J, Lockamy V, Harrison AS. Clinical implementation and failure mode and effects analysis of HDR skin brachytherapy using Valencia and Leipzig surface applicators. Brachytherapy. 2015;14(2):293–9.

15. Skowronek J. Brachytherapy in the treatment of skin cancer: an overview. Postepy Dermatol Alergol. 2015;32(5):362–7.

16. Arenas M, Arguís M, Díez-Presa L, Henríquez I, Murcia-Mejía M, Gascón M, et al. Hypofractionated high-dose-rate plesiotherapy in nonmelanoma skin cancer treatment. Brachytherapy. 2015;14(6):859–65.

17. Ballester-Sánchez R, Pons-Llanas O, Candela-Juan C, Celadá-Álvarez FJ, Barker CA, Tormo-Micó A, et al. Electronic brachytherapy for superficial and nodular basal cell carcinoma: a report of two prospective pilot trials using different doses. J Contemb Brachytherapy. 2016;8(1):48–55.

18. Bhatnagar A. Nonmelanoma skin cancer treated with electronic brachytherapy: results at 1 year. Brachytherapy. 2013;12(2):134–40.

19. Debois JM. Cesium-137 brachytherapy for epithelioma of the skin of the nose: experience with 370 patients. J Belge Radiol. 1994;77(1):1–4.

20. Delishaj D, Laliscia C, Manfredi B, Ursino S. Non-melanoma skin cancer treated with high-dose-rate brachytherapy and Valencia applicator in elderly patients: a retrospective case series. J Contemp Brachytherapy. 2015;7(6):437–44.

21. Guix B, Finestres F, Tello J, Palma C, Martínez A, Guix J, et al. Treatment of skin carcinomas of the face by high-dose-rate brachytherapy and custom-made surface molds. Int J Radiat Oncol Biol Phys. 2000;47(1):95–102.

22. Gauden R, Pracy M, Avery AM, Hodgetts I, Gauden S. HDR brachytherapy for superficial non-melanoma skin cancers. J Med Imaging Radiat Oncol. 2013;57(2):212–7.

23. Köhler-Brock A, Prager W, Pohlmann S, Kunze S. [The indications for and results of HDR afterloading therapy in diseases of the skin and mucosa with standardized surface applicators (the Leipzig applicator)]. Strahlenther Onkol. 1999;175(4):170–4.

24. Paravati AJ, Hawkins PG, Martin AN, Mansy G, Rahn DA, Advani SJ, et al. Clinical and cosmetic outcomes in patients treated with high-dose-rate electronic brachytherapy for non-melanoma skin cancer. Pract Radiat Oncol. 2015;5(6):e659–64.
25. Sedda AF, Rossi G, Cipriani C, Carrozzo AM, Donati P. Dermatological high-dose-rate brachytherapy for the treatment of basal and squamous cell carcinoma. Clin Exp Dermatol. 2008;33(6):745–9.
26. Svoboda VHJ, Kovarik J, Morris F. High dose-rate microselectron molds in the treatment of skin tumors. Int J Radiat Oncol Biol Phys. 1995;31(4):967–72.

Chapter 16
Sarcoma and High-Dose Rate Brachytherapy: Extremity Soft Tissue Sarcoma

Kunal Saigal and Matthew Biagioli

Introduction

- Sarcomas are rare tumors representing <1 % of all adult malignancies.
- These tumors arise from the mesodermal mesenchyme, and therefore can occur in the muscle, fat, fibrous tissues, blood vessels, and supporting cells throughout the body.
- They have a high rate of local recurrence despite aggressive surgical management.

K. Saigal, MD
Department of Radiation Oncology, University of Central Florida College of Medicine, Florida Hospital Cancer Institute, 2501 N. Orange Ave., Suite 181, Orlando, FL 32804, USA
e-mail: Kunal.saigal.md@flhosp.org

M. Biagioli, MD, MSc (✉)
Department of Radiation Oncology, University of Central Florida, College of Medicine, Florida Hospital Cancer Institute, 2501 N. Orange Ave., Suite 181, Orlando, FL 32804, USA
e-mail: Matthew.biagiolo.md@flhosp.org

© Springer International Publishing AG 2017
J. Mayadev et al. (eds.), *Handbook of Image-Guided Brachytherapy*, DOI 10.1007/978-3-319-44827-5_16

■ The addition of radiation therapy to complement surgical resection has greatly altered the treatment paradigm from radical surgery toward a more conservative, function-preserving approach, particularly in extremity soft tissue sarcomas [1–3]

Rationale for Brachytherapy

■ Brachytherapy offers the ability to deliver high doses of radiation therapy to the tumor or tumor bed, while delivering lower doses of radiation to tissues outside the target volume. This can result in reduced treatment sequelae and better functionality.
■ A typical brachytherapy treatment course takes place over 3–7 days, as opposed to 5–6 weeks with external beam techniques, making it far more convenient for patients.
■ Postoperative brachytherapy can be performed while tumor cells are still well oxygenated, thereby delivering a radiobiologic advantage over external beam radiation therapy (EBRT), which must be delayed until adequate wound healing has been achieved.

Goals of Brachytherapy

■ Postoperative radiation therapy is considered in soft-tissue sarcomas if any of the following are present:
  ■ Tumor size > 5 cm
  ■ High-grade histology
  ■ Invasion of superficial fascia
  ■ Close/positive margins
  ■ Locally recurrent disease
■ If complete surgery with a negative margin has been achieved (R0 resection), brachytherapy can be considered as adjuvant monotherapy delivered in the perioperative setting in extremity and superficial trunk sarcomas [4]

- Brachytherapy as monotherapy is often indicated in the setting of a local recurrence with a prior history of external beam radiation therapy to the tumor site to limit volume re-irradiated tissue volume [5]
- In locally recurrent disease which has not been previously irradiated, brachytherapy can be combined with EBRT in the adjuvant setting to optimize local control [6–9]
- In patients with a positive surgical margin brachytherapy can be combined with EBRT [10]

Timing of Brachytherapy

- Brachytherapy is most often delivered in the immediate perioperative setting
- Catheters are placed at the time of tumor resection which facilitates identification of the tumor bed and high-risk areas with multidisciplinary input of surgeon and radiation oncologist
- Treatment is generally delivered over 4–7 days with either an LDR (0.4–0.5 Gy/h) or HDR (2–4 Gy BID) techniques.
- Brachytherapy treatment delivery typically begins 3–5 days after tumor resection to allow for fibroblast proliferation, neovascularization, and wound closure [11]

Pertinent Anatomy for Brachytherapy

- As sarcomas may occur throughout the body, the location of the tumor is paramount to determine the appropriateness of brachytherapy
- Brachytherapy is most often appropriate in cases when the tumor bed is not intimately involving critical blood vessels, nerves, or joints
- Placement of temporary spacers between catheters and surrounding critical structures can optimize the safety and utility of brachytherapy. This can include tissue flaps, gel foam, temporary drains, tissue expanders, etc.

- When identifying the tumor bed, it is critical to consider natural anatomic barriers of spread and conversely, potential seeding of tissues from the current or prior procedures
- Other than the case of superficial tumors with an intact deep fascial plane, the CTV represents a volume rather than a surface. Therefore, a multiplanar implant may be necessary.
- See Fig. 16.1a, b for an example of a chest wall sarcoma after resection and the treatment plan.

Pathology

- See Table 16.1 for histologic subtypes by tissue type.

Rationale for Brachytherapy

Brachytherapy as Monotherapy

- Adjuvant brachytherapy is recommended over observation in high-grade extremity soft tissue sarcomas as per the results of a prospective, randomized clinical trial [12]. For low-grade tumors, LDR brachytherapy did not demonstrate improved local control over wide local excision in a randomized setting
- Limited available published literature suggests similar control rates between HDR and LDR techniques (Tables 16.2 and 16.3)
- Patients with positive surgical margins are likely to benefit from supplemental EBRT in addition to BT (Table 16.3)
- A recent publication by Alektiar et al. suggests improved local control rates with IMRT as compared to brachytherapy despite more adverse pathologic features in patients receiving IMRT [15]. However, this retrospective analysis compares patients treated

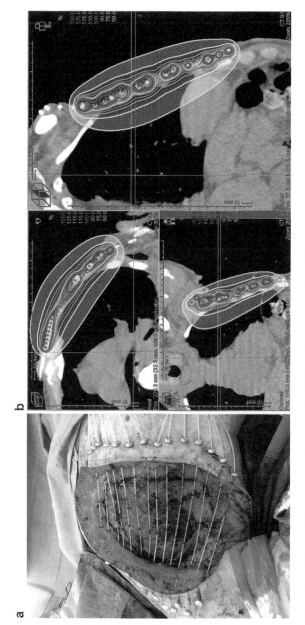

Fig. 16.1. Chest wall sarcoma after resection (**a**) and treatment plan (**b**)

TABLE 16.1 Common histologic subtypes

Tissue type	Common histologic subtypes
Fibrous	Fibrosarcoma
	Malignant fibrous histcytoma
	Desmoid tumor
	Dermatofibrosarcoma protuberans
Muscle	Leiomyosarcoma (smooth muscle)
	Rhabdomyosarcoma (skeletal muscle)
	Spindle cell sarcoma (skeletal muscle)
Synovial	Synovial sarcoma
	Malignant giant cell tumor of tendon sheath
Blood vessels	Angiosarcoma
	Angiomyxoma
	Hemangiopericytoma
	Hemangioendothelioma
	Kaposi's sarcoma
	Lymphangiosarcoma
	Malignant glomus tumor
Peripheral nerves	Malignant peripheral nerve sheath tumor
	Malignant granular cell tumor
	Clear cell sarcoma
	Malignant melanocytic schwannoma
	Primitive neuroectodermal tumors
Bone	Osteosarcoma
Fat	Liposarcoma
Cartilage	Chondrosarcoma

with modern day IMRT with 2D planned LDR brachytherapy from a different era and may not be relevant to modern brachytherapy techniques.

- Results are summarized in Table 16.2

Brachytherapy in Combination with EBRT

- Due to the large, infiltrative nature of soft tissue sarcomas, brachytherapy alone is sometimes not feasible to encompass the entire at-risk volume.

TABLE 16.2 Clinical outcomes of brachytherapy monotherapy in published literature

	Design	Pts	Year	Inclusion	Technique	Follow up	Local control	Note
Monotherapy								
Alektiar et al. [4]	Retrospective	202	2002	STS (70 % >5 cm)	LDR BT (45 Gy)	61 months	84 %	
Pisters et al. [12]	Prospective (randomized)	56	1996	STS	LDR BT (42–45 Gy) observation	76 months	82 %	Benefit of BT limited to high-grade tumors
Chaudhary et al. [13]	Retrospective	152	1998	STS	LDR BT LDR + EBRT	40 months	75 % 71 %	
Itami et al. [8]	Retrospective	25	2010	STS	HDR (6 Gy × 6)	50 months	78 %	Local control (+)margin: 44 % (−)margin: 93 %
Koizumi et al. [14]	Retrospective	16	1999	STS	40–50 Gy in 7–10 fx delivered BID	30 months	50 %	5/8 patients with local failure had (+)margins
Alektiar et al. [15]	Prospective (nonrandomized)	134	2010	STS	LDR (45 Gy) IMRT (median 63 Gy)	46 months	81 % 92 %	Positive margins: IMRT 49 %
							($p = 0.04$)	BT: 20 %

TABLE 16.3 Clinical outcomes of brachytherapy in combination with EBRT in published literature

	Design	Pts	Year	Inclusion	Technique	Follow up	Local control	Note
Combination therapy								
Alektiar [11]	Retrospective	105	1996	STS (70 % >5 cm)	LDR BT (45 Gy)	22 months	82 %	(+)margin LC: BT: 59 %
					LDR BT (15–20 Gy) + EBRT (45 Gy)		90 %	EBRT + BT: 90 %
San Miguel et al. [7]	Retrospective	37	2011	STS	HDR BT (16–24 Gy) + EBRT (45 Gy)	49 months	77 %	
Petera et al. [6]	Retrospective	45	2010	STS	HDR BT (30–54 Gy, 3 Gy BID)	38 months	55 %	
					HDR BT (24 Gy) + EBRT (40–50 Gy)		85 %	
Beltrami et al. [16]	Retrospective	112	2008	STS	LDR BT + EBRT	75 months	87 %	
Andrews et al. [17]	Retrospective	86	2004	STS	LDR BT (10–20 Gy) + EBRT (50 Gy)	69 months	90 %	High-grade LC: 100 % vs. 74 %, $p = 0.09$
					EBRT (59 Gy)		83 %	
Delannes et al. [18]	Retrospective	58	2000	STS	LDR BT (20 Gy) + EBRT (45 Gy)	54 months	89 %	Median tumor size: 10 cm
Schray et al. [19]	Retrospective	63	1990	STS	LDR (15–20 Gy) + EBRT (40–50 Gy)	20 months	96 %	Only one failure in implanted volume
Sharma et al. [20]	Retrospective	52	2015	STS	HDR (4 Gy × 4 BID) + EBRT (50 Gy)	46 months	100 %	HDR started on postop day 3

EB electron beam, *HDR* high dose rate, *SAVI* strut adjusted volume implant, *NR* not reported

- External beam radiation therapy can either be delivered preoperatively or postoperatively. The sequence of EBRT is best determined by tumor size and location. For example, if a tumor is intimately involving neurovascular structures, neoadjuvant therapy can improve resectability. Conversely, for a smaller tumor, adjuvant brachytherapy can be performed and then followed by EBRT if an additional benefit is to be expected
- Results are summarized in Table 16.3

Locally Recurrent Disease

- Brachytherapy can be particularly valuable in the case of locally recurrent disease, especially in the case of prior radiation therapy, as it allows for a much reduced integral dose delivered.
- The use of tissue transfer grafts, mesh, drains, and other spacing devices can greatly reduce doses delivered to previously irradiated tissues with brachytherapy. These spacing devices can often be removed following brachytherapy in a delayed-closure technique. This allows for greater flexibility with the use of brachytherapy, even when previously irradiated critical structures closely approximately the at-risk volume
- A paradigm involving brachytherapy can lead to functional preservation in cases where it would otherwise not be possible, thereby improving patient quality of life.
- Results are summarized in Table 16.4

Selection Criteria

Selection for Implantation

- Candidates for observation

TABLE 16.4 Clinical outcomes of recurrent sarcoma brachytherapy in published literature

	Design	Pts	Year	Inclusion	Technique	Follow up	Local control	Notes
Recurrent STS								
Torres et al. [21]	Retrospective	62	2007	Recurrent STS (all previously irradiated)	WLE vs. WLE+BT (LDR 45–64 Gy)	61 months	51 % overall (nonsignificant difference)	Amputation: 35 % with surgery only vs. 11 % w/BT
Catton et al. [22]	Retrospective	25	1996	Recurrent STS	WLE vs. WLE+BT (LDR 35–65 Gy)	24 months	36 % vs. 100 %	All previously irradiated
Pearlstone et al. [23]	Retrospective	26	1999	Recurrent STS	EBRT+ WLE+BT (LDR mean 47.2 Gy)	16 months	52 %	Complication rate: 19 %
Cambeiro et al. [24]	Retrospective	50	2015	Recurrent STS	WLE+IORT or HDR BT	44 months	54 %	LRC improved in previously un-irradiated pts. (81 % vs. 26 %)

- Small tumors (<5 cm), which are located superficial to the fascia which are resected with wide surgical margins (>2 cm)
- Tumor is located in site where local recurrence would not necessitate loss of function
- Patient is complaint to close surveillance
- Candidates for adjuvant brachytherapy alone
  - Intermediate or high-grade sarcomas which are resected with negative margins (R0)
  - Entire at-risk volume can safely be covered by brachytherapy
  - Existing literature suggests that low-grade tumors may not benefit from adjuvant brachytherapy [12]
- Candidates for adjuvant combination therapy
  - If entire tumor bed cannot be encompassed safely in brachytherapy implant
  - EBRT may be used prior to surgery to improve tumor resectability and function preservation
  - Brachytherapy may be used as boost if margin is uncertain or positive (R1, R2)

Timing of Implant

- Brachytherapy catheters are generally implanted along the tumor bed following surgical resection of the tumor
- Depending upon the implant technique used, treatment can be delivered intraoperatively, immediately (i.e., mesh implant), or postoperatively.
  - When postoperative brachytherapy is used, loading of catheters (LDR) or initiation of therapy (HDR) is often delayed by 5–7 days postoperatively, as this has historically been shown to reduce wound complications [12].
    - LDR: treatment is delivered at 40–50 cGy/h until desired dose is achieved. Common dosages include 15–20 Gy as boost or 45–50 Gy as monotherapy.

- HDR: treatment is delivered at 2–4 Gy/fraction BID (minimum 4–6 h apart) over 2–7 days to achieve total desired dosage (12–20 Gy as boost, 30–54 Gy as monotherapy)
- While conventional teaching has thought this to be necessary to allow for fibroblast proliferation and neovascularization to set in, newer techniques of wound closure may obviate this delay and therefore improve the efficiency of therapy without compromising outcomes or toxicity profiles. These techniques include:
  - Vacuum-assisted wound closure (Fig. 16.2a–c)
  - Tissue transfer flaps
- Intraoperative radiation therapy (IORT) can be a valuable method of delivering focal radiation therapy to the tumor bed. If the treating physician has expertise and this treatment modality is available, it has the unique advantages of direct visualization of the at-risk field and the ability to place shielding agents along adjacent critical structures which may not be possible with implanted brachytherapy techniques.

Medical Operability

- Due to the complexity of tumor resection in STS, patients must typically be able to receive general anesthesia. Regional anesthetic blocks can be considered in special cases
- If a large resection is necessary, special considerations must be made to ensure adequate wound closure, taking into account the negative impact of pre or postoperative radiation therapy
- Preoperative laboratory assessment:
  - Complete blood count (CBC) with platelet count
  - Coagulation profile: PT, PTT, INR
- Postimplant

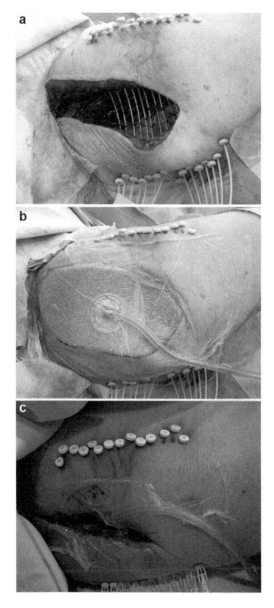

FIG. 16.2. (a–c) Lower extremity tumor bed undergoing wound VAC. Prior to placement (a), after placement (b), and with vacuum applied (c)

- DVT prophylaxis should be considered but must take into account surgical wound and patient lack of mobility. Each patient's risk should be assessed with an individual risk assessment. In cases where deemed appropriate short acting anticoagulation should be utilized.
- It is important to keep open communication with the surgical team and the physical therapy team to ensure that the patient does not participate in movements that might disrupt the catheters' placement.

Image Guidance Utilization

Use of Image Guidance Preprocedure

- Imaging of any soft tissue tumor should begin with conventional radiography.
- A plain radiograph can help to determine if the soft tissue tumor involves bone and to identify vascular calcifications within hemangiomas, ossification within myositis ossificans, and juxta-articular osteocartilaginous masses within synovial osteochondromatosis.
- MRI should follow standard diagnostic plain films, prior to biopsy for appropriate staging and surgical/ implant planning

Types of Image Guidance to Potentially Use and Pros/Cons

- Preoperative MRI provides superior soft tissue contrast, allows multiplanar image acquisition, eliminates exposure to ionizing radiation, obviates the need for ionic contrast agents, and is not associated with streak artifacts, as are seen with computed tomography (CT).
- Multiple investigators have shown that MRI is superior to CT in revealing the extent of soft tissue tumors

and the involvement of adjacent neurovascular structures

■ It is important to note any anatomical compartment breach on MRI prior to resection.

Use of Image Guidance During Procedure

■ As these are open implants performed during a resection intraoperative imaging is not routinely performed.

■ Intraoperative ultrasound with color flow Doppler can be performed to better identify blood vessels particularly if there is concern of arteriole compromise (rare).

■ After removal of the tumor but prior to catheter placement margin status should be obtained via frozen section. This is, however, limited during surgery due to time constraints and sampling error. It is, however, still useful in guidance of further resection or placement of catheters where further resection is not feasible (such as at bone where the periosteum has already been resected or in cases where a large nerve, i.e., sciatic)

■ Intraoperative detection of residual disease during gross total resection using wide-field molecular imaging is currently under evaluation. This imaging uses near-infrared fluorescent probes [25, 26]. This technique is a promising guidance tool for intraoperative catheter placement.

Guidelines for Implantation

Intraoperative CTV Delineation

- ■ CTV should be clipped and drawn that represents a 1–2 cm expansion on the original tumor bed.
- ■ CTV expansion should be limited to less than 1–2 cm where anatomical considerations represent innate barriers to tumor spread such as bone and fascial compartments
- ■ PTV = CTV

Catheter Placement

- ■ In most cases, a single plain implant should be sufficient to appropriately cover the CTV.
- ■ Catheters are typically introduced percutaneously into the tumor bed via a hollow trocar. For this reason it is helpful to use catheters with an appropriately lengthened leader.
- ■ Catheters should be placed in parallel array to each other with a spacing between 1 and 1.5 cm from adjacent catheters assuming Ir-192 brachytherapy source.
- ■ To aid in parallel placement sometimes it is useful to embed or suture catheters onto a vicryl mesh and suture the mesh into the tumor bed. This may be ideal for intrathoracic or intraabdominal tumor beds.
- ■ Catheter placement should extend at least 1 cm beyond the CTV.
- ■ It is important to keep in mind how catheters will move in relation to each other with wound closure. This is particularly important if a primary closure is planned as opposed to a flap or a delayed closure such as a vacuum-assisted closure device.
- ■ Selected orientation of the catheters should take into consideration anatomy as well as planned closure or flap reconstruction.

- Skin entry points of the interstitial catheters should be no less than 1 cm from the CTV.
- Catheters should be anchored down to soft tissue (ideally fascia or muscle) with dissolvable suture such as vicryl.
- If the implant crosses a joint one must be mindful of the joint position as the joint may require immobilization to avoid displacement of the catheters from the time of implant until treatment completion.
- Spacers such as omentum or temporary tissue expanders may be used to displace adjacent organs at risk/normal tissue away from the high dose region immediately adjacent to the catheters. Gel foam can be placed over neurovasculare structures to avoid direct catheter abutment.
- If a drain is used, do not remove until completion of radiation delivery.

Wound Closure

- The wound is typically closed via one of the following techniques: 1. Primary Closure, 2. Skin Flap, 3. Rotational Flap, 4. Free Flap, 5. Vacuum Assisted Closure (VAC) with wound VAC device with subsequent primary closure or flap reconstruction
- If primary closure is performed it is important not to have too much tension on the wound
- Primary wound closure has been associated with wound complications requiring reoperation as high as 12 % [4]
- Staples should ideally be avoided for closure but if used their removal delayed as long as possible
- In cases of re-irradiation where brachytherapy is particularly useful, primary closure and closure with skin grafts should be avoided due to a significantly higher risk of wound complication requiring reoperation [5]. In these cases delayed wound closure with wound VAC and flap reconstruction is preferred.

Immobilization

- When the implant crosses a joint it is important to appropriately immobilize the limb to avoid catheter displacement despite adequate catheter anchoring.
- It is extremely important to communicate with nursing staff and physical therapy team to ensure avoidance of inappropriate patient movements that may disrupt the catheters

Evaluation of Implant

- Ensure appropriate catheter placement distance to avoid potential hot spots
- With primary closure a layered approach is frequently used and care should be taken to not disrupt catheter placement and avoid bunching of catheters
- The outside catheters should be at least 1 cm beyond the intended PTV to ensure dose homogeneity.

Treatment Planning Considerations

Imaging

- 2D planning with fluoroscopy should be avoided. The lack of anatomical detail and appropriate catheter reconstruction in three-dimensions can result in potential hot spots on radiation sensitive structures such as bone and nerves. This may be the reason of reported high rates of bone fractures and >3 grade peripheral nerve damage [10, 27]
- 3D planning with either CT or MRI is the preferred imaging modality for planning due to improved 3D catheter reconstruction and soft tissue delineation.
- With CT planning IV contrast is beneficial in cases for neurovascular bundle identification.

■ MRI planning has the benefit over CT planning with regards to muscle compartment, neurovascular bundle.

■ With MRI planning, CT fusion is typically required for aid in catheter reconstruction as well as surgical clip identification which can prove difficult with MRI alone.

CTV Delineation

■ Final CTV determination should be after final pathology reporting.

■ CTV should be an expansion of 1.5–2 cm on the space that the tumor occupied.

■ The depth of expansion from the plane of the implant should be typically no less than 0.5 cm but consideration for sensitive structures and margin status should be made.

■ Unlike external beam radiation therapy, it is not necessary to include the scar, incision scar, drain site, or the entire muscular compartment.

■ In brachytherapy CTV = PTV

Timing of Initiation of Radiation Treatment

■ In instances where wound closure is performed primarily or with a flap, initiation of treatment should be delayed until postoperative day (POD) 5. Wound complications rate with treatment initiated prior to POD 5 has been reported at 33 % compared with 19 % with treatment initiated at or after POD 5 and 14 % where surgery alone without pre or postoperative radiation [27].

■ When a wound VAC is used, treatment initiation prior to POD 5 is reasonable if the wound edges are appropriately outside of the PTV.

Dose as Monotherapy or in Combination with EBRT

LDR

- Monotherapy LDR dose is 45–50 Gy delivered over 4–6 days; dose-rate is 0.45–0.5 Gy/h
- Postoperative brachytherapy in combination with external beam radiation therapy has been shown to improve local control rates in cases where there is a positive margin [10].
- Combination EBRT and LDR brachytherapy: EBRT 45–50 Gy and brachytherapy 15–20 Gy over 3–4 days with a dose rate of 0.45–0.5 Gy/h.

HDR

- Monotherapy HDR dose 35–36 Gy, dose per fraction is 3.5–3.6 Gy delivered in a bid fashion
- Combination EBRT and HDR brachytherapy: EBRT 45–50 Gy with brachytherapy 12–20 Gy in 2–4 Gy delivered BID over 2–3 days

Toxicity

Toxicity Side Effect Review

- Acute-Skin erythema/desquamation, skin ulceration, infection, seroma, hematoma, wound dehiscence
- Late-Lymph edema, fibrosis, late skin ulceration, soft tissue necrosis, fat necrosis, flap reconstruction devascularization, peripheral neuropathy, osteonecrosis, bone fracture

Management of Brachytherapy Toxicity

- Hematoma can typically be avoided with appropriate operative hemostasis and management of anticoaguative therapy. They can frequently be observed and will resolve over time. Hematomas over 25 cm^3 may require operative evacuation
- Persistent seroma can frequently be conservatively managed with aspiration alone. If conservative management fails the wound may require reoperation.
- Wound infection may require wound reoperation with irrigation and antibiotic treatment
- Skin ulceration scan be first managed with trental and Vitamin E therapy. If conservative management fails then consider hyperbaric oxygen (HO) treatment. In cases where HO is not available or contraindicated then consider reoperation with possible VAC and/or flap reconstruction.
- Peripheral neuropathy can be conservatively managed with oral neurolgics (i.e., gabapentin or like class). In patients at high risk for neuropathy anecdotal evidence may support using glutamine prophylactically.

References

1. Tepper JE, Suit HD. The role of radiation therapy in the treatment of sarcoma of soft tissue. Cancer Invest. 1985;3:587–92.
2. Rosenberg SA, Tepper J, Glatstein E, et al. The treatment of soft tissue sarcomas of the extremities: prospective randomized evaluations of (1) limb-sparing surgery plus radiation therapy compared with amputation and (2) the role of adjuvant chemotherapy. Ann Surg. 1982;196:305–15.
3. Lindberg RD, Martin RG, Romsdahl MM, et al. Conservative surgery and postoperative radiotherapy in 300 adult with soft-tissue sarcomas. Cancer. 1981;47:2391–7.
4. Alektiar KM, Leung D, Zelefsky MJ, et al. Adjuvant brachytherapy for primary high-grade soft tissue sarcoma of the extremity. Ann Surg Oncol. 2002;9:48–56.

5. Finklestein S, Saini A, Ghurani R, Cheong D, Gonzalez R, Johnson D, Zager J, Sondak V, Antonia S, Letson GD, Biagioli MC. High-dose rate brachytherapy re-irradiation for locally recurrent soft-tissue sarcoma. Brachytherapy. 2010;9:S81.

6. Petera J, Soumarova R, Ruzickowa J, et al. Perioperative hyper-fractionated high-dose rate brachytherapy for the treatment of soft tissue sarcomas: multicentric experience. Ann Surg Oncol. 2010;17:206–10.

7. San Miguel I, San Julian M, Cambeiro M, et al. Determinants of toxicity, patterns of failure, and outcome among adult patients with soft tissue sarcomas of the extremity and superficial trunk treated with greater than conventional doses of perioperative high-dose-rate brachytherapy and external beam radiotherapy. Int J Radiat Oncol Biol Phys. 2011;81:e529–39.

8. Itami J, Sumi M, Beppu Y, et al. High-dose rate brachytherapy alone in postoperative soft tissue sarcomas with close or positive margins. Brachytherapy. 2010;9:349–53.

9. Chun M, Kang S, Kim BS, et al. High dose rate interstitial brachytherapy in soft tissue sarcoma: technical aspects and results. Jpn J Clin Oncol. 2001;31:279–83.

10. Alektiar KM, Leung DH, Brennan MF, et al. The effect of combined external beam radiotherapy and brachytherapy on local control and wound complications in patients with high-grade soft tissue sarcomas of the extremity with positive microscopic margin. Int J Radiat Oncol Biol Phys. 1996;36:321–4.

11. Janjan N, Crane C, Delclos M, et al. Brachytherapy for locally recurrent soft-tissue sarcoma. Am J Clin Oncol. 2002;25:9–15.

12. Pisters PW, Harrison LB, Leung DH, et al. Long-term results of a prospective randomized trial of adjuvant brachytherapy in soft tissue sarcoma. J Clin Oncol. 1996;14:859–68.

13. Chaudhary AJ, Laskar S, Badhwar R. Interstitial brachytherapy in soft tissue sarcomas. The Tata Memorial Hospital experience. Strahlenther Onkol 19998;174:522–8.

14. Koizumi M, Inoue T, Yamazaki H, et al. Perioperative fraction-ated high-dose-rate brachytherapy for malignant bone and soft tissue tumors. Int J Radiat Oncol Biol Phys. 1999;43:989–93.

15. Alektiar KM, Brenan MF, Singer S. Local control comparison of adjuvant brachytherapy to intensity-modulated radiotherapy in primary high-grade sarcoma of the extremity. Cancer. 2011; 117:3229–334.

16. Beltrami G, Rudiger HA, Mela MM, et al. Limb salvage surgery in combination with brachytherapy and external beam radiation

for high-grade soft tissues sarcomas. Eur J Surg Oncol. 2008; 34:811–6.

17. Andrews SF, Anderson PR, Eisenberg BL, et al. Soft tissue sarcomas treated with postoperative external beam radiotherapy with and without low-dose-rate brachytherapy. Int J Radiat Oncol Biol Phys. 2004;59:475–80.

18. Delannes M, Thomas L, Martel P, et al. Low-dose-rate intraoperative brachytherapy combined with external beam irradiation in the conservative treatment of soft tissue sarcoma. Int J Radiat Oncol Biol Phys. 2000;47:165–9.

19. Schray MF, Gunderson LL, Sim FH, et al. Soft tissue sarcoma: integration of brachytherapy, resection, and external radiation. Cancer. 1990;66:451–6.

20. Sharma DN, Deo SV, Rath GK, et al. Perioperative high-dose-rate interstitial brachytherapy combined with external beam radiation therapy for soft tissue sarcoma. Brachytherapy. 2015; 14:571–7.

21. Torres MA, Ballo MT, Butler CE, et al. Management of locally recurrent soft-tissue sarcoma after prior surgery and radiation therapy. Int J Radiat Oncol Biol Phys. 2007;67:1124–9.

22. Catton C, Davis A, Bell R, et al. Soft tissue sarcoma of the extremity. Limb salvage after failure of combined conservative therapy. Radiother Oncol. 1996;41:209–14.

23. Pearlstone DB, Janjan NA, Feig BW, et al. Re-resection with brachytherapy for locally recurrent soft tissue sarcoma arising in a previously radiated field. Cancer J Sci Am. 1999;5:26–33.

24. Cambeiro M, Aristu JJ, Moreno Jimenez M, et al. Salvage wide resection with intraoperative electron beam therapy or HDR brachytherapy in the management of isolated local recurrences of soft tissue sarcomas of the extremities and superficial trunk. Brachytherapy. 2015;14:62–70.

25. Mito JK, et al. Intraoperative detection and removal of microscopic residual sarcoma using wide-field imaging. Cancer. 2012;118(21):5320–30.

26. Holt D, et al. Intraoperative near-infrared fluorescence imaging and spectroscopy identifies residual tumor cells in wounds. J Biomed Opt. 2015;20(7):076002.

27. Alektiar K, et al. Morbidity of adjuvant brachytherapy in soft tissue sarcoma of the extremity and superficial trunk. Int J Radiat Oncol Biol Phys. 2000;47(5):1273–9.

Chapter 17

Image-Guided BrachyAblation (IGBA) for Liver Metastases and Primary Liver Cancers

Shyamal Patel, Jens Ricke, and Mitchell Kamrava

Introduction

Liver Metastasis

- Most common liver tumor overall
- Can be detected via liver ultrasound, PET/CT (Fig. 17.1), contrast-enhanced CT, gadolinium-enhanced liver MRI

S. Patel, MD • M. Kamrava (✉)
Department of Radiation Oncology, University of California Los Angeles, 200 UCLA Medical Plaza, Suite B265, Los Angeles, CA 90095, USA
e-mail: patels2010@gmail.com; mkamrava@mednet.ucla.edu

J. Ricke, MD
Department of Radiology and Nuclear Medicine, University of Magdeburg, Leipzigerstr 44, Magdeburg 39120, Germany
e-mail: jens.ricke@med.ovgu.de

© Springer International Publishing AG 2017
J. Mayadev et al. (eds.), *Handbook of Image-Guided Brachytherapy*, DOI 10.1007/978-3-319-44827-5_17

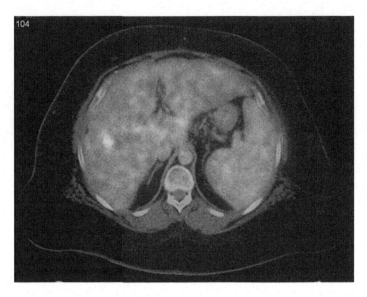

Fig. 17.1. Liver metastasis

- In patients without diffuse metastatic disease, resection is attempted if feasible but often not possible given large tumor size, multiple metastasis, location of metastasis, and patient comorbidities
- In patients with multiple liver metastases, noninvasive treatments favored

HCC/Cholangiocarcinoma

- In cirrhotic patients, hepatocellular carcinoma is the most common liver tumor and cholangiocarcinoma the second most common
- Primary lesions treated with partial hepatectomy +/− liver transplantation or radiofrequency ablation (RFA) with curative intent
- Only 10–20 % of patients are resectable at diagnosis

Recurrent HCC/Cholangiocarcinoma

- Treated with resection if no portal hypertension or elevated bilirubin; otherwise treated with ablation, transarterial chemoembolization, or sorafenib

Nonsurgical Treatment Options

Thermophysical Therapy

- Radiofrequency ablation (RFA)
- Percutaneous ethanol injection (PEI)

Embolization

- Transarterial embolization (TAE)
- Transarterial chemoembolization (TACE)

Selective Internal Radiation Therapy (SIRT)

- Yttrium-90 microspheres (three randomized trials to have results in 2017)

External Beam Radiation Therapy (EBRT)

- Stereotactic body radiation therapy (SBRT) (phase II single-arm studies)

Brachytherapy

- Interstitial high-dose-rate (HDR) (some prospective data but primarily retrospective single-arm studies)

Rationale for Brachytherapy

Potential Limitations of Other Nonsurgical Techniques

- ■ RFA
  - ■ Less effective in terms of local control for larger lesions (>3 cm)
  - ■ Technical challenges for lesions adjacent to hilum/vessels/main bile ducts/bowel because of a combination of heat sink effect limiting efficacy of heating and/or potential injury to organs at risk from overheating
  - ■ No true dosimetry (only have overlapping volumetric spheres of heating/cooling)
- ■ External radiation produces a low-dose "bath" adjacent to target regions and larger margins are needed to account for organ motion
- ■ SBRT is limited by effective liver volume (V_{eff}) constraint (typically ≥700 cm^3 uninvolved normal liver should receive <15 Gy), has lower control rates in lesions >4 cm, and some concern regarding a possible central "no fly zone" similar to lung
- ■ There may be cases where brachytherapy is not possible given technical limitations to being able to actually adequately access the tumor with a percutaneous approach
- ■ Some lesions may also be of a certain size or in a particular location where full dose is not possible given the tolerance of the normal organs at risk
- ■ Patients may have medical comorbidities that preclude them from receiving conscious sedation/anesthesia

Potential Advantages of Brachytherapy

- ■ BT delivers high tumoricidal doses with excellent local control rates even in larger tumors >4 cm
- ■ BT can be delivered to central/hilar locations safely
- ■ Dosimetry to target and organs at risk can be performed
- ■ BT can be utilized in heavily pretreated patients

Timing of Brachytherapy

- Can be used in preoperative, postoperative, definitive, recurrent, or palliative settings
- Typically not done concurrently with chemotherapy

Pertinent Anatomy for Brachytherapy

Structural Anatomy

- Liver divided into four lobes: right (largest), left, caudate, and quadrate
- From nonsurgical standpoint, liver divided by falciform ligament into right and left lobes
- From surgical standpoint, liver divided into right and left lobes by major fissure (Cantlie's line), which runs from gallbladder fossa to the IVC fossa
- Main portal vein divides into right and left branches that interdigitate with three efferent hepatic veins (left, middle, and right), which together divide the liver into segments I–VIII (Couinaud scheme)
- Segments designated in a clockwise fashion starting from the central caudate lobe
- Caudate lobe (segment I); Left lobe (segments II–III); Quadrate lobe (segment IV); Right lobe (segments V-VIII)

Blood Supply and Flow

- Portal vein (75 %) and hepatic arteries (25 %)
- Portal vein carries venous blood drained from GI tract, pancreas, and spleen while hepatic arteries supply arterial blood
- Portal vein and hepatic arteries => liver sinusoids => central veins of hepatic lobules => hepatic veins => IVC

- Each segment has its own vascular inflow and outflow, and can potentially be resected without damaging other segments
- Porta hepatis/hilum—deep fissure in inferior surface of liver through which neurovascular structures (all except hepatic veins) and hepatic ducts enter or leave liver

Bile Production and Drainage

- Hepatocytes => canaliculi => bile ducts => right and left bile hepatic ducts => common hepatic duct => joins with cystic duct from gallbladder to form common bile duct => joined by pancreatic duct to form ampulla of Vater => duodenum via sphincter of Oddi

Procedural Anatomy

- Liver lies under mid-lower right thoracic cage
- Full expiration raises lungs and diaphragm providing better access to liver
- Neurovascular bundle consisting of vein/artery/nerve (VAN) from top to bottom lie underneath each rib and run in subcostal groove within the superior aspect of each intercostal space

Pathology

Metastases

- Most commonly adenocarcinoma from lung, breast, colorectal, or pancreatic origin

HCC

- Classic: well vascularized, wide trabeculae, prominent acinar pattern, small cell changes, cytologic atypia, mitotic activity, vascular invasion, absence of Kupffer cells, loss of reticulin network
- Variants
  - Fibrolamellar—rare, young patients without cirrhosis, better prognosis; tumor cells grow in sheets and trabeculae separated by collagen fibers that are often hyalinized and show characteristic lamellar pattern
  - Sarcomatous—spindle-shaped tumor cells with bizarre anaplastic figures, often with giant cells
  - Scirrhous—diffuse fibrous change often after anti-tumoral treatments; fibrosis along sinusoid-like blood spaces with trabecular atrophy
  - Clear cell—trabecular pattern, characterized by clear glycogen-containing cytoplasm

Cholangiocarcinoma

- Types
  - Intrahepatic [1]
    - Mass forming
    - Periductal infiltrating
    - Intraductal
  - Hilar (formerly "Klatskin")
  - Extrahepatic
- Ninety percent adenocarcinoma, squamous cell carcinoma comprises majority of the rest

Clinical Outcomes with HDR Brachytherapy

- While there arc data using LDR for these types of cases, they are limited. There is more robust literature (including prospective dose escalation studies) with

HDR and so the literature review is focused on HDR experiences only
- One to three year data available supporting use of interstitial HDR BT for:
  - Unresectable HCC
  - Unresectable cholangiocarcinoma
  - Liver metastases from colorectal cancer, breast cancer, gastric cancer, pancreatic cancer, ovarian cancer, renal cell carcinoma
  - Lesions up to 12 cm
  - Lesions adjacent to liver hilum
  - Salvage after recurrence of HCC and cholangiocarcinoma after resection
  - Bridging prior to liver transplantation

Overall Summary of Data

- Liver Metastases: See Tables 17.1, 17.2, and 17.3
  - LC 75–100 % @1 year
  - Dose–response exists for colorectal metastases
- Primary/recurrent HCC: See Table 17.4
  - LC >90 % @1–2 years
- Primary/recurrent cholangiocarcinoma: See Table 17.5
  - LC 50–70 % @1 year

Patient Selection Criteria

- Unresectable primary HCC/cholangiocarcinoma
- Recurrent primary HCC/cholangiocarcinoma
- Metastatic liver lesions: ≤5 intrahepatic metastases and no diffuse extrahepatic spread
- Absence of ascites OR, if present, drainage prior to procedure
- ECOG performance status ≤2
- General lab prerequisites:
  - Child–Pugh class A or B
  - Total serum bilirubin <2 mg/dL

TABLE 17.1 Clinical outcomes with HDR brachytherapy for liver metastasis

Study	Ricke et al. [2]	Ricke et al. [3]	Pech et al. [4]	Ricke et al. [5]	Collettini et al. [6]
Design	CTG IS HDR BT[a] +/− laser-induced thermotherapy (LITT[b]) in patients with mainly liver mets	Phase II trial of CTG IS HDR BT for pts with large liver malignancies or with liver tumors adjacent to liver hilum unfavorable for thermal ablation	Matched-pair analysis comparing CTG IS HDR BT vs. interstitial laser ablation (ILT) for colorectal liver mets	Prospective trial of CTG IS HDR BT via three dose levels for colorectal liver mets	CTG IS HDR BT for metachronous ovarian cancer mets to liver
No. pts/No. lesions	37 pts/36 liver mets, 2 HCC[c]	20 pts/19 liver mets/1 cholangiocarcinoma	18 pts/36 lesions	73 pts/199 lesions	7 pts/12 lesions
Treatment setting/ grouping	21 pts HDR alone, 16 pts HDR after MR-guided LITT; HDR alone for tumors >5 cm or adjacent to CBD/ major vessels not favorable for LITT	Tumors >5 cm (group A) or tumors ≤5 cm and adjacent to liver hilum (group B)	Matching factors: tumor size ≤5 cm and chemotherapy after tumor ablation	98 lesions 15 Gy, 68 lesion 20 Gy, 33 lesions, 25 Gy	Isolated ovarian ca mets to liver

(continued)

TABLE 17.1 (continued)

Study	Ricke et al. [2]	Ricke et al. [3]	Pech et al. [4]	Ricke et al. [5]	Collettini et al. [6]
RT dose	Mean min[a] 17 Gy × 1 (10–20)	Mean min 17 Gy × 1 (12–25 Gy)		15, 20, 25 Gy	Min 15 Gy × 1 (2 fx for 12 cm lesion treated over 4 weeks with CTV divided into two parts)
Lesion size (cm) or tumor volume (cc)	Mean 4.6 (2.5–11)	A: Mean 7.7 (5.5–10.8) B: Mean 3.6 (2.2–4.9)		Median 5 (1–13.5)	1.3–12.0 cm
Median follow-up	6 months	13 months	14 months (3–24)		Mean 15.4 months
Local control/ outcomes	73 % (HDR + LITT) @ 6 months 87 % (HDR alone) @ 6 months	A: 74 % @6 months, 40 % @12 months B: 100 % @6 months, 71 % @12 months All but one local recurrence (diffuse tumor progression) retx successfully with HDR leading to 93 % LC @12 months	HDR: 72 % @ 14 months ILT: 44 % @ 14 months	15 Gy: 65 % 20 Gy: 78 % 25 Gy: 97 % +sig diff between 25 Gy vs. 20 or 15 Gy Mean local recurrence-free survival: 34 months	100 % @15.4 months OS 100 % @12 months, 71 % @24 months

Toxicity	N/V, 2 pts (1 pt with liver failure, possibly 2/2 continued capecitabine use, 1 pt with obstructive jaundice 2/2 tumor edema). Moderate increase in LFTs found in pts treated with both	1 pt with 1 pt with obstructive jaundice 2/2 tumor edema, 1 pt with intra-abdominal hemorrhage, 70 % pts with moderate asymptomatic increase in LFTs		2.5 % occult bleeding, 2.5 % gastric ulcer, 1 % recurrent pleural effusion, 1 % anaphylactic reaction to iodide contrast media	No complications
Findings	IS HDR BT +/− LITT is safe/ effective; however, HDR alone had advantages over combined tx	IS HDR BT can be used to tx large liver lesions as well as those located adjacent to the liver hilum	IS HDR BT achieved better LC than ILT in long-term follow-up for colorectal liver mets	Local tumor control after IS HDR BT demonstrates strong dose dependency	IS HDR BT is safe and valid for treatment of metachronous isolated liver mets from ovarian ca

[a]CT-guided interstitial high-dose-rate brachytherapy
[b]Laser-induced thermal therapy
[c]Hepatocellular carcinoma
[d]Mean minimum dose to planning target volume

TABLE 17.2 Clinical outcomes with HDR brachytherapy for liver metastasis

Study	Wieners et al. [7]	Collettini et al. [8]	Geisel et al. [9]	Collettini et al. [10]	Tselis et al. [11]
Design	Phase II trial of CT-guided IS HDR BT for treatment of liver metastases from breast cancer	CTG IS HDR BT for breast cancer liver mets	CTG IS HDR BT for hepatic mets from gastric ca and gastroesophageal adenoca	CTG IS HDR BT for mets adjacent to liver hilum	CTG IS HDR BT for unresectable primary and secondary centrally located liver tumors
No. pts/No. lesions	41 pts/115 lesions	37 pts/80 mets	8 pts/12 lesions	32 pts/34 lesions	41 pts/50 lesions
Treatment setting/grouping	Unresectable mets	Unresectable mets	12 isolated hepatic mets from lower esophageal and gastric cancers	Liver mets adjacent to the hilum (CBD or hepatic bifurcation ≤5 mm distance) including colorectal/breast/neuroendocrine/pancreatic mets	Primary and secondary unresectable liver tumors; tumors >4 cm located adjacent to liver hilum or bile duct bifurcation
RT dose	Median min 18.5 Gy × 1 (12–25 Gy)	Mean min 15 Gy × 1	6 pts with 1 fx, 2 with 2 fx due to large tumor volume in relation to liver. 20 Gy for 5 pts, 15 Gy for 3 pts; min 15 Gy	Mean min 17 Gy × 1 (15–20 Gy)	Median 20 Gy (7–32) given BID with median fx of 7 Gy (4–10) in 19 pts Median 8 Gy (7–14) given via 1 fx in 22 pts
Lesion size (cm) or tumor volume (cc)	Median 4.6 (1.5–11)	Mean 2.6 (0.8–7.4)	Median 4.6 (1.4–6.8)	Mean 4.3 (1.3–10.7) Mean tumor volume 69 cm^3 (3.1–362)	Tumors >4 cm with median volume of 84 cm^3 (38–1348)

Median follow-up	18 months (1–56)	Mean 11.6 months (3–32)	6.1 months	Mean 18.75 months (3–56)	12 months
Local control/ outcomes	97 % @6 months, 93.5 % @12 months, 93.5 % @18 months	97.4 % @11.6 months	100 % @6 months	88 % @18 months	Primary lesions: 90 % @6 months, 81 % @12 months, 50 % @18 months
	Intra/extrahepatic PFS: 53 % @6 months, 40 % @12 months, 27 % @18 months	Distant PFS 78.6 % @11.6 months	Distant progression 42 %	Distant progression 69 %	Mets: 89 % @6 months, 73 % @12 months, 63 % @18 months
	OS: 97 % @6 months, 79 % @12 months, 60 % @18 months	Median OS 18 months (3–39)		Median OS: 20 month	
Toxicity	One major complication (symptomatic postinterventional bleeding, 1.5 %) and six minor complications (8.7 %)	9 pts had liver capsule pain during procedure, treated with analgesia/local anesthesia. 1 pt had inadvertent skin overdose 2/2 partial dislocation of brachy catheter; severe skin fibrosis developed requiring surgical skin grafting	1 pt developed perihepatic hematoma	1 pt with 8 cm liver met from pancreas developed biliary abscess in treatment zone with cholestasis	Severe side effects in 5 % of interventions with no tx-related deaths
Findings	IS HDR BT safe and effective for breast cancer liver mets	IS HDR BT is safe and effective for breast cancer liver mets	IS HDR BT may be a feasible alternative to resection of liver mets from gastric/ lower esophageal primaries	IS HDR BT is safe and effective for unresectable liver mets close to the liver hilum untreatable by thermal ablation	IS HDR BT is safe and effective for treating central liver tumors and unresectable hepatic lesions

TABLE 17.3 Clinical outcomes with HDR brachytherapy for liver metastasis

Study	Sharma et al. [12]	Geisel et al. [13]	Collettini et al. [14]	Wieners et al. [15]
Design	Prospective trial of CTG IS HDR BT for liver metastases	CTG IS HDR BT for liver mets from renal cell carcinoma	CTG IS HDR BT for unresectable colorectal liver mets	CTG IS HDR BT for liver mets from pancreatic cancer
No. pts/No. lesions Treatment setting/ grouping	10 pts/12 lesions Patients ineligible for surgery or refused surgery	10 pts/16 lesions All pts s/p nephrectomy, 3 pts with extrahepatic mets, 6 pts s/p immunotherapy/ targeted therapy	80 pts/179 lesions Unresectable colorectal liver mets s/p resection of primary lesion	20 pts/49 lesions Liver mets from pancreatic cancer
RT dose	20 Gy×1	20 Gy×1	19.1 Gy (15–20)	Mean min 19 Gy×1 (15–20 Gy)
Lesion size (cm) or tumor volume (cc)	Median 3.8 (2.7–7)	Mean 3.8 (1.0–8.2)	Mean 2.9 (0.8–10.7)	Mean 2.9 (1.0–7.3)
Median follow-up	9 months (3–17)	Mean 21.6 months	Mean 16.9 months	Mean 13.7 months

Local control/outcomes	75 % @12 months PFS: 33 % @12 months	90 % @21.6 months 50 % systemic progression @ mean 19.7 months	88 % @12 months, 81 % @24 months, 68 % @36 months 63 % systemic progression @ median 6 months Tumors >4 cm had higher rate of LF than smaller ones	90 % @13.7 months (44/49 lesions, 17/20 pts) Median PFS: 4.9 months OS: Median 8.6 months 80 % @6 months, 45 % @12 months
Toxicity	Pain (3 pts), Nausea/vomiting (2 pts), asymptomatic pleural effusion (1 pt)	No major/minor complications during treatments	No major complications	Minor complications (pain, fever). Three major complications—postinterventional abscesses
Findings	IS HDR BT for liver tumors is safe and effective	IS HDR BT is viable alternative to hepatic resection of liver mets from renal cell carcinoma in selected patients	IS HDR BT is effective for treatment of unresectable colorectal liver mets	IS HDR BT is safe and effective for liver mets from pancreatic cancer

TABLE 17.4 Clinical outcomes with HDR brachytherapy for primary/recurrent HCC

Study	Collettini et al. [16]	Collettini et al. [17]	Schnapauff et al. [18]	Denecke et al. [19]
Design	CTG IS HDR BT of large (5–7 cm) and very large (>7 cm) HCCs	CTG IS HDR BT for unresectable hepatocellular carcinoma	CTG IS HDR BT as salvage therapy for intrahepatic recurrence of hepatocellular carcinoma after resection	Comparison between CT-guided IS HDR BT and TACE for bridging prior to liver transplantation in HCC
No. pts/No. lesions Treatment setting/ grouping	35 pts/35 lesions 19 large (5–7 cm) tumors, 16 very large (>7 cm); 91 % pts with cirrhosis	98 pts/212 lesions Unresectable hepatocellular carcinoma without metastases	19 pts/48 lesions Salvage treatment of unresectable intrahepatic recurrence after initial surgical resection	12 pts/12 lesions 12 patients with HCC received IS HDR BT for bridging prior to liver transplantation; pts matched by age, sex, number/size of lesions, underlying disease with those undergoing TACE
RT dose	32 pts with 1fx, 3 with 2fx (division of CTV into two parts); min 15 Gy	Mean min 16.5 Gy × 1 with goal 20 Gy (except for 11 large lesions which were divided into two CTVs and treated 6 weeks apart)	Median 20 Gy × 1	Mean 18.9 Gy × 1 (15–25 Gy)

Lesion size (cm) or tumor volume (cc)	Mean 7.1 (5–12); mean CTV was 186 cm³	Mean 5.0 (1.8–12)	Mean 2.5 (0.4–5.7)	3.6 vs. 4.4 (HDR vs. TACE) not sig diff
Median follow-up	Mean 12.8 months	20 months (4–64)	33 months (6–82)	
Local control/ outcomes	93.3 % @12 months (two failures, one in each group) Distant progression: 30 % Mean OS: 15.4 months	92 % @20 month 68 % systemic progression; mean PFS 15 months OS: 80 % @1 year, 62 % @2 years, 46 % @3 years	96 % @33 months Median time to progression was 20 months Median OS after HDR: 50 month	HDR: 90 % @1 year, 90 % @3 years TACE: 86 % @1 year, 70 % @3 years HDR>TACE for tumor necrosis rates
Toxicity	No major/minor complications	No major complications; no radiation-induced liver disease 1 pt had a subcapsular hematoma that resolved spontaneously	One intrahepatic hemorrhage after catheter retraction which spontaneously tamponaded	1 pt had arterial bleeding after retraction of catheters; subsequently underwent coil-embolization of an arterial-portal venous fistula in liver; no tumor seeding

(continued)

Table 17.4 (continued)

Study	Collettini et al. [16]	Collettini et al. [17]	Schnapauff et al. [18]	Denecke et al. [19]
Findings	IS HDR BT is a promising therapy that exceeds indications for thermal ablation	IS HDR BT is effective in achieving local tumor control and should be compared to RFA and TACE in randomized trials	IS HDR BT is a safe and potentially life-prolonging technique in pts with HCC recurrence who have few options	IS HDR BT is comparable and possibly better than TACE for bridging prior to liver transplantation. HCC recurrence not associated with HDR despite possible tumor seeding

TABLE 17.5 Clinical outcomes with HDR brachytherapy for primary/recurrent cholangiocarcinoma

Study	Schnapauff et al. [20]	Kamphues et al. [21]	Mukewar et al. [22]
Design	CTG IS HDR for unresectable intrahepatic cholangiocarcinoma	CTG IS HDR BT for hepatic recurrence of cholangiocarcinoma	Endoscopic nasobiliary HDR BT as a component of neoadjuvant tx for perihilar cholangiocarcinoma
No. pts/No. lesions	15 pts/15 lesions	10 pts/10 lesions	40 pts/40 lesions
Treatment setting/grouping	15 unresectable intrahepatic cholangiocarcinomas	Intrahepatic recurrence after resection of intrahepatic or hilar cholangiocarcinoma that were unresectable	Pts received neoadjuvant chemoRT consisting of 5-FU/capecitabine, 45 Gy EBRT, and nasobiliary HDR BT before liver transplantation
RT dose	1 fx unless very large tumor volume where 2 fx were used (CTV split into two). Median min 20 Gy	Median 20 Gy×1 (reduced to 15–17 Gy due to surrounding tissue in three cases)	9.3–16 Gy in 1–4 fractions delivered over 1–2 days
Lesion size (cm) or tumor volume (cc)	Median 5.25 (1–12) Mean tumor volume 131 cm³ (10–257)	Mean 3.1 (1.1–5.4) Mean tumor volume 23 cm³ (4–85)	
Median follow-up	18 months (1–27)	46 months (12–105)	

(continued)

Table 17.5 (continued)

Study	Schnapauff et al. [20]	Kamphues et al. [21]	Mukewar et al. [22]
Local control/ outcomes	50 % @10 month, 27 % @18 months	70 % @ 46 months (some patients received multiple sessions of BT resulting in 100 % LC)	Nasobiliary brachytherapy catheters displacement seen in 20 % pts (five intraprocedure, three postprocedure). One RT error and one nasobiliary tube kinking occurred
	OS: 40 % @18 months	OS after intrahepatic recurrence: 77 % @ 1 year, 51 % @5 years	
	MS: 14 months		
Toxicity	No major complications	No major complications	Cholangitis (12.5 %), severe abdominal pain (7.5 %), duodenopathy (7.5 %), gastropathy (7.5 %), and both duodenopathy/gastropathy (2.5 %)
Findings	IS HDR BT is safe for tx of unresectable intrahepatic cholangiocarcinoma	IS HDR BT is a safe option for recurrent bile duct cancer and could lead to prolongation of survival	Endoscopic nasobiliary HDR BT is safe and technically feasible in the tx of unresectable perihilar cholangiocarcinoma

- Hemoglobin >10 g/dL
- Leukocytes >3 × 10⁹/L
- Platelets >50,000/μL
- Partial thromboplastin time (PTT) <50 s
- International normalized ratio (INR) <1.5
- Imaging workup of the liver
  - Gadolinium-enhanced MRI and/or
  - Triphasic (arterial/portal venous/delayed phases) contrast-enhanced CT

Use of Image Guidance

- Iterative CT scanning while slowly advancing needles/ catheters (Fig. 17.2)
  - Most accessible, most common method
  - Somewhat time consuming due to frequent exit/ entry into room in between scans
- CT fluoroscopy
  - Provides real-time imaging while advancing needle
  - Quick, efficient
  - Significant exposure to patient and to medical personnel
- MR scanning (iterative vs. fluoroscopy)
  - Provides excellent soft-tissue resolution for needle advancement
  - Somewhat time consuming due to frequent exit/ entry into room in between scans (iterative approach; fluoroscopy avoids this)
  - No radiation exposure to patient or medical personnel
  - Not commonly accessible at most institutions
- Ultrasound
  - Provides good soft-tissue resolution but has learning curve
  - Provides real-time imaging while advancing needle (Fig. 17.3)
  - No radiation exposure to patient or medical personnel

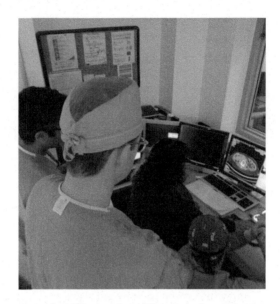

FIG. 17.2. Iterative CT scanning while advancing catheter

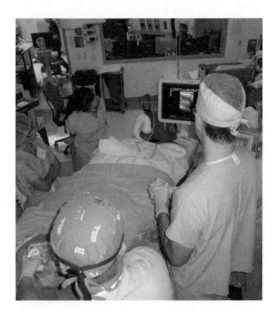

FIG. 17.3. US guidance while advancing catheter

- Commonly accessible, quick, and efficient
- Not all lesions are easily visible on ultrasound

Guidelines for Implantation

Preoperative Considerations

- Hold anticoagulants (NSAIDS, antithrombotics) for 5 days prior to procedure unless the risks of continued anticoagulation outweigh the risk of postinterventional bleeding

Patient Setup and Analgesia

- Patient to lie on imaging table supine, head-first, with right arm raised up and right hand resting underneath head
- Obtain baseline set of vital signs and cycle as needed
- Set up table with sterile drape, local anesthetic, 25 gauge needle, trocar puncture needle, guide wire vascular sheaths, HDR catheters (Fig. 17.4)
- Typically procedure can be done using conscious sedation
- Can start with fentanyl 50 μg IV and titrate in increments of 25 μg as needed as well as midazolam 1 mg IV and titrate in increments of 0.5 mg as needed
- High-risk patients (post-hepatojejunostomy, cholangiocarcinoma, poststenting) can be considered for lifelong metronomic antibiotics

Determine Catheter Entrance Sites

- Use markers on the patient to estimate anticipated catheter insertion sites (Fig. 17.5)
- Perform an initial CT scan to confirm insertion sites and modify if necessary

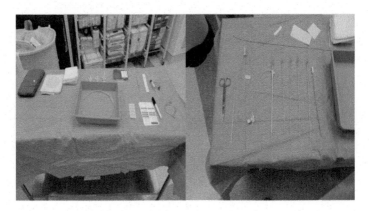

FIG. 17.4. Sterile table setup with trocar puncture needle, guide wire, vascular sheath, and HDR catheters

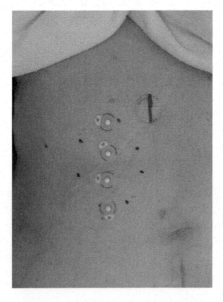

FIG. 17.5. Determining and marking insertion points

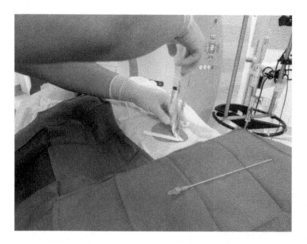

FIG. 17.6. Applying local anesthetic

- After confirming appropriate insertion sites prep and drape
- Apply lidocaine 2 % (or bupivacaine 0.5 % for longer effect duration) SC via a 25 gauge needle over designated spot of catheter insertion (Fig. 17.6)
- Administer more local via a 21 gauge needle in both superficial and deep planes while advancing the needle to the liver capsule using image guidance (CT and/or ultrasound)
- For intercostal needle insertion (anesthetic or catheter), insert percutaneously in mid to lower intercostal space to avoid neurovascular bundle that runs immediately inferior to rib in subcostal groove
- Under image guidance (CT/MRI/US), insert 18-gauge (no clear recommendation but 14-G and thinner have been used) trocar puncture (coaxial) needle to previously anesthetized region adjacent to liver capsule (Fig. 17.7)
- Have patient hold breath at end expiration and then advance needle transhepatically into the lesion

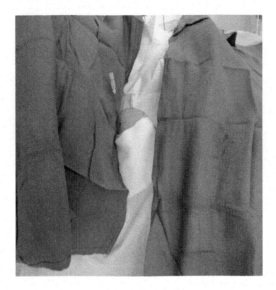

Fig. 17.7. Trocar puncture (coaxial) needle

(breath-hold helps avoid costophrenic recesses and decreases chance of pneumothorax)

- Insert stiff, angiographic guide wire (0.035 Amplatz wire) through trocar needle (Fig. 17.8)
- Remove trocar needle while maintaining guide wire
- Insert 6-F vascular sheath (with hydrophilic coating to reduce pain) over guide wire (Seldinger technique) (Fig. 17.9)
- Remove guide wire while maintaining sheath
- Insert 6-F, 16-G (or thinner) after loading blunt-ended catheter through sheath into tumor (Fig. 17.10)
- Utilize one catheter for ≤2–4 cm diameter tumor (can use more than one; however, typically fewer needles are used in these cases in comparison to more standard 1 cm catheter spacing)
- Repeat catheter insertions until specified lesions are covered adequately

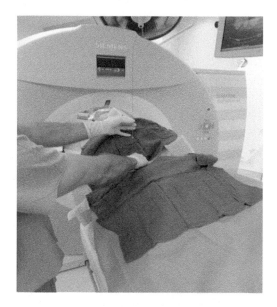

FIG. 17.8. Guide wire (0.035 Amplatz wire) insertion through trocar needle

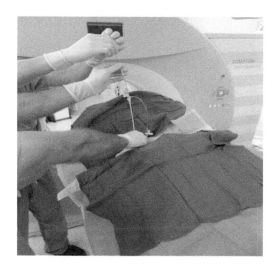

FIG. 17.9. 6-F vascular sheath insertion over guide wire

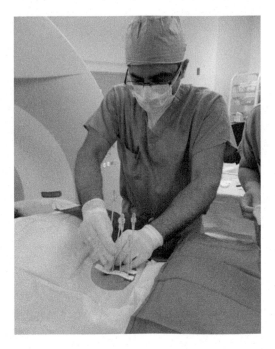

FIG. 17.10. HDR catheter insertion

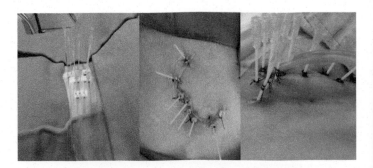

FIG. 17.11. Various techniques for securing catheters to the skin

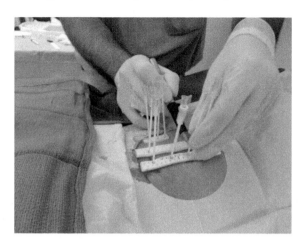

FIG. 17.12. Marking catheters at skin entry point to record depth

- Secure catheters to skin (can use buttons and suture with a drain tie) (Fig. 17.11)
- Mark catheters at skin entry point to serve as a reference for catheter depth between time of CT simulation and HDR treatment (Fig. 17.12)
- Perform a contrast-enhanced CT (or MR) simulation
- After HDR treatment is complete, remove catheters
- Apply a hemostatic, thrombogenic agent (such as a fibrin tissue adhesive or Gelfoam) through each sheath to prevent postinterventional bleeding

Evaluation of Implantation

- For an optimal implant, preplan catheter insertion sites, make a virtual plan, and try to reproduce on day of actual implant
- With experience physicians are typically able to roughly estimate the number and distribution of catheters based on the patients diagnostic imaging

- In general, one to two catheters are used for lesions up to 2–4 cm to limit the number of insertions into the liver. Generally, catheters are evenly distributed and tend to be placed more centrally rather than on the periphery of the tumor so that the radiation isodose can be pulled from the middle of the tumor. This creates a large "hot spot" centrally within the tumor while allowing for rapid dose fall off outside of the tumor

Treatment Planning Considerations

Contours

- GTV = CTV
- Contour visible tumor with enhancing rim on contrast scans including clinically suspicious extent of disease

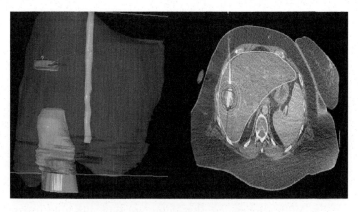

FIG. 17.13. CTV and treatment plan dosimetry

Prescription

- D100 of 20 Gy×1 for metastases, primary/recurrent HCC, and primary/recurrent cholangiocarcinoma if constraints can be met, with minimum dose of 15 Gy and no maximum central dose (Fig. 17.13)
- For larger lesions (>10 cm), consider splitting treatment into two separate areas to be irradiated on two separate visits

Organs at Risk (OAR)

- Uninvolved: liver, spinal cord, right lung, stomach, small bowel (duodenum), kidneys

OAR Constraints

- Liver $V5_{Gy}$ <67 %
- Maximum D_1 cm^3 <15 Gy: Stomach/Small Bowel (Duodenum)/Colon
- Maximum D_1 cm^3 <8 Gy: Spinal Cord
- When irradiating large liver volumes, postinterventional enoxaparin, pentoxifylline, and ursodeoxycholic acid can reduce incidence of radiation-induced liver injury [23]
- If gastric wall/duodenal mucosa D_1 cm^3 ≥10 Gy, prescribe PPI (pantoprazole 40 mg) daily for 6–12 weeks

Toxicity

- Minor: pain, fever, nausea/vomiting, asymptomatic pleural effusion, increase in LFTs
- Serious: subcapsular/intrahepatic hematoma, postinterventional bleeding after catheter retraction (reduce incidence with use of fibrin adhesive/Gelfoam), postin-

terventional abscess, possible duodenopathy/gastropathy depending on area irradiated

Follow-Up

- Liver MRI with gadolinium (or triple phase contrast-enhanced CT) at 6 weeks, 12 weeks, and then every 3 months afterward
- Can assess response based on RECIST (Response Evaluation Criteria in Solid Tumors)
- Systemic imaging as indicated
- If patient has local failure, evaluate for reirradiation with HDR brachytherapy depending on size and location of lesion

References

1. Chung YE, Kim M-J, Park YN, et al. Varying appearances of cholangiocarcinoma: radiologic-pathologic correlation. Radiographics. 2009;29(3):683–700.
2. Ricke J, Wust P, Stohlmann A, et al. CT-guided interstitial brachytherapy of liver malignancies alone or in combination with thermal ablation: phase I-II results of a novel technique. Int J Radiat Oncol Biol Phys. 2004;58(5):1496–505.
3. Ricke J, Wust P, Wieners G, et al. Liver malignancies: CT-guided interstitial brachytherapy in patients with unfavorable lesions for thermal ablation. J Vasc Interv Radiol. 2004;15(11):1279–86.
4. Pech M, Wieners G, Kryza R, et al. CT-guided brachytherapy (CTGB) versus interstitial laser ablation (ILT) of colorectal liver metastases: an intraindividual matched-pair analysis. Strahlenther Onkol. 2008;184(6):302–6.
5. Ricke J, Mohnike K, Pech M, et al. Local response and impact on survival after local ablation of liver metastases from colorectal carcinoma by computed tomography-guided high-dose-rate brachytherapy. Int J Radiat Oncol Biol Phys. 2010;78(2):479–85.
6. Collettini F, Poellinger A, Schnapauff D, et al. CT-guided high-dose-rate brachytherapy of metachronous ovarian cancer metastasis to the liver: initial experience. Anticancer Res. 2011;31(8):2597–602.

7. Wieners G, Mohnike K, Peters N, et al. Treatment of hepatic metastases of breast cancer with CT-guided interstitial brachytherapy—a phase II-study. Radiother Oncol. 2011;100(2):314–9. doi:10.1016/j.radonc.2011.03.005.

8. Collettini F, Golenia M, Schnapauff D, et al. Percutaneous computed tomography-guided high-dose-rate brachytherapy ablation of breast cancer liver metastases: initial experience with 80 lesions. J Vasc Interv Radiol. 2012;23(5):618–26.

9. Geisel D, Denecke T, Collettini F, et al. Treatment of hepatic metastases from gastric or gastroesophageal adenocarcinoma with computed tomography-guided high-dose-rate brachytherapy (CT-HDRBT). Anticancer Res. 2012;32(12):5453–8.

10. Collettini F, Singh A, Schnapauff D, et al. Computed-tomography-guided high-dose-rate brachytherapy (CT-HDRBT) ablation of metastases adjacent to the liver hilum. Eur J Radiol. 2013; 82(10):e509–14.

11. Tselis N, Chatzikonstantinou G, Kolotas C, Milickovic N, Baltas D, Zamboglou N. Computed tomography-guided interstitial high dose rate brachytherapy for centrally located liver tumours: a single institution study. Eur Radiol. 2013;23(8):2264–70.

12. Sharma DN, Thulkar S, Sharma S, et al. High-dose-rate interstitial brachytherapy for liver metastases: first study from India. J Contemp Brachytherapy. 2013;5(2):70–5.

13. Geisel D, Collettini F, Denecke T, et al. Treatment for liver metastasis from renal cell carcinoma with computed-tomography-guided high-dose-rate brachytherapy (CT-HDRBT): a case series. World J Urol. 2013;31(6):1525–30.

14. Collettini F, Lutter A, Schnapauff D, et al. Unresectable colorectal liver metastases: percutaneous ablation using CT-guided high-dose-rate brachytherapy (CT-HDBRT). RöFo. 2014;186(6): 606–12.

15. Wieners G, Schippers AC, Collettini F, et al. CT-guided high-dose-rate brachytherapy in the interdisciplinary treatment of patients with liver metastases of pancreatic cancer. Hepatobiliary Pancreat Dis Int. 2015;14(5):530–8.

16. Collettini F, Schnapauff D, Poellinger A, et al. Hepatocellular carcinoma: computed-tomography-guided high-dose-rate brachytherapy (CT-HDRBT) ablation of large (5-7 cm) and very large (>7 cm) tumours. Eur Radiol. 2012;22(5):1101–9.

17. Collettini F, Schreiber N, Schnapauff D, et al. CT-guided high-dose-rate brachytherapy of unresectable hepatocellular carcinoma. Strahlenther Onkol. 2015;191(5):405–12.

18. Schnapauff D, Collettini F, Hartwig K, et al. CT-guided brachytherapy as salvage therapy for intrahepatic recurrence of HCC after surgical resection. Anticancer Res. 2015;35(1):319–23.
19. Denecke T, Stelter L, Schnapauff D, et al. CT-guided interstitial brachytherapy of hepatocellular carcinoma before liver transplantation: an equivalent alternative to transarterial chemoembolization? Eur Radiol. 2015;25(9):2608–16.
20. Schnapauff D, Denecke T, Grieser C, et al. Computed tomography-guided interstitial HDR brachytherapy (CT-HDRBT) of the liver in patients with irresectable intrahepatic cholangiocarcinoma. Cardiovasc Intervent Radiol. 2012;35(3):581–7.
21. Kamphues C, Seehofer D, Collettini F, et al. Preliminary experience with CT-guided high-dose rate brachytherapy as an alternative treatment for hepatic recurrence of cholangiocarcinoma. HPB (Oxford). 2012;14(12):791–7.
22. Mukewar S, Gupta A, Baron TH, et al. Endoscopically inserted nasobiliary catheters for high dose-rate brachytherapy as part of neoadjuvant therapy for perihilar cholangiocarcinoma. Endoscopy. 2015;47(10):878–83.
23. Seidensticker M, Seidensticker R, Damm R, et al. Prospective randomized trial of enoxaparin, pentoxifylline and ursodeoxycholic acid for prevention of radiation-induced liver toxicity. PLoS One. 2014;9(11):e112731.

Chapter 18
Central Nervous System Brachytherapy

A. Gabriella Wernicke, Shoshana Taube, Andrew W. Smith, and Bhupesh Parashar

Introduction

- This chapter will discuss application of brachytherapy using Cesium-131 radioactive isotope in the treatment of brain metastases.
- Brain metastases occur in about 20–40 % of cancers, and instances are increasing due to improvements in primary cancer therapies that extend the patients survival.
- The two radioactive isotopes used for central nervous system brachytherapy are Iodine-125 (I-125) [1–3] and Cesium-131 (Cs-131) [4, 5].

A.G. Wernicke, MD, MS (✉) • B. Parashar, MD
Department of Radiation Oncology, New York Presbyterian Hospital/Weill Cornell Medicine,
525 E 68th Street, New York, NY 10021, USA
e-mail: gaw9008@med.cornell.edu; bup9001@med.cornell.edu

S. Taube, BA
Bar Elan Medical School, Ber Sheva, Israel
e-mail: shotaube@gmail.com

A.W. Smith, BA
University of Rochester School of Medicine and Dentistry,
601 Elmwood Avenue, Box 379, Rochester, NY 14642, USA
e-mail: andreww_smith@urmc.rochester.edu

© Springer International Publishing AG 2017   539
J. Mayadev et al. (eds.), *Handbook of Image-Guided Brachytherapy*, DOI 10.1007/978-3-319-44827-5_18

Rationale for Brachytherapy

- Maximally safe neurosurgical tumor resection is considered a standard part of treatment for brain metastases; however, surgery alone offers inadequate local control.
  - When surgery is combined with radiation therapy, local recurrence rates diminish [6].
- Large metastases (i.e., greater than 3 cm in diameter) or irregularly shaped brain metastases often require both surgical resection and adjuvant radiation therapy.
  - Adjuvant Whole Brain Radiation Therapy (WBRT) unnecessarily exposes healthy brain tissue to radiation. This can cause cognitive and/or neurological deficits and may limit the patient's treatment options in the case of new metastases or tumor recurrence [7].
  - Adjuvant treatment with External Beam Radiation Therapy (EBRT) to large tumor cavities or cavities of irregular shape presents a challenge in developing of a treatment plan with a high degree of conformality [8–10].
- Brachytherapy can be implemented to a cavity of any size and/or shape, thus tumor cavities may receive more conformal radiation coverage with intraoperative brachytherapy than with EBRT [11].
  - This maximizes the dose to the surgical cavity and potential microscopic tumor cells while minimizing normal brain tissue exposure.
  - Intraoperative brachytherapy with the isotope I-125 increased the local control of the tumor cavity, but is also associated with high rates of radiation necrosis.
- Intraoperative brachytherapy is performed at the time of neurosurgical resection thereby eliminating the delay between surgery and adjuvant EBRT.

- Allowing for immediate radiation treatment to be delivered, potentially overcoming tumor cell repopulation.
- Additionally, there is a convenience to the patients that they only have to come into the hospital for one procedure.

Goal of Brachytherapy: Definitive, Postoperative, Salvage

- The goal of brachytherapy is to precisely target the radiotherapy treatment to the tumor cavity and microscopic tumor cells that may have remained after resection or surround the resection cavity.
- CNS brachytherapy is always performed following either neurosurgical tumor resection or biopsy of the tumor.
- Radioactive seeds are implanted at the time of neurosurgical resection or biopsy.
  - In addition to the advantage of the immediate delivery of radiation therapy, this option is more convenient for the patients.
- Brachytherapy is an option for treating metastases upon initial diagnosis [4].
- Intraoperative brachytherapy may also be used as salvage treatment for singular or multiply recurrent disease [5].

Pertinent Anatomy for Brachytherapy

- See Fig. 18.1: Post-op MRI-1 was taken 1–2 days following surgery. Post-op MRI-2 was taken 1 month following surgery, and Post-op MRI-3 was taken 3 months following surgery.

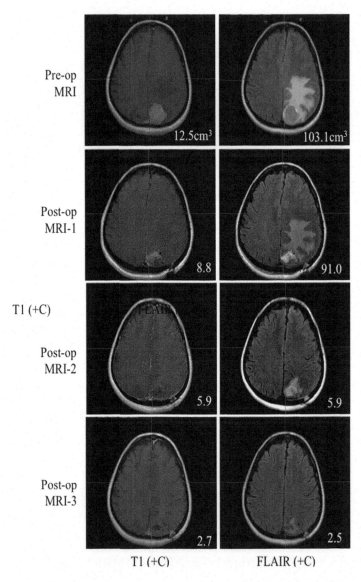

FIG. 18.1. Pre- and Post-op MRIs. Post-op MRI-1 was taken 1–2 days following surgery. Post-op MRI-2 was taken 1 month following surgery, and Post-op MRI-3 was taken 3 months following surgery

- See Fig. 18.2a, b. Preoperative tumor (a) and 2-month postoperative resection cavity with brachytherapy seeds (b).
- See Fig. 18.3a–e. (a) Pre-Op. (b) Post-Op. (c) 1 month. (d) 3 month. (e) 5 month.

Pathology

Typical Pathology

- Common primary malignancies treated with intra-operative brachytherapy include: non-small cell lung cancer, breast cancer, melanoma, renal cell carcinoma (clear cell), pancreatic cancer, and gastric cancer.
- Small cell lung cancer metastases to the brain are generally treated with WBRT, not with intraoperative brachytherapy.

Rationale for Brachytherapy

- Local recurrence (Table 18.1)
- Disease-free survival (Table 18.2)

Selection Criteria

Selection for Implantation and Clinical Guidelines to Judge Readiness for Implantation

- Ability to tolerate neurosurgery (KPS/ECOG and clinical evaluation).
- Expected survival greater than or equal to 6 months.
- Surgery is indicated for alleviation of symptoms or resolution of midline shift.
- Target metastases are greater than or equal to 2.5 cm in diameter. In our practice, we do not have a maximum size exclusion with a caveat that the metastasis is resectable.

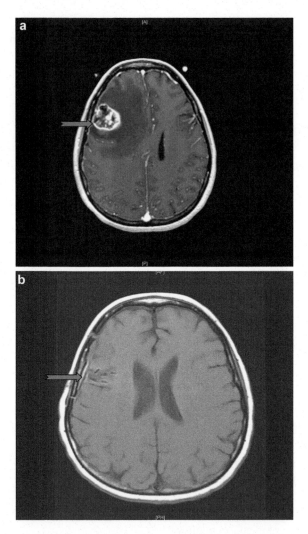

Fig. 18.2. Preoperative tumor (**a**) and 2-month postoperative resection cavity with brachytherapy seeds (**b**)

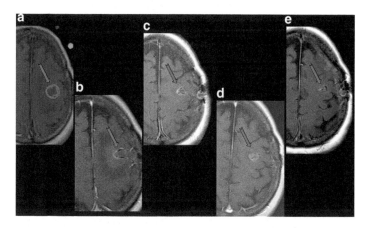

FIG. 18.3. Tumor MRIs. (a) Pre-op. (b) Post-op. (c) 1 month Post-op. (d) 3 month Post-op. (e) 5 month Post-op

- There are four or less metastases to the brain, one of which is eligible for neurosurgical resection.
- Cumulative historical radiation dose to brain and/or treatment area must be less than 60 Gy.
- Primary malignant disease does not need to be controlled prior to receiving brachytherapy.
- Patients who: have unresectable disease, are not surgical candidates, or have metastases less than 2.5 cm may best be managed by focal EBRT techniques such as stereotactic radiosurgery.

When to Implant (Post EBRT, During EBRT)

- Implantation occurs at the time of neurosurgical resection or biopsy.
- SRS or EBRT to additional lesions distant to implantation site may be performed as long as cumulative radiation dose remains below toxic levels.

Table 18.1 Published results of brachytherapy for brain metastases

First author	Type of implant using I-125 isotope	Number and type of patients	Use of adjuvant WBRT	Crude local FFP (%)	Median survival (months)	Necrosis (%)
Bernstein	Temporary	10 Recurrent	No	60	10.5	30
Bogart	Permanent	15 New	No	80	14	0
Dagnew[a]	Permanent	26 New	No	96	17.8	8
McDermott	Temporary	5 New	Yes (4/5)	–	68.2	10
		25 Recurrent	No	–	13.9	
Ostertag	Temporary	38 New	Yes	89	17	0
		34 New	No	91	15	
		21 Recurrent	No	95	6	
Rogers	Temporary[b]	54 New	No	82–87	9.3	20
Schulder	Permanent	1 New	No	82	9	15
		12 Recurrent	No			
Zamorano	Temporary	16 Recurrent	No	–	10.2	–
Current series	Permanent	19 New	No	95	12.0	26
		21 Recurrent	No	90	7.3	19

[a]This series included 11 of the patients reported in the current series
[b]This series used I-125 solution rather than seeds as in all the other series
WBRT Whole brain radiotherapy, *FFP* Freedom from progression, *I-125* Iodine-125
Used with permission from Huang K, Sneed PK, Kunwar S, et al. Surgical resection and permanent iodine-125 brachytherapy for brain metastases. J Neurooncol 2009;91:83–93

References

Bernstein M, Laperriere N, Leung P, et al. Interstitial brachytherapy for malignant brain tumors: preliminary results. Neurosurgery. 1990;26:371–9; Discussion 379–80

Bogart JA, Ungureanu C, Shihadeh E, et al. Resection and permanent I-125 brachytherapy without whole brain irradiation for solitary brain metastasis from non-small cell lung carcinoma. J Neurooncol. 1999;44:53–7

Dagnew E, Kanski J, McDermott MW, et al. Management of newly diagnosed single brain metastasis using resection and permanent iodine-125 seeds without initial whole-brain radiotherapy: a two institution experience. Neurosurg Focus. 2007;22:E3

McDermott MW, Cosgrove GR, Larson DA, et al. Interstitial brachytherapy for intracranial metastases. Neurosurg Clin N Am. 1996;7:485–95

Ostertag CB, Kreth FW. Interstitial iodine-125 radiosurgery for cerebral metastases. Br J Neurosurg. 1995;9:593–603

Rogers LR, Rock JP, Sills AK, et al. Results of a phase II trial of the GliaSite radiation therapy system for the treatment of newly diagnosed, resected single brain metastases. J Neurosurg. 2006;105(3):375–84

Schulder M, Black PM, Shrieve DC, et al. Permanent low-activity iodine-125 implants for cerebral metastases. J Neurooncol. 1997;33:213–21

Zamorano L, Yakar D, Dujovny M, et al. Permanent iodine-125 implant and external beam radiation therapy for the treatment of malignant brain tumors. Stereotact Funct Neurosurg. 1992;59:183–92

TABLE 18.2 Disease-free survival

Treatment	Mean survival	12-month survival rate (%)
Surgery + Cs-131	15.5	50
Surgery + WBRT (10 fx)	11.4	49
WBRT (10 fx)	9	31

Medical Operability: Anesthesia Consent, Guidelines for CBC, Anticoagulation

- Standard preoperative clearance requirements

Image Guidance Utilization

Use of Image Guidance Pre-procedure

- A preoperative MRI is performed determining location, size, and operability.
- If patients are unable to undergo MRI scans, preoperative CT scans may be performed instead.

Types of Image Guidance to Potentially Use and Pros/Cons

- While preoperative MRI determines preoperative tumor size, it may not effectively estimate size of the surgical cavity immediately after resection due to post-resection cavity collapse.
- As a result, preoperative MRI may overestimate the number of seeds required to deliver adequate radiation to the postoperative cavity.
- Intraoperative modification of the treatment plan using a nomogram may be necessary to adjust for cavity dynamics.

Use of Image Guidance During Procedure

- Intraoperative stereotactic MRI is an option to obtain a more precise real-time cavity dimensions in the face of changing cavity size after resection.
- However, measurement of the cavity by the surgical team using a standard surgical ruler is often sufficient to determine cavity diameter and represents a more cost-effective strategy to adjust treatment plans in the operating room.

Intraoperative Images

- See Fig. 18.4a–c: Resection cavity (a), Cs-131 seeds (b), and Surgicel® (Ethicon, Somerville, NJ, USA) and Tisseel® (Deerfield, IL, USA) (c).

Guidelines for Implantation

Pre-procedure Advice: Exam Findings, Procedural Positioning, Exam Assessment

- Preoperative MRI delineates tumor boundaries and is used for treatment planning.
- Cavity diameter, as measured by the preoperative scan, is used to determine the number of seeds used for implantation according to institutional nomograms.
- Preoperative neurocognitive status should be quantified by the Karnofsky performance status scale and/or ECOG performance in addition to the Mini-Mental Status Examination.
- Quality of Life Assessment should be performed prior to the procedure and subsequently at the patients follow-up appointments to track patient progress after surgery and implantation.

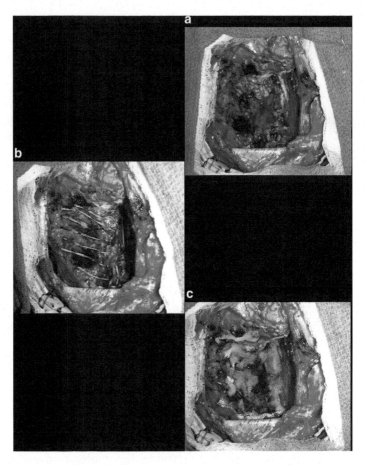

FIG. 18.4. Intraoperative images. (**a**) Resection cavity. (**b**) Cs-131 seeds. (**c**) Surgicel® (Ethicon, Somerville, NJ, USA) and Tisseel® (Deerfield, IL, USA) (**c**)

Procedure Tips

■ Individual seeds are connected by a suture and implanted as a group in a tangential pattern along the surgical cavity, causing the cavity to be lined like barrel staves or parallel tracks along the walls of the resection cavity.

- The tensile strength of the barrel stave seed placement technique maintains a certain degree of outward pressure on the cavity, thus limiting the incidence of cavity collapse.
- The seeds are then covered with Surgicel® in order to prevent seed migration.
- Tisseel® is also added to further prevent seed migrations and to stabilize cavity by resisting cavity shrinkage and collapse.
- A post-implant CT should be performed within 48 h following the procedure.

Verification of Brachytherapy with Visual and Imaging

- Seed placement is initially verified visually by the radiation oncologist directly after implantation by the neurosurgical team.
- Postoperative imaging with CT scan is used to determine dose distribution and follow-up MRI is used to evaluate seed placement, recurrent disease, edema, and toxicity.

Evaluation of Implantation

Distribution of Implant

- At the time of implantation, the neurosurgeon and radiation oncologist directly observe implant distribution to ensure uniform seed placement.
- CT scans are performed within 2 days of surgery to record seed placement, evaluate dose distribution, and detect potential seed migration.
- Follow-up CT scans on postoperative day 14 and postoperative day 30 evaluate seed placement and dose distribution as the postsurgical cavity begins to collapse.

■ Postsurgical cavity collapse is commonly seen with the removal of brain metastases, but the most significant collapse occurs after brachytherapy seeds are no longer active.

Review Imaging Real Time or When a Change Is Needed

■ Tumor cavity size may change during surgery as compared to preoperative imaging measurements.
■ The surgical team measures the tumor cavity after resection and before seed implantation, and treatment planning is adjusted in real time to match the new cavity size.

Treatment Planning Considerations

Optimal Brachytherapy Dose Rx (Table 18.3)

■ Isotope: Cs-131: Rx Dose: 80 Gy at a 0.5 cm from surface of cavity
  ■ Seed spacing varies between 7 and 10 mm.

TABLE 18.3 Optimal brachytherapy dose prescription

Cavity diameter (cm)	Activity/ seed (U)	Cavity surface area (cm²)	Total activity (U)	# Seeds
5	2.44	78.5	134.4	55
4	2.44	50.3	87.4	36
3	2.44	28.3	68.4	28
2	2.44	12.6	34.2	14

Use of Image Guidance for Target Volume Delineation

■ Patients receive a postoperative CT scan 24–48 h after surgery to evaluate dosimetry and ensure proper seed position.
■ Scans are transferred to dose planning software and each seed is identified on the CT slices.

Optimization of Target Volume: Point Based, Volume Based

■ The volume implant is to be precalculated based on preoperative data on tumor size and the institutional physics nomogram and was adjusted real time for the resulting intracavitary volume of the resected metastasis.
■ The 10-cm, suture-stranded ^{131}Cs seeds (0.5-cm inter-seed spacing) are cut into smaller lengths per the nomogram, and placed as a permanent volume implant along the cavity in a tangential pattern to maintain a 7- to 10-mm spacing between seeds [4].

Dose Distributions

■ See Fig. 18.5.

Toxicity

Toxicity Side Effect Review: Common, Rare

■ Common side effects include but are not limited to:
  ■ surgical site infection
  ■ postoperative seizure
  ■ postoperative edema

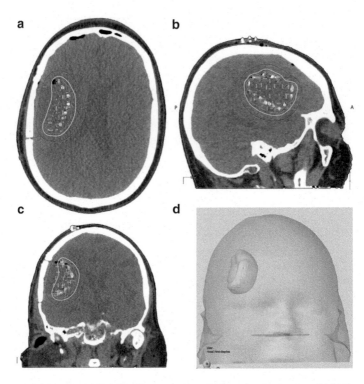

FIG. 18.5. Dose distribution: computed tomography scans of 131Cs brachytherapy seeds in the postoperative resection cavity. (**a**) Axial plane. (**b**) Sagittal plane. (**c**) Coronal plane. (**d**) Three-dimensional radiation cloud from the 80-Gy isodose line

- headache
- local alopecia
- radiation necrosis
- temporary neurological deficits
- Rare side effects include but are not limited to:
  - seed migration
  - cognitive changes
  - permanent neurological deficits

Management of Brachytherapy Toxicity According to Disease Site

- Postoperative edema and headaches are generally managed with corticosteroids.
- Asymptomatic radiation necrosis can be managed with corticosteroids, hyperbaric oxygen, antiplatelet medications, or oral Vitamin E.
- Severe and symptomatic radiation necrosis may require re-operation and debridement of necrotic tissue.
- Postoperative seizures may be managed with anti-epileptics drugs.
- Seed migration may require surgical removal if the seeds are radioactive when migration is discovered. Migration of inert seeds may be managed expectantly if the patient is asymptomatic. If the migrated see are causing the patient symptoms, then the seed should be removed.

References

1. Petr MJ, McPherson CM, Breneman JC, et al. Management of newly diagnosed single brain metastasis with surgical resection and permanent I-125 seeds without upfront whole brain radiotherapy. J Neurooncol. 2009;92:393–400.
2. Ruge MI, Suchorska B, Maarouf M, et al. Stereotactic 125iodine brachytherapy for the treatment of singular brain metastases: closing a gap? Neurosurgery. 2011;68:1209–18. Discussion 1218–1209.
3. Ruge MI, Kickingereder P, Grau S, et al. Stereotactic biopsy combined with stereotactic (125)iodine brachytherapy for diagnosis and treatment of locally recurrent single brain metastases. J Neurooncol. 2011;105:109–18.
4. Wernicke AG, et al. Phase I/II study of resection and intraoperative ccsium-131 radioisotope brachytherapy in patients with newly diagnosed brain metastases. J Neurosurg. 2014;121: 338–48.

5. Wernicke AG, Smith AW, Taube S, Yondorf M, Trichter S, Nedialkova L, Sabbas A, Christos P, Ramakrishna R, Pannullo S, Stieg P, Schwartz T. Cesium-131 brachytherapy for recurrent brain metastases offers durable salvage treatment for previously irradiated patients. J Neurosurg. 2016;1–8 [Epub ahead of print].

6. Soffietti R, Kocher M, Abacioglu UM, et al. A European Organisation for Research and Treatment of Cancer phase III trial of adjuvant whole-brain radiotherapy versus observation in patients with one to three brain metastases from solid tumors after surgical resection or radiosurgery: quality-of-life results. J Clin Oncol. 2013;31:65–72.

7. Chang EL, Wefel JS, Hess KR, et al. Neurocognition in patients with brain metastases treated with radiosurgery or radiosurgery plus whole-brain irradiation: a randomised controlled trial. Lancet Oncol. 2009;10:1037–44.

8. Molenaar R, Wiggenraad R, Verbeek-de Kanter A, et al. Relationship between volume, dose and local control in stereotactic radiosurgery of brain metastasis. Br J Neurosurg. 2009; 23:170–8.

9. Sneed PK, Mendez J, Vemer-van den Hoek JG, et al. Adverse radiation effect after stereotactic radiosurgery for brain metastases: incidence, time course, and risk factors. J Neurosurg. 2015;123:373–86.

10. Shaw E, Scott C, Souhami L, et al. Single dose radiosurgical treatment of recurrent previously irradiated primary brain tumors and brain metastases: final report of RTOG protocol 90-05. Int J Radiat Oncol Biol Phys. 2000;47:291–8.

11. Yang R, Wang J, Zhang H. Dosimetric study of Cs-131, I-125, and Pd-103 seeds for permanent prostate brachytherapy. Cancer Biother Radiopharm. 2009;24:701–5.

Chapter 19
Lung Brachytherapy

Justin Mann, Alex Herskovic, Jonathan Chen,
A. Gabriella Wernicke, and Bhupesh Parashar

Introduction

- In 2015, the estimated incidence for lung cancer is 221,200, accounting for 13 % of all new cancer diagnoses with 158,040 estimated deaths, making lung cancer the leading cause of cancer death for men and women in the United States [1]
- The standard of care for early-stage NSCLC is surgical resection; however, only a small proportion (approximately 20 %) of newly diagnosed patients present at this stage
- Radiation therapy is one of the primary modalities in the treatment of lung cancer and may be used with curative or palliative intent

J. Mann, MD (✉) • A. Herskovic, MD • J. Chen, MD, PhD
A.G. Wernicke, MD, MS • B. Parashar, MD (✉)
Department of Radiation Oncology, New York Presbyterian Hospital/Weill Cornell Medicine, 525 E 68th Street, New York, NY 10021, USA
e-mail: jum9094@nyp.org; alh9074@nyp.org; joc2037@nyp.org; gaw9008@med.cornell.edu; bup9001@med.cornell.edu

© Springer International Publishing AG 2017
J. Mayadev et al. (eds.), *Handbook of Image-Guided Brachytherapy*, DOI 10.1007/978-3-319-44827-5_19

Rationale for Brachytherapy

- Delivers high-dose radiation in a conformal manner. Recurrent endobronchial disease may be responsible for up to 60 % of mortality from post-obstructive pneumonia, sepsis, and respiratory failure in this setting; therefore, the option of brachytherapy in this setting is an important one
- Enables delivery of high-dose radiation in a previously irradiated site in the lung
- Ease of treatment delivery since patient does not need to come daily for weeks
- Could potentially be an application that can be combined with surgery without any additional visits to the hospital for radiation, e.g., interstitial lung implant for sublobar resection
- If a surgical procedure carries a risk of close or positive surgical margins, there is a role for interstitial brachytherapy, where the radioactive source is placed directly into the targeted lung tissue

Goal of Brachytherapy

- Deliver highly conformal radiation dose for recurrent disease
- Deliver radiation to minimize toxicity to normal tissues
- Adjuvant treatment for suboptimal surgical resection

Timing of Lung Brachytherapy

- Interstitial brachytherapy is used usually at the time of sublobar resection. It can also be used for high risk surgical resections, where there is a suspicion that surgery may not clear out microscopic disease

- Interstitial brachytherapy may also be used to areas of suspected positive or close surgical margins such as in the bronchial stump area or high risk chest wall resections
- Endobronchial brachytherapy is commonly used for palliation of symptoms. High-dose rate (HDR) intra-luminal brachytherapy allows for placement of a radioactive source next to a centrally located tumor (within 5–10 mm) and may be used in conjunction with surgery, external beam radiation therapy (EBRT), or alone

Pertinent Anatomy for Lung Brachytherapy

- The trachea divides at the carina forming the left and right mainstem bronchi which further divide into secondary or lobar bronchi, smaller bronchi, and bronchioles until they connect to alveoli. Each segment has its own pulmonary arterial branch and thus, the bronchopulmonary segment is a portion of lung supplied by its own bronchus and artery
- In general, each lung has ten segments: the upper lobes contain three segments, the middle lobe/lingula two, and the lower lobes five. Bilaterally, the upper lobes have apical, posterior and anterior segments, and the lower lobes superior (apical) and four basal segments (anterior, medial, posterior and lateral). The middle lobe on the right has two segments: medial and lateral (easy to remember—middle lobe, medial and lateral)
- The lingula on the left is part of the left upper lobe and is the equivalent of the middle lobe on the right, and hence it has two segments, but is divided into superior and inferior segments
- Regarding brachytherapy application, the target is typically defined as the tumor bed or gross tumor, which can be identified on imaging as the site of cancer requiring resection or the bronchial tumor obstructing

the airway and causing post-obstructive symptoms respectively
- Organs at risk include:
  - Lung: Prescription dose is usually at 0.5 cm from the implant site and normal lung is usually spared
  - Chest wall: Excluded from PTV unless involved by tumor or at risk
  - Heart and blood vessels: Cardiac sparing and blood vessel sparing is increasingly emphasized although this is a concern mostly with interstitial implant and not with endobronchial brachytherapy. The chance of major toxicity is usually low given the highly conformal nature of interstitial implants
  - Bronchus: The endobronchial tissue is at a risk of sloughing, stenosis, and fistula especially in previously irradiated patients

Dose Distribution of the Implanted Seeds in the Right Lung

See Fig. 19.1.

Placement of Brachytherapy Catheter in RLL

See Fig. 19.2. Red arrow points to radio-opaque catheter tip. Blue arrow points to bronchial radiolucent silicone stent.

Pathology

- Interstitial implants are mostly used in resectable non-small cell cancers such as adenocarcinoma, squamous cell cancers, large cell and occasional resected small cell carcinoma
- Palliative brachytherapy is used in all non-small cell and small cell histologies

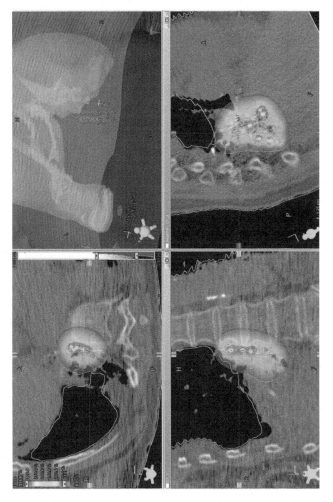

FIG. 19.1. Dose distribution of the implanted seeds in the right lung

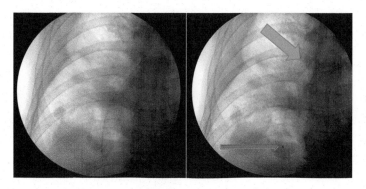

FIG. 19.2. Placement of brachytherapy catheter in RLL. *Red arrow* points to radio-opaque catheter tip. *Blue arrow* points to bronchial radiolucent silicone stent

- Interstitial implants can also be used in sarcomas or other high risk but rare histologies of the thoracic region

Rationale for Lung Brachytherapy

Local recurrence: Lung brachytherapy has been shown to reduce local recurrence and improve disease-free survival. However, most studies have failed to show an improvement in overall survival.

Evidence: See Tables 19.1 and 19.2.

Selection Criteria

Selection Criteria for Endobronchial Brachytherapy

- Patients must be able to tolerate bronchoscopy and have no bleeding disorders
- Palliation of obstructive symptoms secondary to large endobronchial tumors not amenable to further external beam radiation therapy or surgery

TABLE 19.1 Selected randomized trials assessing endobronchial brachytherapy

Author, Year	Patients	Treatment arms	Survival	Response	Fatal hemoptysis rate
Niemoeller et al. [2], 2013	142 total Arm 1: 60 Arm 2: 82	Randomized 1: EBB 14.4 Gy/2 fractions at 1 cm over 3 weeks 2: EBB 15.2 Gy/4 fractions at 1 cm weekly	One-year survival 11.4 % versus 21.1 % (n.s.)	Significantly higher mean time of local control with 14.4 Gy in 2 fractions (median 12 vs. 6 weeks; $p \leq 0.015$)	Fatal hemoptysis 18 %
Huber et al. [3], 1995	93 total Arm 1: 44 Arm 2: 49	Randomized 1: EBB 15.2 Gy/4 fractions at 1 cm weekly 2: EBB 14.4 Gy/2 fractions at 1 cm over 3 weeks	One-year survival 11.4 % versus 20.4 % (n.s.)	No significant difference in local control between arms	Fatal hemoptysis 20 %

(continued)

TABLE 19.1 (continued)

Author, Year	Patients	Treatment arms	Survival	Response	Fatal hemoptysis rate
Huber et al. [4], 1997	98 total Arm 1: 42 Arm 2: 56	Randomized 1: EBRT 60 Gy 2: EBB 4.8 Gy/1 fraction at 1 cm, followed by EBRT 60 Gy, followed by EBB 4.8 Gy/1 fraction at 1 cm	Median survival 28 weeks versus 27 weeks (n.s.); Trend toward survival with squamous histology in Arm 2 (40 vs. 33 weeks, $p=0.09$)	Trend toward local control benefit for arm 2 (12 weeks vs. 21 weeks, $p=0.052$); Significant when limited to squamous histology	Fatal hemoptysis 15.3 % versus 20.8 % (n.s.)
Mallick et al. [5], 2006	45 total Arm 1: 15	Randomized 1: EBRT 30 Gy/10 fractions followed by EBB 16 Gy/2 fractions at 1 cm weekly	NR	ORR for dyspnea was 90.7 %; cough, 84.5 %; hemoptysis, 94.1 %; and obstructive pneumonia, 82.7 %	Fatal hemoptysis 2 %
	Arm 2: 15	2: EBRT 30 Gy/10 fractions followed by EBB 10 Gy/1 fraction at 1 cm		Median time to symptom relapse was 4–8 months	
	Arm 3: 15	3: EBB 15 Gy/1 fraction at 1 cm			

| Langendijk et al. [6], 2001 | 98 total
Arm 1: 47
Arm 2: 48 | Randomized
1: EBRT 30 Gy or 60 Gy
2: Same EBRT with EBB 15 Gy/2 fractions at 1 cm, weekly | Median survival 8.5 months versus 7.0 months (n.s.) | ORR for dyspnea was 37 % versus 46 % ($p = 0.29$)
Palliation favored subset of patients with tumor obstructing the main bronchus | Fatal hemoptysis 13 % |
| Sur et al. [7], | 65 total | Randomized
All patients received palliative EBRT of 30 Gy/10 fractions, 36 Gy/18 fractions or 40 Gy/20 fractions followed by:
Arm 1: EBB 12 Gy/2 fractions at 1 cm weekly
Arm 2: EBRT 20 Gy/10 fractions | One-year survival 29.7 % versus 29.4 % ($p > 0.05$) | Median duration of symptom-free survival was 77 versus 129 days ($p < 0.05$), favoring the EBRT arm. | NR |

(continued)

TABLE 19.1 (continued)

Author, Year	Patients	Treatment arms	Survival	Response	Fatal hemoptysis rate
Stout et al. [8], 2000	99 total Arm 1: 49 Arm 2: 50	Randomized 1: EBB 15 Gy/1 fraction at 1 cm 2: EBRT 30 Gy/8 fractions	One-year survival 22 % versus 38 % ($p = 0.04$) favoring EBRT arm	Gain in overall survival with EBRT versus EBB and good symptom response in both arms; however, 51 % of EBB patients required EBRT, while only 28 % of EBB patients required EBRT	Fatal hemoptysis 8 % versus 6 % (n.s.)
Chella et al. [9], 2000	29 Arm 1: 15 Arm 2: 14	Randomized 1: Nd:YAG laser 2: Nd:YAG followed by EBB 15 Gy/3 fractions at 0.5 cm, weekly	Median survival 7.4 months versus 10.3 months (n.s.)	Statistically significant improvement in period free from disease progression (2.2 vs. 7.5 months, $p < 0.05$) and period free from symptoms (2.8 vs. 8.5 months, $p < 0.05$)	No cases of fatal hemoptysis

EBB endobronchial brachytherapy, *EBRT* external beam radiation therapy, *Gy* gray, *NR* not reported, *n.s.* Nonsignificant, *ORR* overall response rate

TABLE 19.2 Selected trials assessing interstitial brachytherapy for stage I NSCLC

Author, Year	Patients	Treatment arms	Survival	Local control
Fernando et al. [10], 2004	291 patients	Retrospective 167 patients underwent lobar resection 64 patients underwent sublobar resection alone 60 patients underwent sublobar resection with brachytherapy (iodine 125 implant; prescribed dose of 100–120 Gy at 0.5 cm)	No difference	Among sublobar resection arms, addition of brachytherapy significantly decreased LR incidence of 11 patients (17.2 %) versus 2 patients (3.3 %), $p=0.12$
Santos et al. [11], 2003	203 patients	Retrospective 102 patients underwent sublobar resection alone 101 patients underwent sublobar resection with brachytherapy (iodine 125 implant; prescribed dose of 100–120 Gy at 0.5 cm)	No difference	Local recurrence significantly greater in sublobar resection alone arm (18.6 % vs. 2 %, $p=0.0001$)
Lee et al. [12]. 2003	35 patients	Retrospective 35 patients underwent sublobar resection with brachytherapy (iodine 125 implant; prescribed dose of 100–120 Gy at 0.5 cm)	Five-year survival 47 %	Two patients had local recurrence at the resection margin

(continued)

Table 19.2 (continued)

Author, Year	Patients	Treatment arms	Survival	Local control
Parashar et al. [13], 2015	272 patients	Retrospective 97 patients underwent stereotactic body radiation therapy 123 patients underwent wedge resection 52 patients with suspected close or positive margins (high-risk) underwent wedge resection with brachytherapy (cesium 131 mesh or "double-suture" method; prescribed dose of 80 Gy at 0.5 cm)	No difference among wedge resection arms; Lower survival in SBRT arm	Wedge resection with brachytherapy equivalent to wedge resection in terms of local control, despite high-risk, showing possible benefit to brachytherapy
ACOSOG Z4032 [10], 2014	222 patients	Randomized 114 patients underwent sublobar resection 108 patients underwent sublobar resection with brachytherapy (iodine 125 sutures or mesh implant; prescribed dose of 100 Gy at 0.5–0.7 cm)	Three-year survival 71 % in both arms (No difference)	14 % versus 16.7 % local recurrence rate ($p = 0.59$) For positive staple line cytology, local recurrence-free rate was 90 % in brachytherapy arm versus 75 % ($p = 0.47$), which was the strongest trend favoring brachytherapy arm in reducing local recurrence

NSCLC non-small cell lung cancer

- Patients that fail other bronchoscopic ablative techniques including Nd: YAG laser, endobronchial cautery, argon laser, cryotherapy, or stenting [14]
- Patient-related factors include significant endobronchial disease causing obstructive symptoms, tumors protruding into the lumen versus extrinsic tumors causing mass effect and compression on the airway
- Candidates may be medically inoperable patients secondary to poor pulmonary status, unable to tolerate EBRT, have a history of previous EBRT, and unable to receive additional dose, and their life expectancy should be greater than 3 months, in order to see benefit of treatment [15]
- Tumor-related factors include biopsy-proven lesion without ulceration of major vascular involvement and the ability to move the catheter through and past the tumor [16]
- A passage through the obstruction should be feasible; otherwise, one should be made via debridement, laser, or electrocautery. This should be done in a procedure prior to the actual brachytherapy catheter placement

Selection Criteria for Interstitial Brachytherapy

- Patients believed to be at high risk for local recurrence after surgical resection because of suboptimal surgery or if there is concern for incomplete resection or close margins
- Volume implant suitability based on CT imaging, taking into account tumor location, size, and surrounding organs at risk [15]

Image Guidance Utilization

Use of Image Guidance Pre-procedure

- The two main functions of pre-procedure imaging are selecting which patients are suitable for brachytherapy and treatment planning
- CT imaging is one of the most commonly used modalities. Determination of tumor size, shape, and position relative to other structures (e.g., vessels) is helpful in both the selection and planning aspects
- CT imaging plays a greater role in patient selection for implant brachytherapy. The tumor location and size are defined, and the positions of organs at risk are determined
- In contrast, the presence of endoluminal disease suitable for brachytherapy is typically determined at bronchoscopy
- CT imaging is still recommended to determine whether there is a significant extrabronchial extent of the tumor, in which case brachytherapy may be chosen as a boost to EBRT or held in reserve for future relapse [15]
- Additionally, minimizing the time that elapses and potential movement of the patient between pre-procedure imaging and the procedure helps maximize the utility of pre-procedure imaging

Types of Image Guidance to Potentially Use and Pros/Cons

- Pre-planning imaging has shifted from radiographic imaging to CT, and, to a lesser extent, MRI
- Ultrasound and fluoroscopy are used in other sites like gynecological and prostate malignancies, but for lung brachytherapy, CT, and bronchoscopy are the primary modalities of imaging
- Fluoroscopy can be used during endobronchial procedures as mentioned below

Use of Image Guidance During Procedure

- Imaging during the procedure is important to ensure proper placement based on planning. Endobronchial brachytherapy will require bronchoscopy for direct visualization of the tumor
- The bronchoscope is used to traverse the tumor, ensuring that the tip passes distal to the entire volume of the endobronchial mass
- Videotaping of the bronchoscopy is recommended
- Documenting the proximal and distal end of the tumor relative to a fixed landmark can be used in planning. Fluoroscopy should be done continuously during withdrawal of the bronchoscope to ensure immobilization of the catheter
- Real-time imaging is less important with implant placement, which often relies on pre-procedure imaging and actual tactile and anatomic information encountered during the operation. Catheters can be placed using image guidance [17]

Use of Image Guidance After Procedure

- Post-procedure imaging is equally as important. It confirms the proper positioning of seeds and/or catheters and guards against both improper placement as well as mobilization from natural movement of the patient
- Movement of brachytherapy applicators has been documented from a few mm up to a few cm [18, 19]. Intraluminal applicators are believed to be the most susceptible to movement
- Some have theorized that circumferential movement of the catheter within the airway lumen can contribute to dose variations as well as hot spots along the bronchial mucosa
- However, attempts at mechanical devices (balloons, sheaths, cages) to fix the catheter centrally in the lumen [20, 21] have not yet been widely adopted

- Although fluoroscopy can be used [22], the ABS guidelines from 2015 recommend CT imaging to identify the applicator position. This is believed to be a superior modality for determining the proximity to organs at risk, particularly blood vessels, which may result in decreased complications like massive hemoptysis [23]
- Comparison of two- versus three-dimensional planning demonstrated that reference doses with 100 % coverage of PTV were 31 % higher with three-dimensional than with two-dimensional planning, in addition to minimizing doses to critical normal tissues [24]
- Another study showed an improvement in 90 % isodose coverage from 15–35 % to 85–100 % using CT target definition [25]
- Post-procedure imaging after interstitial implant helps determine the adequacy of coverage of tumor bed and need for adjuvant external beam radiation if coverage is inadequate

Guidelines for Implantation

Endobronchial Brachytherapy Guidelines for Implantation

- The presence of endoluminal disease suitable for endobronchial brachytherapy is determined via bronchoscopy. CT imaging is still recommended to help determine if there is significant extrabronchial extent of tumor
- If there is extensive extrabronchial extent, EBRT may be recommended first with brachytherapy reserved for a boost. It is recommended that the tumor is photographed on bronchoscopy to aid in brachytherapy planning
- As part of the pre-brachytherapy assessment, a narrow bore brachytherapy tube should be passed at least 1–2 cm distal to the tumor. This tube should have markings 1 cm apart. These markings are used to

determine the length of the tumor and thus the length of the area to be treated

■ For patient for whom multiple fractions are planned, the use of mini-tracheostomies has been described to decrease the requirement for multiple bronchoscopies [26]

■ After a narrow bore brachytherapy tube has been placed and the size and location of the tumor has been determined, the tube should be firmly secured to the nostril with tape

■ A marker wire should be placed in the tube to identify the location of the tumor accurately. For a carinal or subcarinal lesion, two catheters may be used, one in each bronchus, to give a cumulative dose to the central area

■ A CT scan is obtained after catheter insertion for treatment planning. Proximity to OARs, especially to major blood vessels, can be determined. This is useful in designing a dose distribution that can decrease the chances of major hemoptysis

■ It is important to treat the patient in the same position as the CT scan. Of important note, Ir-192 has typically been the radioisotope of choice for endobronchial brachytherapy

Permanent Implant Interstitial Brachytherapy Guidelines for Implantation

■ Imaging and exam findings which might make a patient appropriate for a permanent implant include the following:
  ■ Limited pulmonary function which excludes a patient from lobectomy
  ■ Hilar tumors adherent to major vessels with no clearance for safe dissection
  ■ Tumors unresectable because of extension into the trachea, esophagus, aorta, or other such vital structures

- Preoperative CT imaging and treatment planning can be used for volume implant dose estimation
- If the surgeon is concerned that tumor resection will be incomplete or margins will likely be positive, then the patient should be consented for intraoperative interstitial brachytherapy ahead of the surgical procedure
- I-125 or Cs-131 are radioisotopes which may be used for this procedure. They are commercially available in metal pellets that come in a vicryl suture. The pellets are placed 1 cm along the suture. The radial dose distribution for I-125 and Cs-131 are similar although their half-lives differ. Therefore, the technical placement of the seeds is similar for both radioisotopes
- Before the surgical procedure, the number of seeds which likely will be needed should be determined. This depends on the size of the area to be covered. The area to be covered may be tumor bed, or it may include unresectable gross tumor as well
- In the operating room, the strands are typically sutured 1 cm apart from each other in parallel lines across the tumor bed and/or residual tumor

Remote Afterloading Interstitial Brachytherapy

- Interstitial brachytherapy with temporary catheters placed in the target area with subsequent remote afterloading of radioactive sources is another approach
- The target volume is determined at the time of surgery to be an area at high risk of recurrence or potential area of positive margins
- Afterloading catheters are placed in the operating room either directly into unresectable tumor tissue or across the surface of a tumor bed
- After placement of catheters in the operating room, a CT scan is obtained for treatment planning purposes. A plan is designed, and the patient is typically brought

to a brachytherapy suite where the remote afterloading takes place
- The radioactive sources are afterloaded into the catheters 3–5 days after surgery to allow for some degree of tissue healing first

Treatment Planning Considerations

Endobronchial Brachytherapy Treatment Planning Considerations

- HDR endobronchial brachytherapy may be delivered in a single fraction, in once weekly fractions, or as a fractionated treatment with a single catheter insertion as long as there are at least 6 h between fractions
- Pulsed-dose rate (PDR) brachytherapy has also been described although it requires the catheter to be in place for longer [15]
- Depending on the diameter of the bronchus, position of the catheter, or curvature of the catheter, the dose to the bronchial mucosa may be very high. Bronchial mucosal dose is important because a high dose to this area may increase the chances of hemoptysis
- Placement methods have been described to ensure that the catheter is placed as centrally within the bronchial lumen as possible [20, 21]
- Prescribing to a radius of 4 mm has been suggested to be safer than prescribing to a larger radius [27]. On the other hand, use of a fixed prescription point may result in underdosing of the gross tumor volume
- CT target definition has been shown to improve the 90 % isodose coverage of the tumor to ranges of 85–100 % coverage, as compared to only 15–35 % coverage with 2D planning methods [25]
- Target volume coverage consists of the gross tumor with margin. Margin sizes vary, but a margin of 1 cm could typically be used

- Doses to OARs can also be determined with CT planning
- Different dose prescriptions for endobronchial brachytherapy have been described
- For palliation, doses of 15 Gy in one fraction, 15 Gy in three fractions at weekly intervals, and 14.4 Gy in 2 fractions with a 3-week interval have been described [8, 9, 28]
- The 15 Gy in three fraction scheme was added to Nd: YAG laser resection of tumor

Permanent Implant Interstitial Brachytherapy Treatment Planning Considerations

- I-125 has been used most often for interstitial lung brachytherapy. A dose of 80–120 Gy at the 0.5–1.0 cm wedge line has been used with success and minimal toxicity [12, 29–31]. I-125 emits therapeutic energies from 22.1 keV to 35.5 keV
- The seeds are placed 10 mm apart in a line. The seeds are contained within a vicryl suture which holds them together; each line contains a suture that is itself sutured to the tumor bed. Alternatively, the seeds can be sutured to a vicryl mesh, and the mesh can then be sutured to the tumor bed
- Vicryl mesh with Cesium-131 seeds embedded for a lung interstitial permanent implant (Fig. 19.3)
- Cs-131 is a newer source in clinical practice; however, no standard prescriptions have yet been established although 80 Gy has been used [13]. Cs-131 emits therapeutic energies in the 20–30 keV range
- It is important to note that in clinical practice the surgical bed or tumor to which the radioisotopes are sutured will rarely be completely flat. Instead, the implant is more often times curved
- Dose penetration will be asymmetric for a curved implant compared to a flat implant [32]

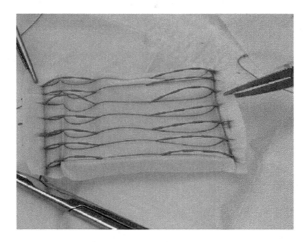

Fig. 19.3. Vicryl mesh with Cesium-131 seeds embedded for a lung interstitial permanent implant

- Isodoses on the convex side tend to be drawn toward the implant, reducing the range of the prescription isodose line. On the concave side, there is a focusing with enhanced penetration of the isodose lines. These can be used for a therapeutic advantage by placing the concave side so that it encompasses the area most at risk for disease recurrence
- For permanent interstitial implants, a postoperative CT scan is essential to determine dosimetry
- Determining dose distribution in these patients is especially important in patients who may receive further EBRT or brachytherapy at a later time
- Postoperative CT dosimetry scans also aid in determining the quality of the implant and can help the practitioner to ensure quality in future implants

Remote Afterloading Interstitial Brachytherapy

- As opposed to a permanent interstitial implant, remote afterloading of HDR sources allows a plan to be designed that optimizes the position of the implant. Dwell times across the catheters can be modified to increase dose to the target volume and decrease dose to OARs
- Malfunctions in the implant, such as movement of a catheter requiring the removal of that catheter, can be compensated for by changing the dwell times of radioactive sources in adjacent catheters and optimizing the plan
- In LDR Ir-192 temporary implants, a minimal peripheral dose of 3000 cGy is prescribed and is supplemented with 4500–5000 cGy of EBRT
- In HDR Ir-192 temporary remote afterloading implants, a minimal peripheral dose of 1000 cGy is delivered in 3–4 min and the afterloading catheters are removed following the treatment [14]

Toxicity

- Most studies report complications of at least 5 % all the way up to 40 %, which can occur as early as hours to days to weeks following treatment [23, 33, 34]
- Perioperative toxicity is rare and mainly relating to the procedure itself including anesthesia, bronchoscopy, and catheter insertion complications
- These are usually reported in up to 5 % of procedures and include hemoptysis, pneumothorax, pneumonia, arrhythmia, cardiac arrest, and other complications of anesthesia [33]
- Older age and multiple risk factors such as chronic obstructive pulmonary disease, hypertension, and cardiac arrhythmias are risk factors for early complications [34]

- Toxicities from treatment include radiation bronchitis, esophagitis, fibrous-tracheal malacia, persistent cough, and endobronchial mycosis; however, the most critical toxicities secondary to endobronchial brachytherapy are fatal hemoptysis, tracheoesophageal fistulas, bronchospasm, and bronchial stenosis [35]
- A Cancer Care Ontario meta-analysis of the role of EBB showed fatal hemoptysis rates ranging from 7 to 22 % [36]. Fatal hemoptysis is thought to occur due to the close proximity between major blood vessels and the HDR applicator; however, it is controversial as to whether this occurs secondary to treatment, disease progression, or a combination of the two
- The Manchester group's series of 406 patients is one of the largest published experiences of EBB, demonstrating a fatal hemoptysis rate of 7.9 % with most events occurring between 9 and 12 months [37]
- They showed that doses greater than 15 Gy, previous laser treatment, a second EBB fraction, concurrent EBRT, and longer overall survival were significantly associated with massive hemoptysis
- Other risk factors found to be associated with fatal hemoptysis include volume of disease, irradiated volume length, and dose per fraction [38]

References

1. American Cancer Society. Cancer facts & figures 2015. Atlanta: American Cancer Society; 2015.
2. Niemoeller OM, Pöllinger B, Niyazi M, et al. Mature results of a randomized trial comparing two fractionation schedules of high dose rate endoluminal brachytherapy for the treatment of endobronchial tumors. Radiat Oncol. 2013;7:8.
3. Huber RM, Fischer R, Hautmann H, et al. Palliative endobronchial brachytherapy for central lung tumors. A prospective, randomized comparison of two fractionation schedules. Chest. 1995;107:463–70.
4. Huber RM, Fischer R, Hautmann H, et al. Does additional brachytherapy improve the effect of external irradiation?

A prospective, randomized study in central lung tumors. Int J Radiat Oncol Biol Phys. 1997;38:533–40.

5. Mallick I, Sharma SC, Behera D. Endobronchial brachytherapy for symptom palliation in non-small cell lung cancer—analysis of symptom response, endoscopic improvement and quality of life. Lung Cancer. 2007;55:313–8.

6. Langendijk H, de Jong J, Tjwa M, et al. External irradiation versus external irradiation plus endobronchial brachytherapy in inoperable non-small cell lung cancer: a prospective randomized study. Radiother Oncol. 2001;58:257–68.

7. Sur R, Donde B, Mohuiddin M, et al. Randomized prospective study on the role of high dose rate intraluminal brachytherapy (HDRILBT) in palliation of symptoms in advanced non-small cell lung cancer (NSCLC) treated with radiation alone [abstract]. Int J Radiat Oncol Biol Phys. 2004;60:S205.

8. Stout R, Barber P, Burt P, et al. Clinical and quality of life outcomes in the first United Kingdom randomized trial of endobronchial brachytherapy (intraluminal radiotherapy) vs. external beam radiotherapy in the palliative treatment of inoperable non-small cell lung cancer. Radiother Oncol. 2000;56:323.

9. Chella A, Ambrogi MC, Ribechini A, et al. Combined Nd-YAG laser/HDR brachytherapy versus Nd-YAG laser only in malignant central airway involvement: a prospective randomized study. Lung Cancer. 2000;27:169–75.

10. Fernando HC, Landreneau RJ, Mandrekar SJ, et al. Impact of brachytherapy on local recurrence rates after sublobar resection: results from ACOSOG Z4032 (Alliance), a phase III randomized trial for high-risk operable non-small-cell lung cancer. J Clin Oncol. 2014;32(23):2456–62.

11. Santos R, Colonias A, Parda D, et al. Comparison between sublobar resection and 125Iodine brachytherapy after sublobar resection in high-risk patients with Stage I non-small-cell lung cancer. Surgery. 2003;134(4):691–7.

12. Lee W, Daly BD, Dipetrillo TA, et al. Limited resection for non-small cell lung cancer: observed local control with implantation of I-125 brachytherapy seeds. Ann Thorac Surg. 2003;75(1):237–42.

13. Parashar B, Port J, Arora S, et al. Analysis of stereotactic radiation vs. wedge resection vs. wedge resection plus Cesium-131 brachytherapy in early stage lung cancer. Brachytherapy. 2015; 14(5):648–54.

14. Nag S, Kelly JF, Horton JL, Komaki R, Nori D. Brachytherapy for carcinoma of the lung. Oncology (Williston Park). 2001;15(3): 371–81.

15. Stewart A, Parashar B, Patel M, et al. American Brachytherapy Society consensus guidelines for thoracic brachytherapy for lung cancer. Brachytherapy. 2016;15(1):1–11.
16. Ernst A. Principles and practice of interventional pulmonology. New York: Springer; 2013.
17. Sharma DN, Rath GK, Thulkar S, et al. Computerized tomography guided percutaneous high-dose-rate interstitial brachytherapy for malignant lung lesions. J Cancer Res Ther. 2011;7:174–9.
18. King CG, Stockstill TF, BLoomer WD, et al. Point dose variations with time in brachytherapy for cervical carcinoma. Abstr Med Phys. 1993;19:777.
19. Thomadsen BR, Shahabi S, Stitt JA, et al. High dose rate intracavitary brachytherapy for carcinoma of the cervix: the Madison System: II. Procedural and physical considerations. Int J Radiat Oncol Biol Phys. 1992;24:349–57.
20. Kennedy MP, Jimenez CA, Chang J, et al. Optimisation of bronchial brachytherapy catheter placement with a modified airway stent. Eur Respir J. 2008;31:902–3.
21. Marsiglia H, Baldeyrou P, Lartigau E, et al. High-dose-rate brachytherapy as sole modality for early-stage endobronchial carcinoma. Int J Radiat Oncol Biol Phys. 2000;47:665–72.
22. Liu L, Bassano DA, Prasad SC, et al. On the use of C-arm fluoroscopy for treatment planning in high dose rate brachytherapy. Med Phys. 2003;30:2297–302.
23. Hara R, Itami J, Aruga T, et al. Risk factors for massive hemoptysis after endobronchial brachytherapy in patients with tracheobronchial malignancies. Cancer. 2001;92(10):2623–7.
24. Sawicki M, Kazalski D, Lyczek J, et al. The evaluation of treatment plans in high-dose-rate endobronchial brachytherapy by utilizing 2D and 3D computed tomography imaging methods. J Contemp Brachytherapy. 2014;6:289–92.
25. Lycek J, Kazalski D, Kowali K, et al. Comparison of the GTV coverage by PTV and isodose of 90% in 2D and 3D planning during endobronchial brachytherapy in the palliative treatment of patients with advanced lung cancer. Pilot study. J Contemp Brachytherapy. 2012;4:113–5.
26. Kishi K, Yoshimasu T, Shirai S, et al. Usefulness of minitrachoesotmy and torque controlled insertion of applicator in fractionated endobronchial brachytherapy. Br J Radiol. 2006;79:522–5.
27. Gay HA, Allison RR, Downie GH, et al. Toward endobronchial Ir-192 high-dose-rate brachytherapy therapeutic optimization. Phys Med Biol. 2007;52:2987–99.

28. Ferstl A, Fischer R, Hautmann H, et al. Simultaneous chemotherapy and high dose rate brachytherapy (HDRBT) in the treatment of locally advanced non-small cell lung cancer. Eur Respir J. 1997;10 Suppl 25:198.

29. D'Amato TA, Galloway M, Syzdlowski G, et al. Intraoperative brachytherapy following thoracoscopic wedge resection of stage I lung cancer. Chest. 1998;114:1112–5.

30. Fleischman EH, Kagan AR, Streeter OE, et al. Iodine 125 interstitial brachytherapy in the treatment of carcinoma of the lung. J Surg Oncol. 1992;49:25–8.

31. Trombetta MG, Colonias A, Malishi D, et al. Tolerance of the proximal aorta using intraoperative iodine-125 interstitial brachytherapy in cancer of the lung. Brachytherapy. 2008;7: 50–4.

32. Cormack RA, Holloway CL, O'Farrell D, et al. Permanent planar iodine-125 implants: the dosimetric effect of geometric parameters for idealized source configurations. Int J Radiat Oncol Biol Phys. 2007;69:1310–5.

33. Skowronek J, Piorunek T, Kanikowski M, et al. Definitive high-dose-rate endobronchial brachytherapy of bronchial stump for lung cancer after surgery. Brachytherapy. 2013;12:560–6.

34. Zaric B, Perin B, Jovelic A, et al. Clinical risk factors for early complications after high-dose-rate endobronchial brachytherapy in the palliative treatment of lung cancer. Clin Lung Cancer. 2010;11:182.

35. Perez CA, Brady LW, editors. Principles and practice of radiation oncology. 2nd ed. Philadelphia: JB Lippincott Co; 1992:50–63. pp. 114–23.

36. Ung YC, Yu E, Falkson C, et al. The role of high-dose-rate brachytherapy in the palliation of symptoms in patients with non-small-cell lung cancer: a systematic review. Brachytherapy. 2006;5(3):189–202.

37. Gollins SW, Ryder WD, Burt PA, et al. Massive haemoptysis death and other morbidity associated with high dose rate intraluminal radiotherapy for carcinoma of the bronchus. Radiother Oncol. 1996;39:105–16.

38. Ozkok S, Karakoyun-celik O, Goksel T, et al. High dose rate endobronchial brachytherapy in the management of lung cancer: response and toxicity evaluation in 158 patients. Lung Cancer. 2008;62(3):326–33.

Appendix A: Consent Forms

Appendix A1. Anesthesia Consent Form.

ANESTHESIA CONSENT

I understand that anesthesia is necessary for the procedure or operation that my physician has scheduled. The anesthesia will be administered by a physician member of the Department of Anesthesiology & Pain Medicine, a Certified Registered Nurse Anesthetist (CRNA) or an anesthesia resident (physician in specialist training). I understand that nurse anesthetists and residents always work under the supervision of an anesthesiologist (licensed anesthesia doctor).

I agree to receive the following forms of anesthesia that may be appropriate for my procedure or surgery.

☐ **General Anesthesia:** Administration of anesthetic medications by intravenous injection and inhalation, resulting in a temporary state of unconsciousness.

☐ **Regional Anesthesia** (nerve block, spinal or epidural anesthesia): Numbing medications are injected close to major nerves. This causes a temporary loss of feeling and movement in the part of the body where the procedure or treatment will be performed. You will be awake but unable to feel pain.

☐ **Monitored Anesthesia Care (MAC):** The anesthesia provider will administer medications to calm your nerves, sedate you and treat any pain or discomfort, but you will not necessarily be completely asleep. The anesthesia team will monitor blood pressure, oxygenation, heart rate and mental state, supplementing sedation and pain medication as needed.

Because of unforeseen conditions, anesthesia techniques such as placing breathing tubes, performing nerve blocks or invasive monitors may be technically difficult and may require another technique. I consent to an alternative type of anesthesia, if necessary, as deemed appropriate by the anesthesia team.

RISKS:

I understand there are potential risks and complications to anesthesia. These include but are not limited to:

Allergic/adverse reaction to the anesthesia, sore throat, nausea and/or vomiting, vocal cord injury, eye injury, backache, headache, pain, infection, localized swelling and or redness, muscle aches, loss of limb function, aspiration, awareness under anesthesia, nerve injury, loss of sensation, pneumonia, wrong site for injection of anesthesia, seizure, bleeding, blood clot, inability to reverse the effects of anesthesia, paralysis, blindness, heart failure, heart attack, brain damage, coma, and death.

I understand that accidental oral or dental injury is a known risk of anesthesia and that the anesthesia provider cannot be held responsible for injuring teeth, gums, lips, tongue, crowns, fillings, partials, or dentures. I understand that unforeseen problems can occur at any time during the procedure and anesthetic.

I also understand that the following additional risks may occur in connection with the anesthesia proposed for me:

_____

_____

ALTERNATIVES:
The alternatives to sedation, analgesia, or anesthesia include undergoing the planned procedure without intravenous or regional anesthesia or analgesia (for example, with local anesthesia alone, if feasible) or re-evaluating the need for the planned procedure with my physician.

I have informed the anesthesia provider of all my known allergies. I have informed the anesthesia provider of all medications I am currently taking, including prescriptions, over-the-counter remedies, herbal therapies, and any other nutritional supplements.

My signature below constitutes my acknowledgement that the proposed administration of anesthesia has been satisfactorily explained to me and that I have all of the information which I desire about the anesthesia. I have been given an opportunity to ask any questions that I might have.

| Date | Time | PATIENT OR PATIENT'S LEGAL REPRESENTATIVE |

RELATIONSHIP OF REPRESENTATIVE TO PATIENT
(If applicable)

| Date | Time | PHYSICIAN/PROVIDER | PI Number |

INTERPRETER (if applicable)

Appendix A.2: Conscious sedation consent form.

CONSENT TO OPERATION, PROCEDURES, BLOOD
TRANSFUSION AND ADMINISTRATION OF ANESTHESTICS
Page 1 of 4

1. I herby authorize _____, and any associates or assistants as may be selected by him/her to perform the following operation(s) or procedure(s) (this description should include the **SIDE** and **SITE** of the procedure): **Conscious Sedation** _____

2. I understand that UCDMC is a teaching institution and that the associates or assistants involved in the operation(s) or procedure(s) may include residents, fellows, medical students or other allied healthcare professionals. I authorize that such associates or assistants perform portions of the operation(s) or procedure(s) under the direction of the physician(s) identified in paragraph 1, above.

3. I understand that _____ will be present during the key portions of the operation(s) or procedure(s) and at all other times will be immediately available or will ensure another qualified surgeon is immediately available.

4. The operation(s) or procedure(s) has been explained to me by _____.

5. I have been informed that there are significant risks, such as severe loss of blood, blood clots, infection, cardiac arrest, and other untoward consequences, that are involved in the performance of any surgical procedure that can lead to death or permanent or temporary disability or complete or partial disability. I have been made aware of certain risks, consequences and significant side effects that are associated with the operation(s) or procedure(s) described in paragraph 1. These include but are not limited to: seizure, abnormal heart rhythm, bleeding, bruising, headache, injection site pain, no pain relief or worsened pain, infection, temporary or permanent nerve damage, temporary or permanent paralysis, temporary or persistent mood changes, trouble sleeping, temporary or persistent hallucinations, confusion, impaired senses (disorientation and confusion), impaired judgement, impaired motor coordination, mood or emotional changes including exaggerated sense of well-being (euphoria) and psychosis, spastic jerking movements, increased muscle tone, muscular tremors, reduced clarity of awareness of the environment (delirium), psychological disconnection from surroundings, high or low blood pressure, amnesia, loss of emotional control, depression, fatal respiratory problems, allergic or life threatening anaphylactic reaction, other less common temporary or permanent medication side effects, other less common temporary or permanent neurological complications and death.

I understand that the risks described above are the most common risks and other more remote risks may be associated with this operation(s) or procedure(s).

CONSENT TO OPERATION, PROCEDURES, BLOOD TRANSFUSION
AND ADMINISTRATION OF ANESTHETICS – Page 1 of 4

A6040 (12/13)-E

6. I understand that the practice of medicine and surgery is not an exact science, and I acknowledge that no guarantees or assurances have been made to me concerning the results of the chosen operation(s) or procedure(s).

7. The medically acceptable alternative(s) in treating such condition(s) has been explained to me and I understand it and the risks and benefits to be: ALTERNATIVE: not to do the procedure today and to continue with your current method of pain management. RISK/BENEFITS: Your current level of pain and function may remain the same or may worsen.

8. **IF TRANSFUSION IS A REASONABLE POSSIBILITY:** My doctor discussed with me that there is a reasonable possibility that a transfusion of blood or blood products may be necessary. I received a copy of The Patient's Guide to Blood Transfusion brochure describing my transfusion options (unless I have a life-threatening emergency or medical contraindications). My doctor has discussed the risks, benefits and alternatives of the transfusion of blood and blood products with me. I have also learned about the option of pre-donating my own blood. I consent to the transfusion of blood or blood products,as my doctor may order, in connection with the operation(s) or procedure(s) discussed in this form.

9. I consent to the administration of sedation and/or anesthetics as may be considered necessary or advisable. I have been advised that there are certain risks associated with anesthetics that may include allergic reactions and/or drug intolerances, cardiac arrest and brain damage.

10. I recognize that, during the course of the operation or procedure, unforeseen conditions may necessitate other procedures, which are in addition to, or different from those described in paragraph 1. I understand that it may be difficult or impractical to obtain my consent for those procedures. I authorize the above-named health care provider his/her assistant, or his/her designees, to performsuch procedures.

11. I authorize the pathologist, at his or her discretion, to retain, preserve, use, or dispose of any tissues, organs, bones, bodily fluid or medical devices that may be removed during the operation(s) or procedure(s). I understand that such specimens may be used for research, as permitted by federal and state law. I understand right or entitlement in any research or research product using or derived from the specimens.

588   Appendix A: Consent Forms

12. I understand that there may be health care industry representatives or other visitors present, with the approval of UCDMC, during my operation(s) or procedure(s) for purposes of medical observation or to provide technical support. I authorize those individuals to be present.

13. I have been informed whether my health care provider has, or had within the previous 12 months, a substantial compensation arrangement, investment interest or research interest with a business whose supplies, products or devices will be used in my operation/procedure. Specifically, he/she has informed me that these interests are:

☐ None
☐ As follows (details supplied by physician): _____
_____
_____

14. I understand that if an implantable device is used, information regarding the device and my Social Security Number may be reported to the device manufacturer, if requested, and as required by federal law.

15. I understand that I have the right to refuse this operation(s) or procedure(s) at anytime. I further understand that the explanations I have received may not be exhaustive and all-inclusive and that other more remote risks may be involved. However, the information that I have received is sufficient for me to consent to the operation or procedure described above. I have had full opportunity to ask questions concerning my condition, the authorized operation(s) or procedure(s), the alternatives, and the risks and consequences associated with it. All my questions have been answered to my satisfaction.

16. **I have read and understand the above consent. I acknowledge the risks, benefits and alternatives associated with the operation(s) or procedure(s). The likelihood of achieving the goals of the operation(s) or procedure(s) and the potential problems with recuperation have been explained to me and I wish to proceed with the operation(s) or procedure(s) described above.**

Title . . . .
Name of Patient:
Date of Birth:
        Place Label Here

_____ _____   _____
DATE TIME   PATIENT OR PATIENT'S REPRESENTATIVE

                     _____
                     RELATIONSHIP OF REPRESENTATIVE TO PATIENT
                     (if applicable)

_____ _____   _____
DATE TIME   PHYSICIAN / PROVIDER   PI NUMBER

                     _____
                     INTERPRETER (if applicable)

Unforeseen circumstances require changing the individual practitioners involved in conducting the surgery or a change in the operation(s) or procedure(s) listed above. Please identify:_____
_____
_____

_____ _____   _____
DATE TIME   PATIENT OR PATIENT'S REPRESENTATIVE

                     _____
                     PHYSICIAN / PROVIDER   PI NUMBER

Appendix A.3 : Consent to gynecologic brachytherapy.

UNIVERSITY OF CALIFORNIA, DAVIS
MEDICAL CENTER
SACRAMENTO, CALIFORNIA
**CONSENT TO HIGH DOSE RATE BRACHYTHERAPY
FOR GYNECOLOGIC CANCER**
Page 1 of 5

1. I herby authorize _____, and any associates or assistants as may be selected by him/her to perform the following operation(s) or procedure(s) (this description should include the **SIDE** and **SITE** of the procedure):

   ☐ High dose rate intracavitary brachytherapy for gynecologic cancer   **Number of Treatments:_____**

   ☐ High dose rate interstitial brachytherapy for gynecologic cancer   **Number of Treatments:_____**

   SITE:_____   SIDE:_____

   ☐ **If NO site or side determination is needed** *(check box)*

2. I understand that UCDMC is a teaching institution and that the associates or assistants involved in the operation(s) or procedure(s) may include residents, fellows, medical students or other allied healthcare professionals. I authorize that such associates or assistants perform portions of the operation(s) or procedure(s) under the direction of the physician(s) identified in paragraph 1, above.

3. I understand that _____ will be present during the key portions of the operation(s) or procedure(s) and at all other times will be immediately available or will ensure another qualified surgeon is immediately available.

4. The operation(s) or procedure(s) has been explained to me by _____.

5. I have been informed that there are significant risks, such as severe loss of blood, blood clots, infection, cardiac arrest, and other untoward consequences, that are involved in the performance of any surgical procedure that can lead to death or permanent or temporary disability or complete or partial disability. I have been made aware of certain risks, consequences and significant side effects that are associated with the operation(s) or procedure(s) described in paragraph 1. These include but are not limited to:

   Side effects during and after procedure: nausea, abdominal discomfort, abdominal pain, loose stools, blood in the stool, rectal urgency, rectal narrowing, rectal ulcer, rectal fistula requiring surgery, rectal bleeding,

UNIVERSITY OF CALIFORNIA, DAVIS
MEDICAL CENTER
SACRAMENTO, CALIFORNIA
CONSENT TO HIGH DOSE RATE BRACHYTHERAPY
FOR GYNECOLOGIC CANCER
Page 2 of 5

decreased blood counts, diarrhea, change in bowel habits, bladder irritation causing urgency, frequency, burning with urination, bladder infection, bladder inflammation, decreased bladder capacity, blood in the urine, vaginal irritation, vaginal narrowing, vaginal shortening, vaginal dryness, pain with intercourse, vaginal bleeding and spotting, vaginal bleeding after intercourse, vaginal discharge, vaginal tissue necrosis, vaginal fistula requiring surgery, skin redness, skin tanning, skin breakdown, skin itching, skin irritation, tenderness, pain, swelling, loss of pubic hair, fatigue, pelvic fracture, nerve damage, leg swelling.

Reproductive risks: If you are a woman of child bearing potential, you must use an adequate form of contraception prior to and during radiation. If you are pregnant, you may not undergo radiation and if you become pregnant, the radiation will be discontinued. If you become pregnant, you must notify your doctor immediately.

Infertility risks: If you are a premenopausal woman, the brachytherapy form of radiation will render your ovaries nonfunctional and you will become post-menopausal. You may need to take a medication due to this process after the radiation therapy as prescribed by your doctor. You will not be able to become pregnant after the radiation due to the radiation effect on your ovaries. The radiation to the uterus will not allow expansion for childbirth and therefore you will be unable to carry a child to term and you cannot be a surrogate mother.

Radiation can also cause the formation of a secondary cancer in the field of radiation several years after treatment.

I understand that the risks described above are the most common risks and other more remote risks may be associated with this operation(s) or procedure(s).

6. I understand that the practice of medicine and surgery is not an exact science, and I acknowledge that no guarantees or assurances have been made to me concerning the results of the chosen operation(s) or procedure(s).

7. The medically acceptable alternative(s) in treating such condition(s) has been explained to me and I understand it and the risks and benefits to be:

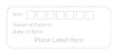

UNIVERSITY OF CALIFORNIA, DAVIS
MEDICAL CENTER
SACRAMENTO, CALIFORNIA
**CONSENT TO HIGH DOSE RATE BRACHYTHERAPY
FOR GYNECOLOGIC CANCER**
Page 3 of 5

ALTERNATIVE: Not to do the brachytherapy and be observed, consider other methods of radiation, or continue with current method of pain management.

RISK/BENEFIT: Your cancer may not be controlled and you may experience bleeding, pain or even death.

8. **IF TRANSFUSION IS A REASONABLE POSSIBILITY:** My doctor informed with me that there is a reasonable possibility that a transfusion of blood or blood products may be necessary. My doctor has discussed the risks, benefits and alternatives of the transfusion of blood and blood products with me. I received a copy of The Patient's Guide to Blood Transfusion brochure describing my transfusion options (unless I have a life-threatening emergency or medical contraindications). I have also learned about the option of pre-donating my own blood. I consent to the transfusion of blood or blood products, as my doctor may order, in connection with the operation(s) or procedure(s) discussed in this form.

9. I consent to the administration of sedation and/or anesthetics as may be considered necessary or advisable. I have been advised that there are certain risks associated with anesthetics that may include allergic reactions and/or drug intolerances, cardiac arrest and brain damage.

10. I recognize that, during the course of the operation or procedure, unforeseen conditions may necessitate other procedures, which are in addition to, or different from those described in paragraph 1. I understand that it may be difficult or impractical to obtain my consent for those procedures. I authorize the above-named health care provider his/her assistant, or his/her designees, to perform such procedures.

11. I authorize the pathologist, at his or her discretion, to retain, preserve, use, or dispose of any tissues, organs, bones, bodily fluid or medical devices that may be removed during the operation(s) or procedure(s). I understand that such specimens may be used for research, as permitted by federal and state law. I understand that I have no property ownership or interest in such specimens or data derived from those specimens and no right or entitlement in any research or research product using or derived from the specimens.

UNIVERSITY OF CALIFORNIA, DAVIS
MEDICAL CENTER
SACRAMENTO, CALIFORNIA
**CONSENT TO HIGH DOSE RATE BRACHYTHERAPY
FOR GYNECOLOGIC CANCER**
Page 4 of 5

12. I understand that there may be health care industry representatives or other visitors present, with the approval of UCDMC, during my operation(s) or procedure(s) for purposes of medical observation or to provide technical support. I authorize those individuals to be present.

13. I have been informed whether my health care provider has, or had within the previous 12 months, a substantial compensation arrangement, investment interest or research interest with a business whose supplies, products or devices will be used in my operation/procedure. Specifically, he/she has informed me that these interests are:

    ☐ None

    ☐ As follows (details supplied by physician): _____

    _____
    _____
    _____

14. I understand that if an implantable device is used, information regarding the device and my Social Security Number may be reported to the device manufacturer, if requested, and as required by federal law.

15. I understand that I have the right to refuse this operation(s) or procedure(s) at anytime. I further understand that the explanations I have received may not be exhaustive and all-inclusive and that other more remote risks may be involved. However, the information that I have received is sufficient for me to consent to the operation or procedure described above. I have had full opportunity to ask questions concerning my condition, the authorized operation(s) or procedure(s), the alternatives, and the risks and consequences associated with it. All my questions have been answered to my satisfaction.

16. **I have read and understand the above consent. I acknowledge the risks, benefits and alternatives associated with the operation(s) or procedure(s). The likelihood of achieving the goals of the operation(s) or procedure(s) and the potential problems with recuperation have been explained to me and I wish to proceed with the operation(s) or procedure(s) described above.**

**CONSENT TO HIGH DOSE RATE BRACHYTHERAPY FOR
GYNECOLOGIC CANCER – PAGE 4 of 5**

A7131-1 (3/16)

595 Appendix A: Consent Forms

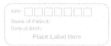

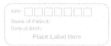

UNIVERSITY OF CALIFORNIA, DAVIS
MEDICAL CENTER
SACRAMENTO, CALIFORNIA
**CONSENT TO HIGH DOSE RATE BRACHYTHERAPY
FOR GYNECOLOGIC CANCER**
Page 5 of 5

DATE   TIME   PATIENT OR PATIENT'S REPRESENTATIVE

                   RELATIONSHIP OF REPRESENTATIVE TO PATIENT
                   (if applicable)

DATE   TIME   PHYSICIAN / PROVIDER   PI NUMBER

                   INTERPRETER (if applicable)

Unforeseen circumstances require changing the individual practitioners involved in conducting the surgery or a change in the operation(s) or procedure(s) listed above. Please identify:_____
_____
_____

DATE   TIME   PATIENT OR PATIENT'S REPRESENTATIVE

                   PHYSICIAN / PROVIDER   PI NUMBER

Appendix B: Brachytherapy Quality Assurance Checklists

© Springer International Publishing AG 2017   595
J. Mayadev et al. (eds.), *Handbook of Image-Guided
Brachytherapy*, DOI 10.1007/978-3-319-44827-5

Appendix B.1: HDR Daily QA Check.

Department of Radiation Oncology
Policy and Procedures
HDR Daily Quality Assurance Check

Introduction

These checks will be performed on all treatment days before the first treatment. Results will be recorded on the GammaMed HDR Daily Check Sheet, and the completed sheets will be filed in the HDR Daily QA notebook.

I. GammaMed Unit Checks

    A. *Source Positioning and Indexing*. Insert a a strip of GaFchromic film into the GammaMed Perma-Doc Phantom. Connect the Perma-Doc to channel 1 of the indexer. Deliver Perma-Doc plan. Develop film and verify that the center of the exposed areas and the tungsten wires match to within 1 mm. Date and initial the film and file with the GammaMed HDR Daily Check Sheet.

    B. *Treatment Unit Selection Switches.* Turn the key switch to Gamma Knife and verify that treatment can not be initiated. Turn the key switch to HDR and the toggle switch to Nucletron and verify that treatment can not be initiated.

    C. *Key Tests*

        1. *Power key switch.* Turn the Power key on the control console to the horizontal position. Verify that all indicators on the control console flash briefly and an audible signal sounds. Verify that the following lights remain lit: Mains and Battery (in the Power section), Normal (in the Mode section), and Safe (in the Source section). If the source key in the afterloader keypad is in the locked position, the Locked light on the control console will flash.

        2. *Source key switch.* With the source key switch on the afterloader keypad in the locked position, verify that the treatment can not be initiated.

    D. *Source Guide Tube Misconnection*. Insert a source guide tube incorrectly into the indexer head and verify that treatment can not be initiated.

    E. *Interrupt Button*. Press the Interrupt Button while the source is extended. Verify that an audible alarm sounds and the source returns to the safe. After the source has returned, verify the Interrupted light on the control console is on, the Radiation light is off, the Source Out light is off, the Source Safe light is on, and the Started light is flashing. Verify the message "Warning: Interrupt Manual" appears on the control PC.

F. *Door Interlock*. Open the treatment room door while the source is extended. Verify that an audible alarm sounds and the source returns to the safe. After the source has returned, verify the Door light on the control console is on, the Interrupted light is on, the Radiation light is off, the Source Out light is off, the Source Safe light is on, and the Started light is flashing. Verify the message "Warning: Interrupt Door" appears on the control PC.

G. *Emergency Return Switch* (control room wall). Press the Emergency Return Switch while the source is extended. Verify that an audible alarm sounds on both the control console and the control PC, the Alarm light on the control console flashes, and the source returns to the safe. After the source has returned, verify the Radiation light on the control console is off, the Source Out light is off, the Source Safe light is on, and the Started light is a steady green. Verify the message "Warning: Emergency Manual" appears on the control PC. Pull out button on Emergency Return Switch, press Alarm Reset on the control console.

H. *Timer Check treatment*. Use a calibrated stopwatch to measure the actual dwell time not including travel time. Measured time should be +3% of programmed dwell time.

   1. The GammaMed console will scale the dwell time with decay of the source, so the programmed dwell time will not be the same day-to-day.

   2. Stopwatch may be calibrated in-house using a stopwatch with calibration tracing to NIST.

I. *UPS Backup Power*. With the source extended, switch off power to the UPS (Uninterruptible Power Supply) by pulling the power plug connecting the UPS unit to the wall outlet. Verify that the UPS maintains power to the control PC to abort treatment and retract source. Plug UPS back in, and continue with remaining treatment fraction.

II. Other Checks

   A. Procedures. Confirm that operating instructions are available and the emergency procedures are posted in the console room.

   B. Emergency pig. Confirm that the emergency source pig and long-handled forceps are in the treatment room.

   C. Closed circuit TV. Verify proper functioning of the closed circuit TV system and monitors.

D. Radiation Monitor Lights. With the source extended, verify that the lights on the radiation monitors in the treatment room and in the console room are flashing.

E. GammaMed Radiation Indicator Lights. With the source extended, verify that the Radiation indicator lights on the afterloader keypad and on the control console are lit.

F. Beam On Light. With the source extended, verify that the Beam On light by the treatment door is on.

III. Radiation Survey

A. Survey meter. Record the number and calibration due date of the survey meter used. The same survey meter should be used for the recorded survey of the day's patients.

B. Perform Survey Meter Daily Response Check Procedure to verify meter is operating correctly.

IV. Machine Problems

A. Inform Physics if any of the above is not within specifications. If this occurs, print a copy of the Treatment Delivery Report and give to Physics.

B. Any malfunctions of the device will be reported immediately to Physics.

C. **TREATMENT SHALL NOT PROCEED UNTIL REPAIRS ARE COMPLETED AND ALL CHECKS ARE WITHIN SPECIFICATIONS.** Until then:

1. The machine will be turned off and remain off except for repair and testing.

2. Keys will be given to Physics or Clinical Engineering and remain in their custody until the device is released for clinical use.

3. A sign stating the machine is not to be used clinically will be posted on the console.

V. Physicist Review

A. The Daily Check Sheet will be reviewed by an HDR Authorized Medical Physicist within 15 days. The physicist will initial and date the sheet.

Appendix B.2: HDR Daily Check Sheet

GammaMed HDR Daily Check Sheet

Tests Performed By:_____   Date: _____

Physics check by: _____   Date:_____

I.   GAMMAMED UNIT CHECKS

☐   a.   Source positioning and indexing

☐   b.   UPS backup power: unplug UPS while source is extended during PermaDoc test

☐   c   Treatment unit selection switches

☐   d   Key tests

☐   1. Power key

☐   e   2. Source key

☐   f   Source guide tube misconnection

☐   g   Interrupt Button

☐   h   Door interlock

☐   i   Emergency Return switch

☐   j   Timer Accuracy: programmed = _____ s; meas = _____ s   (spec=$\pm 3\%$)

II.   OTHER CHECKS

☐   a.   Operating and emergency procedures in console room

☐   b.   Emergency pig and forceps

☐   c.   Closed circuit TV

☐   d.   Radiation monitor lights

☐   e.   GammaMed radiation indicator lights (afterloader & control console)

☐   f.   Beam on light

III.   RADIATION SURVEY

a.   Survey meter used:
Meter #:_____   Cal Due Date: _____

☐   b.   Daily Response Check (should read between 0.5 and 2 mR/hr on x1 scale at Gamma Knife shielding doors)

Inform Physics if any of the above is not within specifications. Any malfunctions of the device should be reported immediately to Physics.

TREATMENT SHALL NOT PROCEED UNTIL REPAIRS ARE COMPLETED AND ALL CHECKS ARE WITHIN SPECIFICATIONS. Turn off unit, give keys to Physics or Clin Eng, and post sign on treatment console.

Appendix B.3 General HDR Brachytherapy Procedure

Department of Radiation Oncology
General HDR Brachytherapy Procedure

1. Introduction

1.1. This document presents an overview. Additional and more specific procedure-related procedures and their related check sheets exist in separate documents.

2. General

2.1. The treatment room will be closed when unattended and locked on days when there are no scheduled procedures.

2.2. The GammaMed unit is currently housed in the same treatment room as the Gamma Knife; therefore, Increased Controls requirements governing access to that room will be followed.

2.3. The keys to operate the GammaMed will be kept in the lockbox when not in use.

2.4. The console room will be closed and locked when unattended.

2.5. The Emergency Procedures will be posted in the GammaMed console room.

3. Classification of patients

3.1. The types of treatment can be classified into the categories listed below, depending on the imaging, simulation, and treatment planning requirements. The Pre-Simulation, Simulation, and Treatment Planning procedures will vary depending on the treatment category.

3.1.1. Category A treatment plans are determined by the fixed geometry of the applicator, and a standard pre-calculated "standard" plan can be used. They do not require patient simulation although a pre-treatment imaging may be performed to verify applicator position. An example is a vaginal cylinder case.

3.1.2. Category B treatments involved a once-time insertion of applicators or cathethers but are treated for more than one fraction. These patients require only a single simulation and treatment plan. An example is a SAVI case.

3.1.3. Category C treatments require insertion of applicators/catheters and a treatment plan for each fraction. An example is a tandem-and-ring case.

4. Simulation

4.1. Category A patients (see Section III) do not require simulation. If simulation is performed, the steps for Category B or C patients will be followed.

4.2. Category B and C patients

    4.2.1. Patient identification will be verified by two methods before catheter/applicator insertion.

    4.2.2. Catheters and/or applicators will be inserted under the supervision of the Radiation Oncologist.

    4.2.3. After catheter/applicator insertion, the patient will be placed on the imaging unit table in as close as possible to the treatment position.

    4.2.4. Marker cables will be inserted into each catheter or applicator as needed.

    4.2.5. Imaging will be performed as needed for insertion verification and treatment planning.

5. Treatment Planning

  5.1. "Standard" plans

    5.1.1. Existing "standard" plans that have already undergone a second check do not need to be checked again before being used for treatment.

    5.1.2. A new "standard" plan must undergo a second check before it can be used for treatment.

    5.1.3. A new "standard" plan must also undergo an additional second check within 30 days.

  5.2. Pre-treatment patient-specific plans

    5.2.1. Imaging information from simulation will be transferred into the treatment planning system.

    5.2.2. A treatment plan shall be produced by qualified Physics or Dosimetry staff in accordance with the written directive signed by the Radiation Oncologist.

    5.2.3. For plan documentation, the electronic charting procedure will be followed.

    5.2.4. The treatment planner with complete the dosimetry QCL in MOSAIQ.

    5.2.5. An Authorized Medical Physicist not involved in the treatment planning will check the plan before treatment is given. The Physicist will treatment approve the plan, export it to the treatment unit and complete the physics 2nd check QCL in MOSAIQ.

6. Pre-Treatment

6.1. For each patient treatment, the pre-treatment procedures in the document GammaMed HDR Treatment Check Procedure will be performed and the results recorded on the GammaMed HDR Treatment Check Sheet.

6.2. If necessary, patient plan parameters will be imported into the control PC.

6.3. The Therapist will select the proper treatment plan on the control PC and print the Planned Treatment Report.

6.4. When the patient is in the room alone, the patient will be continually monitored using the closed circuit TV systems and the intercom.

7. Treatment

7.1. A procedural pause will be executed prior to initiation of treatment.

7.2. No one other than the patient will be allowed in the room when the afterloader is activated.

7.3. The Authorized User (Radiation Oncologist) will be in direct supervision of the GammaMed operator during treatments.

7.4. The Authorized User (Radiation Oncologist) and the Authorized Medical Physicist will be physically present during treatment per NRC guidelines, i.e. within hearing distance of a "normal" voice.

7.5. The patient will be continually monitored using the closed circuit TV systems and the intercom.

7.6. In case of emergency, the procedure in the document GammaMed HDR Emergency Procedures will be followed.

8. Post-Treatment

8.1. The Therapist and physicist will perform the post-treatment procedures in the document GammaMed HDR Treatment Check Procedure and record the results on the GammaMed HDR Treatment Check Sheet

9. Quality Assurance and New Source Calibration

9.1. A full calibration is defined as including performing all tests as defined in the GammaMed HDR Monthly Quality Assurance Procedure.

9.2. A full calibration will be performed by an Authorized Medical Physicist prior to patient treatment:

9.2.1. Before first medical use of the HDR unit.

9.2.2. After reinstallation of the unit in a new location

9.2.3. After each source exchange

9.2.4. Following repair of the unit that includes source removal or major repair of components associated with the source exposure assembly

9.3. The procedures specified in the document GammaMed HDR Monthly Quality Assurance Procedure will be performed once per calendar month.

9.4. The manufacturer's recommended preventative maintenance schedule will be followed and records of the preventative maintenance will be maintained.

10. Training

10.1. All users of the system will received emergency procedure training before being allowed to operate the system and will receive refresher training at least once each calendar year thereafter. Training will be documented.

11. Medical Emergency/Death

11.1. In the event of a medical emergency or death involving an HDR patient or human research subject, the Authorized User (Radiation Oncologist) and the Radiation Safety Officer or his/her designee shall be notified as soon as possible.

11.2. All other applicable standard procedures will also be followed.

Appendix B.4 Brachytherapy Patient Treatment Verification

Department of Radiation Oncology
Brachytherapy Patient Treatment Verification Procedure

Introduction

These procedures will be performed for each patient treatment. The results will be recorded on the GammaMed HDR Treatment Check Sheet and completed sheets will be added to the patient's chart.

I. Pretreatment checks

    A. Patient ID. The patient will be identified before being connected to the afterloader. Because the patient may be sedated from applicator insertion, it may not be possible for the patient to respond; therefore, more passive methods of identification such as photo ID may be used. Such patients will have already been identified by two methods by staff before applicator insertion.

    B. Patient name. Verify the correct patient name on the Planned Treatment Report.

    C. Date and time. Verify the correct date and time on the Planned Treatment Report.

    D. Source strength. Verify the correct current source strength on the Planned Treatment Report by comparison to the printed decay tables.

    E. Dwell positions. Verify the number of channels and the number of dwell positions per channel in the Planned Treatment Report agrees with the plan printout.

    F. Planned dwell times. Verify the planned dwell times for each position agree with the plan printout.

    G. Total scaled Curie-seconds. Multiply the current source strength and the total scaled seconds from the Planned Treatment Report to determine the total scaled Curie-seconds. Compare to the total Curie-seconds in the plan printout. Should agree within $\pm 1\%$.

    H. Signatures. The Authorized User (Radiation Oncologist) will verify the patient name and treatment delivery information and will sign the Planned Treatment Report as confirmation of his/her review. The Authorized Medical Physicist and therapist will sign the Planned Treatment Report as confirmation of his/her review.

    I. Intercom and TV monitors. Verify that the intercom and closed circuit TV between the treatment and console rooms are functional for two-way communication.

    J. SAVI pre-tx checksheet. For SAVI patients only, verify that the pre-treatment checksheet has been completed and the attending physician has signed the sheet as required.

K. Guide tube integrity. Check each source guide tube for kinks and other defects.

L. Guide tube/applicator length. Connect the applicators/catheters to source guide tubes. Use the length gauge to check each guide tube/applicator for the correct length.

M. Connection to indexer. The the Physicist and Authorized User physician will confirm that the applicator/catheters are connected to the correct channels on the afterloader, according to the plan printout.

N. Probe extension. For all implants with cylinders, measure the probe extension at insert and after treatment. Notify physics if difference exceeds > 0.1 cm. Expected value for cylinders is 9.25 cm.

O. Written directive in MOSAIQ approved by Radiation Oncologist. The Therapist and the Physicist will confirm that a prescription for the treatment exists in MOSAIQ and has been approved by an attending Radiation Oncologist.

P. Pre-treatment survey. Record the number and calibration due date of the survey meter. Use the same survey meter as used for the Daily Check. Before treatment, survey the patient at approximately the position of the implant. If the radiation level is > 1 mR/hr, record the reading and provide an explanation (e.g. patient had a recent Nuclear Medicine study).

Q. Authorized users. Confirm that the Radiation oncologist and Physicist standing by for the treatment, and the Radiation oncologist approving the prescription, are on the list posted in the HDR control room as Authorized Users for HDR.

R. A procedural pause will be executed prior to initiation of treatment, per departmental policy.

II. Post-Treatment Checks

A. Treatment delivery. Confirm that the total delivered seconds equals the total scaled seconds

B. Post-treatment survey. Immediately after treatment, survey the patient at the same position as previously. If the radiation level is above that measured pre-treatment, confirm the reading with the other survey meter, then implement emergency procedures and record the reading on the Treatment Check Sheet.

C. SAVI expansion tool. For SAVI patients only, confirm that the tool is removed from the SAVI device after treatment.

D. Treatment Delivery Planned Treatment Report. Print and initial the Treatment Delivery Planned Treatment Report and put it in the patient's chart.

E. Treatment recorded in MOSAIQ. Confirm the treatment was entered manually into MOSAIQ.

Appendix B.5 HDR Procedural Pause: Example GYN Brachytherapy

HDR Brachytherapy Procedural Pause

- Patient Name
- Procedure Type
- Implant #/#
- Fraction #/#
- Rx: _____ Gy to _____
- Bladder fill (Y/N)
- BB removed (Y/N)
- MD signed plan (Y/N)
- Physicist signed plan (Y/N)
- All staff are out of the HDR room
- Does anyone have any concerns prior to proceeding?

Appendix B.6 HDR Treatment Check Sheet

GammaMed HDR Treatment Check Sheet

Initial all lines

Treatment date:
Plan name:

Therapist	Pre-Treatment General Checks
	Intercom and CCTV functional
	Pre-treatment Tolerance <1 mR/hr survey:_____mR/hr Survey meter #:_____ Cal due date: _____ ***If radiation level is > 1 mR/hr, give explanation: _____
	Confirm Radiation Oncologist and Physicist are authorized for HDR
	Cylinder diameter was checked on CT vs. prescription

Therapist	Physicist	Treatment Plan Checks	
		Patient name correct	on Planned Treatment Report
		Date and time correct	
		Source strength correct	
		Total scaled Curie-seconds are correct	
		Dwell position and times correct	
		Signatures of RadOnc, Physicist and RTT	
		RadOnc approved prescription	in MOSAIQ
		RadOnc and physicist approved plan pdf	

Therapist	Physicist	Patient Checks	
		Patient identified by two methods	
		Guide tube integrity	
		Guide tube/applicator length	
		Connection to indexer channel correct	
		Pre-treatment check sheet complete (SAVI and surface applicator only)	
		SAVI expansion tool in place	For SAVI only
		Probe extension at insert ____cm Probe extension after Tx ____cm Physics notified if difference >0.1 cm	All implants with cylinders; 9.25 cm expected for standard cylinder
		Procedural pause at time:	

Therapist	Post-Treatment Checks
	Treatment delivered as planned
	Post treatment survey: ____ **mR/Hr** *** If post-Tx reading > pre-Tx reading, confirm reading then implement emergency procedures ***
	SAVI Expansion tool removed
	Treatment delivery report printed
	Treatment recorded and charged in MOSAIQ

In case of error or treatment emergency, document error(s) and total treatment interruption time:

Appendix B.7 Emergency HDR Procedure

Department of Radiation Oncology
Emergency Procedure HDR

1. The following emergency equipment shall always be present in the treatment room during treatment: Emergency Container; Long-handled forceps; Pliers.
2. The following procedure shall be followed in case the source fails to retract to the safe within the device.
3. The Radiation Therapist shall depress the INTERRUPT button on the treatment console and/or the Emergency Return button on the wall of the console room. If the source retracts, go to step 12; otherwise, proceed to step 4.
4. The Radiation Physicist shall enter the treatment room with a survey meter.
5. The Physicist shall press the Emergency Return button on the afterloader. If the source retracts, go to step 12; otherwise, proceed to step 6.
6. The Physicist shall pull the handle out of the hand crank at the back of the afterloader and turn the crank in the direction of the arrow until a distinct resistance is noticeable or the room radiation level is safe. If the source retracts, go to step 12; otherwise proceed to step 7.
7. The Physician shall remove the applicator from the patient, ensuring that the radiation is confined to the applicator. The Physician or Physicist shall insert the applicator containing the source into the Emergency Container using a long forceps.
8. The Physician and/or Physicist shall IMMEDIATELY assist the patient from the room.
9. The Physicist or the Therapist shall survey the patient and confirm that the dose rate is at background level.
10. The Physicist shall ensure that the applicator and source are safely stored inside the emergency container.
11. The Physicist shall ensure that all personnel have left the treatment room. (S) he shall close the door, lock it, and mark it **NO ENTRY**.
12. The Therapist shall retain the treatment data printout.
13. The Physicist shall notify the manufacturer and the instituional Health Physics.

Appenidx B.8 Image Guided Brachytherapy Suite Design

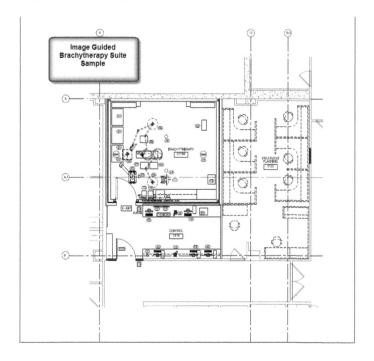

ID	Resp	Equipment	MT	Weight	Height	Width	Depth	BTU	Utilities	Anchorage	Comments
1	OFOI	Storage Cabinet	M					NA			
2	OFOI	Brachytherapy Unit	M					NA	P,D		
3	OFOI	Procedure table	M					NA			
4	OFCI	Procedure light w/monitor	C	268					P,D		
5	OFCI	Procedure Light	C	129					P		
6	OFCI	Documentation Boom	C	445					P,D,O,A		
7	OFOI	Propac	M					NA	P		1
8	OFOI	Anesthesia Cart	M					NA			
9	OFOI	Nurse Cart	M					NA			
10	OFOI	PC	M					1200	P,D		1
11	OFOI	WOW	M					1200	P,D		2
12	OFOI	Bio Hazard Trash Can	M					NA			
13	OFOI	Trash Can	M					NA			
14	OFCI	Blanket warmer	M	256	25	26	23	2250	P		3
15	OFOI	Brachy. Control	M					1200	P,D		
16	OFOI	Intercom	M					150	P,D		
17	CFCI	CCTV Monitor	W					150	P,D		
18	OFOI	Desk Phone	M					NA	D		
19	OFOI	PC Workstation	M					1200	P,D		
20	OFOI	Eclipse	M					1200	P,D		
21	OFOI	Ipod Dock & amplifier	M					NA	P,D		
22	CFCI	CCTV Camera	C					NA	P,D		4
23	OFOI	Wireless Access Point	C					NA	P,D		4
24	CFCI	Speaker	C					NA	D		
25	OFOI	Printer	M						P,D		
26	OFOI	Nurse Call	M						P,D		

RESPONSIBILITY MATRIX
OFOI = Owner Furnished, Owner Installed
OFCI = Owner Furnished, Contractor Installed
CFCI = Owner Furnished, Contractor Installed

MOUNTING
M = Mobile
F = Floor
C = Ceiling
W = Wall

COMMENTS
1. Located on documentation Boom
2. Wireless connection
3. On mobile stand
4. Power over Ethernet

UTILITIES
W = Water, see plumbing drawings
P = Power, see electrical drawings
D = Data cable, See Electrical Drawings
O = Oxygen, see Plumbing Drawings
A = Air, See Plumbing Drawings

Index

© Springer International Publishing AG 2017   611
J. Mayadev et al. (eds.), *Handbook of Image-Guided
Brachytherapy*, DOI 10.1007/978-3-319-44827-5

Printed by Printforce, the Netherlands